ICSA Book Series in Statistics

Series Editors
Jiahua Chen
Department of Statistics
University of British Columbia
Vancouver
Canada

Ding-Geng (Din) Chen
University of North Carolina
Chapel Hill, NC, USA

More information about this series at http://www.springer.com/series/13402

Ding-Geng (Din) Chen • Jeffrey Wilson

Editors

Innovative Statistical Methods for Public Health Data

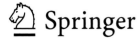 Springer

Editors
Ding-Geng (Din) Chen
School of Social Work
University of North Carolina
Chapel Hill, NC, USA

Jeffrey Wilson
Arizona State University
Tempe, AZ, USA

ISSN 2199-0980 ISSN 2199-0999 (electronic)
ICSA Book Series in Statistics
ISBN 978-3-319-18535-4 ISBN 978-3-319-18536-1 (eBook)
DOI 10.1007/978-3-319-18536-1

Library of Congress Control Number: 2015946563

Springer Cham Heidelberg New York Dordrecht London

Printed on acid-free paper

Springer International Publishing AG Switzerland is part of Springer Science+Business Media (www.springer.com)

To my parents and parents-in-law who value higher-education and hard-working, and to my wife, Ke, my son, John D. Chen, and my daughter, Jenny K. Chen, for their love and support. This book is also dedicated to my passion to the Applied Public Health Statistics Section in American Public Health Association!

Ding-Geng (Din) Chen, Ph.D.

To my grandson, Willem Wilson-Ellis, and my three daughters, Rochelle, Roxanne, and Rhonda for their continued love and support. To the graduate statistics students at Arizona State University present and past for their direct and indirect support.

Jeffrey Wilson, Ph.D.

Preface

This book was originated when we were become part of the leadership of the Applied Public Health Statistics Section (https://www.apha.org/apha-communities/member-sections/applied-public-health-statistics) in the American Public Health Association. Professor Chen was the Chair-Elect (2012), Chair (2013), and Past-Chair (2014) while Professor Wilson was the Chair-Elect (2011), Chair (2012) and Past-Chair (2013). In addition, Professor Wilson has been the Chair of the Editorial Board of the American Journal of Public Health for the past 3 years and a member for 5 years. He has been a reviewer for the journal and a contributor to Statistically Speaking.

During our leadership of the Statistics Section, we also served as APHA Program Planners for the Section in the annual meetings by organizing abstracts and scientific sessions as well as supporting the student paper competition. During our tenure, we got a close-up view of the expertise and the knowledge of statistical principles and methods that need to be disseminated to aid the development and growth in the area of Public Health. We were convinced that this can be best met through the compilation of a book on the public health statistics.

This book is a compilation of present and new developments in statistical methods and their applications to public health research. The data and computer programs used in this book are publicly available so the readers have the opportunity to replicate the model development and data analyses as presented in each chapter. This is certain to facilitate learning and support ease of computation so that these new methods can be readily applied.

The book strives to bring together experts engaged in public health statistical methodology to present and discuss recent issues in statistical methodological development and their applications. The book is timely and has high potential to impact model development and data analysis of public health research across a wide spectrum of the discipline. We expect the book to foster the use of these novel ideas in healthcare research in Public Health.

The book consists of 15 chapters which we present in three parts. Part I consists of methods to model clustered data; Part II consists of methods to model incomplete or missing data; while Part III consists of other healthcare research models.

Part I, Modelling Clustered Data, consists of five chapters. Chapter 1 is on Methods for Analyzing Secondary Outcomes in Public Health Case–Control Studies. This chapter unlike what is common does not deal with the analysis of the association between the primary outcome and exposure variables but deals with the association between secondary outcomes and exposure variables. The analysis of secondary outcomes may suffer from selection bias but this chapter presents and compares a design-based and model-based approach to account for the bias, and demonstrates the methods using a public health data set.

Chapter 2: Controlling for Population Density Using Clustering and Data Weighting Techniques When Examining Social Health and Welfare Problems. This chapter provides an algebraic weight formula (Oh and Scheuren 1983), in path analysis to elucidate the relationship between underlying psychosocial mechanisms and health risk behaviors among adolescents in the 1998 NLSY Young Adult cohort. The oversampling of underrepresented racial/ethnic groups is controlled by mathematically adjusting the design weights in the calculation of the covariance matrices for each cluster group while comparing non-normalized versus normalized path analysis results. The impact of ignoring weights leading to serious bias in parameter estimates with the underestimation of standards errors is presented.

Chapter 3: On the Inference of Partially Correlated Data with Applications to Public Health Issues. This chapter provides several methods to compare two Gaussian distributed means in the two-sample location problem under the assumption of partially dependent observations. For categorical data, tests of homogeneity for partially matched-pair data are investigated. Different methods of combining tests of homogeneity based on Pearson Chi-square test and McNemar chi-squared test are investigated. In addition, several nonparametric testing procedures which combine all cases in the study are introduced.

Chapter 4: Modeling Time-Dependent Covariates in Longitudinal Data Analyses. This chapter discusses the effect of the time-dependent covariates on response variables for longitudinal data. The consequences of ignoring the time-dependent nature of variables in models are discussed by considering various common analysis techniques, such as the mixed-modeling approach or the GEE (generalized estimating equations) approach.

Chapter 5: Solving Probabilistic Discrete Event Systems with Moore-Penrose Generalized Inverse Matrix Method to Extract Longitudinal Characteristics from Cross-Sectional Survey Data. This chapter presents the Moore-Penrose (M-P) generalized inverse matrix theory as a powerful approach to solve an admissible linear-equation system when the inverse of the coefficient matrix does not exist. This chapter reports the authors' work to systemize the Probabilistic Discrete Event Systems modeling in characterizing health risk behaviors with multiple progression stages. The estimated results with this approach are scientifically stronger than the original method.

Part II, Modelling Incomplete or Missing Data, consists of four chapters. Chapter 6: On the Effect of Structural Zeros in Regression Models. This chapter presents an extension of methods in handling sampling zeros as opposed to structural zeros when these zeros are part of the predictors. They present updated approaches and illustrate the importance of disentangling the structural and sampling zeros in alcohol research using simulated as well as real study data.

Chapter 7: Modeling Based on Progressively Type-I Interval Censored Sample. In this chapter, several parametric modeling procedures (including model selection) are presented with the use of maximum likelihood estimate, moment method estimate, probability plot estimate, and Bayesian estimation. In addition, the model presentation of general data structure and simulation procedure for getting progressively type-I interval censored sample are presented.

Chapter 8: Techniques for Analyzing Incomplete Data in Public Health Research. This chapter deals with the causes and problems created by incomplete data and recommends techniques for how to handle it through multiple imputation.

Chapter 9: A Continuous Latent Factor Model for Non-ignorable Missing Data. This chapter presents a continuous latent factor model as a novel approach to overcome limitations which exist in pattern mixture models through the speci-fication of a continuous latent factor. The advantages of this model, including small sample feasibility, are demonstrated by comparing with Roy's pattern mixture model using an application to a clinical study of AIDS patients with advanced immune suppression.

In Part III, we present a series of Healthcare Research Models which consists of six chapters. Chapter 10: Health Surveillance. This chapter deals with the application of statistical methods for health surveillance, including those for health care quality monitoring and those for disease surveillance. The methods rely on techniques borrowed from the industrial quality control and monitoring literature. However, the distinctions are made when necessary and taken into account in these methods.

Chapter 11: Standardization and Decomposition Analysis: A Useful Analytical Method for Outcome Difference, Inequality and Disparity Studies. This chapter deals with a traditional demographic analytical method that is widely used for com-paring rates between populations with difference in composition. The results can be readily applied to cross-sectional outcome comparisons as well as longitudinal studies. While SDA does not rely on traditional assumptions, it is void of statistical significance testing. This chapter presents techniques for significance testing.

Chapter 12: Cusp Catastrophe Modeling in Medical and Health Research. This chapter presents the cusp catastrophe modeling method, including the general principle and two analytical approaches to statistically solving the model for actual data analysis: (1) the polynomial regression method for longitudinal data and (2) the likelihood estimation method for cross-sectional data. A special R-based package "cusp" is given for the likelihood method for data analysis.

Chapter 13: On Ranked Set Sampling Variation and Its Applications to Public Health Research. This chapter presents the ranked set sampling as a cost-effective alternative approach to traditional sampling schemes. This method relies on a small fraction of the available units. It improves the precision of estimation. In RSS, the desired information is obtained from a small fraction of the available units.

Chapter 14: Weighted Multiple Testing Correction for Correlated Endpoints in Survival Data. In this chapter, a weighted multiple testing correction method for correlated time-to-event endpoints in survival data, based on the correlation matrix estimated from the WLW method is presented. Simulations are conducted to study the family-wise type I error rate of the proposed method and to compare the power performance of the proposed method to the nonparametric multiple testing methods such as the alpha-exhaustive fallback fixed-sequence and the weighted Holm-Bonferroni method when used for the correlated time-to-event endpoints.

Chapter 15: Meta-Analytic Methods for Public Health Research. This chapter presents an overview of meta-analysis intended for public health researchers to understand how to apply and interpret. Emphasis is focused on classical statistical methods for estimation of the parameters of interest as well as recent development in research in meta-analysis.

As a general note, the references for each chapter are at the end of the chapter so that the readers can readily refer to the chapter under discussion. Thus, each chapter is self-contained.

We would like to express our gratitude to many individuals. First, thanks to Hannah Bracken, the Associate Editor in Statistics from Springer (http://link.springer.com) and Professor Jiahua Chen, the Co-Editor of Springer/ICSA Book Series in Statistics (http://www.springer.com/series/13402) for their professional support in the book. Special thanks are due to the authors of the chapters.

We welcome any comments and suggestions on typos, errors, and future improvements about this book. Please contact Professor Ding-Geng (Din) Chen (DrDG.Chen@gmail.com) and Professor Jeffrey Wilson (jeffrey.wilson@asu.edu).

Chapel Hill, NC, USA   Ding-Geng (Din) Chen
Tempe, AZ, USA   Jeffrey Wilson
July 2015

Contents

Contributors

Lynn A. Agre Department of Statistics and Biostatistics, Rutgers University, New Brunswick, NJ, USA

N. Andrew Peterson School of Social Work, Rutgers University, New Brunswick, NJ, USA

Haim Bar Department of Statistics, University of Connecticut, Storrs, CT, USA

James Brady Rutgers University, New Brunswick, NJ, USA

Aimin Chen Department of Environmental Health, University of Cincinnati, Cincinnati, OH, USA

Ding-Geng (Din) Chen School of Social Work, University of North Carolina, Chapel Hill, NC, USA

Xinguang (Jim) Chen Department of Epidemiology, University of Florida, Gainesville, FL, USA

Ronald D. Fricker, Jr. Virginia Tech., Blacksburg, VA, USA

Enas Ghulam Department of Environmental Health, University of Cincinnati, Cincinnati, OH, USA

Ofer Harel Department of Statistics, University of Connecticut, Storrs, CT, USA

Hua He Department of Biostatistics and Computational Biology, University of Rochester Medical Center, Rochester, NY, USA

Nan Jiang Department of Mathematical Sciences, University of South Dakota, Vermillion, SD, USA

Trent L. Lalonde Department of Applied Statistics and Research Methods, University of Northern Colorado, Greeley, CO, USA

Feng Lin Department of Electrical and Computer Engineering, Electric-drive Vehicle Engineering, Wayne State University, Detroit, MI, USA

Yu-Jau Lin Department of Applied Mathematics, Chung-Yuan Christian University, Chung-Li, Taiwan

Christopher Lindsell Department of Emergency Medicine, University of Cincinnati, Cincinnati, OH, USA

Y.L. Lio Department of Mathematical Sciences, University of South Dakota, Vermillion, SD, USA

Yan Ma Department of Epidemiology and Biostatistics, George Washington University, Washington, DC, USA

Valerie Pare Department of Statistics, University of Connecticut, Storrs, CT, USA

Susan M. Pinney Department of Environmental Health, University of Cincinnati, Cincinnati, OH, USA

Mark Reiser School of Mathematical and Statistical Sciences, Arizona State University, Tempe, AZ, USA

Steven E. Rigdon Department of Biostatistics, Saint Louis University, St. Louis, MO, USA

Hani M. Samawi Department of Biostatistics, Jiann-Ping Hsu College of Public Health, Georgia Southern University, Statesboro, GA, USA

Elizabeth D. Schifano Department of Statistics, University of Connecticut, Storrs, CT, USA

Wan Tang Department of Biostatistics and Computational Biology, University of Rochester Medical Center, Rochester, NY, USA

Robert Vogel Department of Biostatiatics, Jiann-Ping Hsu College of Public Health, Georgia Southern University, Statesboro, GA, USA

Jichuan Wang Department of Epidemiology and Biostatistics, The George Washington
University School of Medicine, Children's National Medical Center, Washington, DC, USA

Kesheng Wang Department of Biostatistics and Epidemiology, East Tennessee State University, Johnson City, TN, USA

Wenjuan Wang Department of Biostatistics and Computational Biology, University of Rochester Medical Center, Rochester, NY, USA

Changchun Xie Division of Epidemiology and Biostatistics, Department of Environmental Health, University of Cincinnati, Cincinnati, OH, USA

Jun Zhang Bayer Healthcare Pharmaceuticals Inc., Whippany, NJ, USA

Wei Zhang Department of Epidemiology and Biostatistics, George Washington University, Washington, DC, USA

Part I
Modelling Clustered Data

Methods for Analyzing Secondary Outcomes in Public Health Case–Control Studies

Elizabeth D. Schifano, Haim Bar, and Ofer Harel

Abstract Case–control studies are common in public health research. In these studies, cases are chosen based on the primary outcome but there are usually many other related variables which are collected. While the analysis of the association between the primary outcome and exposure variables is generally the main focus of the study, the association between secondary outcomes and exposure variables may also be of interest. Since the experiment was designed for the analysis of the primary outcome, the analysis of secondary outcomes may suffer from selection bias. In this chapter we will introduce the problem and the potential biased inference that can result from ignoring the sampling design. We will discuss and compare a design-based and model-based approach to account for the bias, and demonstrate the methods using a public health data set.

1 Introduction

Case–control studies are very common in public health research, where conducting a designed experiment is not feasible. This may happen, for example, if assigning subjects to certain treatments is unethical. Particularly in these situations, researchers have to rely on observational studies, in which groups having different outcomes are identified and compared. The example used in this chapter is a typical one—subjects are classified based on an outcome, in this instance a (binary) cancer status, and the goal of the case–control analysis is to identify factors that are associated with this outcome. In the context of our example, the 'controls' are the cancer-free subjects and the 'cases' are the cancer patients.

While the main focus in such studies is on the primary outcome (e.g., cancer status), there is substantial interest to take advantage of existing large case–control studies to identify if any exposure variables are associated with *secondary* outcomes that are often collected in these studies. In particular, secondary outcome analyses are now becoming popular in genetic epidemiology, where the interest is in studying associations between genetic variants and human quantitative traits using data

E.D. Schifano • H. Bar • O. Harel (✉)
Department of Statistics, University of Connecticut, Storrs, CT 06269, USA
e-mail: elizabeth.schifano@uconn.edu; haim.bar@uconn.edu; ofer.harel@uconn.edu

© Springer International Publishing Switzerland 2015
D.-G. Chen, J. Wilson (eds.), *Innovative Statistical Methods for Public Health Data*,
ICSA Book Series in Statistics, DOI 10.1007/978-3-319-18536-1_1

collected from case–control studies of complex diseases (Lettre et al. 2008; Sanna et al. 2008; Monsees et al. 2009; Schifano et al. 2013). For example, in the lung cancer genome-wide association study conducted in Massachusetts General Hospital (MGH), several continuous measures of smoking behavior were collected from both cases and controls (Schifano et al. 2013). In a secondary outcome analysis, one is interested in identifying genetic variants (single nucleotide polymorphisms, or SNPs) that are associated with smoking behavior while accounting for case–control ascertainment. Since the subjects from the case–control study were sampled based on lung cancer status (primary disease outcome), careful attention is warranted for inferences regarding the secondary smoking outcomes, because the case–control sample might not represent a random sample from the population as the cases have been over-sampled. Consequently, the population association of the genetic variant with a secondary outcome can be distorted in a case–control sample, and analysis methods that ignore or improperly account for this sampling mechanism can lead to biased estimates of the effect of the genetic variant on the secondary outcome.

One of the most common and simple approaches for analyzing secondary quantitative traits involves performing the analysis on the control subjects only. This strategy is appropriate only when the disease is rare, in which case the control sample can be considered an approximation to a random sample from the general population. Because the information from the cases is totally ignored, however, this method is generally inefficient. Alternatively, one may attempt to analyze cases and controls separately, or treat case–control status as a predictor in the regression model of the secondary outcome. However, each of these methods may result in erroneous conclusions, as the association between a secondary outcome and an exposure variable in the case and control samples can be different from the association in the underlying population.

Other analysis methods have been proposed to explicitly account for case–control ascertainment and eliminate sampling bias. To study the effect of exposure (such as a genetic variant) on a secondary outcome, Lin and Zeng (2009) proposed a likelihood-based approach, reflecting case–control sampling by using a likelihood conditional on disease status. Extensions and generalizations of the Lin and Zeng (2009) likelihood framework may be found in Wei et al. (2013) and Ghosh et al. (2013). Tchetgen Tchetgen (2014) proposed a general model based on a careful re-parameterization of the conditional model for the secondary outcome given the case–control outcome and regression covariates that relies on fewer model assumptions. In this chapter, we focus on comparing two popular methods, namely, inverse probability weighting (IPW) (Robins et al. 1994) and propensity score matching (PSM) (Rosenbaum and Rubin 1983). These two approaches can be thought of more generally as *design-based* and *model-based* approaches, respectively. In the *design-based* approach, one obtains the probability of selecting a subject from a certain cohort from the sampling distribution of the primary outcome, while in the *model-based* approach, one obtains estimates for the selection probability using a statistical model. In the model-based approach one fits a logistic regression model in which the response is the primary outcome, and the log-odds are assumed to be a linear combination of several explanatory variables. The two approaches differ in the way that the probability that a subject is included in the study is computed, and in the way these probabilities are used in the analysis of the secondary outcome, but both aim to compensate for the over-sampling of one group (i.e., the cases).

We use a subset of the MGH lung cancer case–control data to illustrate the two methods for analyzing secondary outcomes. In Sect. 2 we describe the data in more detail, while in Sects. 3 and 4 we describe the various design-based and model-based techniques for analyzing such data. We demonstrate these methods in Sect. 5 and conclude with a brief discussion in Sect. 6.

2 Data Example: Genetic Association with Smoking Behavior in a Lung Cancer Case–Control Study

The case–control study is a large ongoing study of the molecular epidemiology of lung cancer, which began in 1992 at MGH. The study was reviewed and approved by the Institutional Review Boards of MGH and the Harvard School of Public Health. The cases consisted of adults who were diagnosed with lung cancer, and the controls were recruited from friends and spouses of the patients. Several demographic variables were recorded, as well as multiple genetic variants (SNPs). In our analysis below we only include Caucasian subjects who smoked at some point in their life, and we only use the following variables: cancer status (the primary outcome), sex (binary; male = 0, female = 1), age (continuous), education (binary; less than college degree = 0, at least a college degree = 1), average number of cigarettes smoked per day (CPD), the first three principal components (pc1–pc3) which account for population substructure, and the SNP rs1051730 (chromosome 15), which has previously been found to be associated with risk for lung cancer (Amos et al. 2008; VanderWeele et al. 2012). We further restricted the data set to subjects which had complete data (no missing data in any of the aforementioned variables). For more information regarding the study, refer to VanderWeele et al. (2012) and Schifano et al. (2013).

The total number of cases and controls in our data set are 733 and 792, respectively. There are 770 males and 755 females in the data, and the sample has a mean age of 62.1, with standard deviation 11.4. There are 76 subjects with at least a college degree. We assume an additive model for the SNP, where the SNP is coded as the number of copies of the C allele (C allele frequency = 0.604; T allele frequency = 0.396). The distribution of CPD and square root of CPD are shown in Fig. 1.

We consider the square root of CPD ($\sqrt{CPD}$) as the secondary outcome, and we wish to test whether it is associated with the SNP. The structure of the investigated relationship between variables can be summarized as in Fig. 2, where Y represents

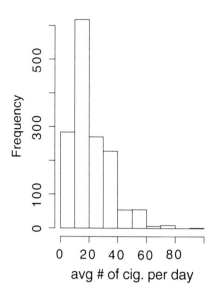

Fig. 1 The distribution of CPD and $\sqrt{CPD}$

Fig. 2 Structure of variables
in secondary outcome
analysis

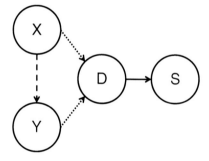

the secondary outcome ($\sqrt{CPD}$), X represents the exposure variable (SNP), D is a
binary disease indicator ($D = 1$ for cases, $D = 0$ for controls), and S is a binary
sampling indicator ($S = 1$ if sampled in the case–control data set, $S = 0$ if not
sampled in the case–control data set). We are interested in detecting the dashed
association between X and Y (the SNP and the smoking habits), but both X and Y
may be associated with disease status D, which, in turn, influences who gets sampled
in the case–control data set ($S = 1$). In general, if Y is associated with D, then the
simple analysis techniques of analyzing cases and controls separately, or treating
case–control status as a predictor in the regression model of the secondary outcome
will yield invalid results (Lin and Zeng 2009). Since smoking is associated with
lung cancer, one must take the sampling mechanism into account.

3 Design-Based Approach to Secondary Outcome Analysis

The idea behind IPW is as follows. Consider a sample of n subjects and the linear model $y_i = \mathbf{x}_i^T \boldsymbol{\beta} + \epsilon_i$, $i = 1, \ldots, n$, where $\boldsymbol{\beta}$ is a vector of regression coefficients, and ϵ_i are independent random errors. In matrix form, we write $Y = \mathbf{X}\boldsymbol{\beta} + \boldsymbol{\epsilon}$, and we assume $E[Y|\mathbf{X}] = \mathbf{X}\boldsymbol{\beta}$ in the population. In general, we can estimate the coefficients $\boldsymbol{\beta}$ by solving an estimating equation such as

$$\frac{1}{n} \sum_{i=1}^{n} u_i(\boldsymbol{\beta}) = 0 .$$

If $E[u_i(\boldsymbol{\beta})] = 0$ for the true $\boldsymbol{\beta}$, then the estimating equation is unbiased for estimating $\boldsymbol{\beta}$. For instance, in a *randomly selected* cohort of size n from the population, the estimating equation

$$\frac{1}{n} \sum_{i=1}^{n} \mathbf{x}_i(y_i - \mathbf{x}_i^T \boldsymbol{\beta}) = 0$$

is unbiased for estimation of $\boldsymbol{\beta}$. If, instead, the n observations consist of n_0 controls and n_1 cases ($n_0 + n_1 = n$), consider the equation

$$\frac{1}{n} \sum_{i=1}^{n} s_i \mathbf{x}_i(y_i - \mathbf{x}_i^T \boldsymbol{\beta}) = 0 \tag{1}$$

which includes the sampling indicator s_i for each subject. Clearly $s_i = 1$ for all n subjects in the case–control sample. Using the law of iterated expectations, it can be shown that (1) is not unbiased in general. However, by including the IPW $w_i = 1/Pr(s_i = 1|d_i)$, the estimating equation

$$\frac{1}{n} \sum_{i=1}^{n} \frac{s_i}{Pr(s_i = 1|d_i)} \mathbf{x}_i(y_i - \mathbf{x}_i^T \boldsymbol{\beta}) = 0$$

is unbiased provided that the probability of selection into the study depends solely on the disease status. Note that weighting the observations in this manner can be inefficient (Robins et al. 1994). However, the simplicity of the model makes it amenable to extensions which can gain power in other ways (e.g., in the joint analysis of multiple secondary outcomes (Schifano et al. 2013)).

4 Model-Based Approach to Secondary Outcome Analysis

In case–control studies the 'treatment' (disease status) and the inclusion in the study are not independent. Consequently, covariates that are associated with the disease might also be associated with the probability (propensity) that a subject is selected for the study. This is in contrast to randomized trials, where the randomization implies that each covariate has the same distribution in both treatment and control (for large samples). This balance is key to unbiased estimation of covariate effects in controlled experiments. Thus, in observational studies, the estimates of effect for covariates which are not balanced across treatments are likely to be biased, and may lead to incorrect conclusions.

PSM (Rosenbaum and Rubin 1983; Abadie and Imbens 2006) is a method which attempts to achieve balance in covariates across treatments by matching cases to similar controls, in the sense that the two have similar covariate values. More formally, recall our previous notation where D is the disease indicator, and X is a set of predictors which may affect $Pr(D = 1)$ and the secondary outcome, Y. Denote the potential outcome $Y(d)$, so that $Y(1)$ is the outcome for cases and $Y(0)$ is the outcome for controls. Of course, we only observe one of $Y(0)$ or $Y(1)$. Denote the propensity score by $p(X) = Pr(D = 1|X)$. Rosenbaum and Rubin (1983) introduced the assumption of 'strong ignorability,' which means that given the covariates, X, the potential outcomes $Y(0)$ and $Y(1)$ are independent of the treatment. More formally, strong ignorability is satisfied if the following conditions hold:

$$D \perp\!\!\!\perp Y(0), Y(1)|X \text{ almost surely.}$$

$$p(D = 1|X = x) \in [p_L, p_U] \text{ almost surely, for some } p_L > 0 \text{ and } p_U < 1.$$

The first condition is referred to as 'unconfoundedness,' and the second condition is called the 'overlap' condition. For certain relaxations of these assumptions, see, for example, Abadie and Imbens (2006).

Rosenbaum and Rubin (1983) proved that D and X are independent, conditional on the propensity scores, $p(X)$. Thus, if the strong ignorability assumption is reasonable, then by adjusting for the difference in the distribution of X between treated and untreated, the propensity matching method results in a data set which 'mimics' a randomized trial.

Matching algorithms have many configurable parameters which lead to different matchings. For example, one may choose to match multiple controls to each case, or require more stringent matching criteria. The search method for the matched controls can also be selected from a number of algorithms (for example, nearest neighbor, exact match, etc.) For more information about matching algorithms and configurations, refer to Ho et al. (2011). Regardless of the choices of the matching algorithm or parameters, to use the PSM method one has to perform the following steps:

1. Run logistic regression with the treatment (case/control) as response, and a set of covariates which are assumed to be associated with the response. Use the predicted probabilities from the regression model, $\hat{p}_i$, or the log-odds, $\log \frac{\hat{p}_i}{1-\hat{p}_i}$, as propensity scores.
2. Match every case with a control which has a similar propensity score. Discard any subject (case or control) for which no match is found.

3. Check that the data set which consists of matched pairs is balanced for each covariate.
4. Perform the multivariate statistical analysis on the matched data set.

In the context of our example, in the last step we fit a regression model in which $\sqrt{CPD}$ is the response variable, but instead of using the complete data set, we use a smaller data set which consists of matched pairs.

5   Data Analysis

Recall from Sect. 2 that we are interested in the effect of a genetic variant (rs1051730) on smoking habits ($\sqrt{CPD}$). First, we fit a logistic regression model for the primary outcome variable (cancer status). The results which are summarized in Table 1 suggest that the risk for lung cancer increases as the average number of cigarettes smoked daily increases. The risk also increases with age, and for subjects who have a college degree. Additionally, the risk for lung cancer decreases for increasing numbers of the C allele (or increases for increasing numbers of the T allele).

Since both the genetic variant and smoking behavior are associated with the primary disease outcome, we need to account for selection bias when testing the association between the genetic variant and the secondary smoking outcome. Let us first check if such association exists between the genetic variant and the secondary outcome without accounting for the potential selection bias problem.

We fit a linear regression model with $\sqrt{CPD}$ as the response variable. The results are summarized in Table 2, and they suggest that the genetic variant is, indeed, associated with smoking behavior. It would *appear* that the same variant which is strongly associated with lung cancer is also associated with heavy smoking, and that may be, at least in part, why those individuals end up with the disease. In the following subsections we describe how we use the IPW and PSM methods to test whether $\sqrt{CPD}$ is associated with this genetic variant. We show that when selection bias is accounted for, this genetic variant is not associated with the smoking variable.

Table 1 A logistic regression model fitting the primary outcome (disease status)

	Estimate	Std. error	z value	Pr(> |z|)
(Intercept)	−5.08	0.44	−11.46	0.00
sqcigavg	0.45	0.04	10.46	0.00
rs1051730	−0.32	0.08	−3.88	0.00
Age	0.05	0.01	9.23	0.00
Sex	0.16	0.12	1.33	0.18
Education	1.11	0.28	3.94	0.00
pc1	−4.05	2.58	−1.57	0.12
pc2	0.13	2.58	0.05	0.96
pc3	−7.61	2.49	−3.06	0.00

Covariate *sqcigavg* represents $\sqrt{CPD}$

Table 2 A regression model fitting the secondary outcome ($\sqrt{CPD}$), without any adjustment for selection bias

	Estimate	Std. error	t value	Pr($> |t|$)
(Intercept)	4.87	0.23	21.49	0.00
rs1051730	−0.13	0.05	−2.44	**0.01**
Age	0.01	0.00	1.65	0.10
Sex	−0.62	0.07	−8.21	0.00
Education	−0.29	0.17	−1.71	0.09
pc1	3.38	1.69	2.00	0.05
pc2	−2.38	1.68	−1.41	0.16
pc3	0.57	1.62	0.35	0.73

Table 3 A regression model fitting the secondary outcome ($\sqrt{CPD}$), using the inverse probability weights to adjust for selection bias

	Estimate	Std. error	Wald	Pr($> |W|$)
(Intercept)	5.04	0.29	298.38	0.00
rs1051730	−0.12	0.08	2.65	0.10
Age	−0.00	0.00	0.77	0.38
Sex	−0.61	0.11	32.53	0.00
Education	−0.55	0.28	3.86	0.05
pc1	4.46	2.51	3.16	0.08
pc2	−0.77	2.50	0.09	0.76
pc3	2.47	2.25	1.20	0.27

5.1 Inverse Probability Weights

One way to account for selection bias is to weight observations based on the probability that a subject is sampled in the case–control data set. As described in Monsees et al. (2009), we use the function `geeglm` in the R (R Core Team 2014) package `geepack` (Højsgaard and Halekoh 2005) in order to perform the IPW analysis. For n_1 case subjects and n_0 control subjects ($n_0 + n_1 = n$), the weight to be applied to cases is $1/Pr(S = 1|D = 1) \propto \pi/p_{n_1}$ where $\pi = 0.000745$ is the disease prevalence (VanderWeele et al. 2012) and $p_{n_1} = n_1/(n_0 + n_1)$ is the proportion of cases in the data set, and the weight for controls is $1/Pr(S = 1|D = 0) \propto (1 - \pi)/(1 - p_{n_1})$. Table 3 contains the results of the IPW analysis. The effect of genetic variant rs1051730 on $\sqrt{CPD}$, after adjusting for covariates in the IPW model is -0.1229 ($z = 2.65, p = 0.103$). Only the sex and education variables are associated with the smoking behavior at the 0.05 level when applying the IPW.

Note that in this data set, the weights are proportional to $(1 - \pi)/(1 - p_{n_1}) = 1.92407$ for the controls and $\pi/p_{n_1} = 0.00155$ for the cases. This illustrates how the IPW procedure down-weights the cases and up-weights the controls to reflect the true population structure.

5.2 Propensity Score Matching

A model-based approach for accounting for the selection bias is to compute individual propensity scores based on a logistic regression model, applied to the disease status, and then match case and control pairs. Under the 'strong ignorability' assumption, this process can create a data set in which predictor variables are balanced across the two treatment groups.

There are several implementations of the PSM algorithm. Here, we use the `MatchIt` package (Ho et al. 2011) in R. The matching algorithms have many options. Here we use the 'nearest neighbor' criterion, which, as the name suggests, attempts to find the closest control to each case. To do that, one has to define a distance between observations. For example, suppose that each observation is associated with k variables, then it may be viewed as a point in a k-dimensional Euclidean space, and then take the Euclidean distance between pairs of points. Then, to ensure that matched pairs are sufficiently similar to each other, one can set the 'caliper parameter' to a small value, say, 0.01. The caliper serves as a threshold, so that if no control is found to be close enough to a case observation, then the case observation is dropped, and is not included in the matched-pairs data set. This results in a smaller data set, but the variables in the subsequent analysis are much more balanced across the two groups. For more information about PSM options, see Ho et al. (2011).

The matching algorithm yields 519 pairs, so 273 controls and 214 cases were dropped in order to improve the balance between the two groups. Increasing the caliper will increase the number of matches, but some controls will be less similar to their matching cases. Table 4 shows the results from a linear regression model, using the same response and predictor variables as in Table 3, applied to the matched-pairs data set.

As was the case with IPW, the genetic variant is no longer significantly associated with the smoking variable at the 0.05 level. The sex and education variables remain significantly associated with the smoking variable, $\sqrt{CPD}$.

Note that the estimates obtained from the two methods are quite similar, except for the second and third population substructure covariates (pc2 and pc3). This could be a result of using different weighting methods. In addition to the sex and education

Table 4 A regression model fitting the secondary outcome ($\sqrt{CPD}$), using the propensity score matching method to adjust for selection bias

	Estimate	Std. error	t value	$\Pr(> |t|)$
(Intercept)	5.20	0.31	17.04	0.00
rs1051730	−0.07	0.07	−1.05	0.29
Age	−0.00	0.00	−0.05	0.96
Sex	−0.63	0.09	−6.85	0.00
Education	−0.49	0.24	−2.01	0.04
pc1	4.49	2.08	2.16	0.03
pc2	−4.10	2.08	−1.97	0.05
pc3	1.70	1.95	0.87	0.38

Table 5 A summary of the differences between the case and control groups, using the original data set

	Means treated	Means control	SD control	Mean diff.	eQQ Med	eQQ Mean	eQQ Max
Distance	0.53	0.43	0.15	**0.10**	0.10	0.10	0.11
rs1051730	1.12	1.29	0.68	**−0.16**	0.00	0.16	1.00
Age	65.19	59.21	11.56	**5.98**	5.95	6.02	14.61
Sex = 0	0.54	0.47	0.50	**0.07**	0.00	0.07	1.00
Sex = 1	0.46	0.53	0.50	**−0.07**	0.00	0.07	1.00
Education = 1	0.07	0.03	0.16	**0.05**	0.00	0.05	1.00
pc1	−0.00	0.00	0.02	**−0.00**	0.00	0.00	0.02
pc2	−0.00	0.00	0.02	**−0.00**	0.00	0.00	0.02
pc3	−0.00	0.00	0.02	**−0.00**	0.00	0.00	0.01

The eQQ Med, Mean, and Max columns provide the corresponding summary statistics of the empirical quantile–quantile function, of Treated vs. Control

Table 6 A summary of the differences between the case and control groups, using the matched-pairs data set, after applying the propensity score matching method to adjust for selection bias

	Means treated	Means control	SD control	Mean diff.	eQQ Med	eQQ Mean	eQQ Max
Distance	0.49	0.49	0.13	**0.00**	0.00	0.00	0.00
rs1051730	1.22	1.21	0.69	**0.01**	0.00	0.02	1.00
Age	62.77	62.89	9.93	**−0.13**	0.62	0.68	2.63
Sex = 0	0.55	0.51	0.50	**0.03**	0.00	0.03	1.00
Sex = 1	0.45	0.49	0.50	**−0.03**	0.00	0.03	1.00
Education = 1	0.04	0.03	0.18	**0.00**	0.00	0.00	1.00
pc1	0.00	0.00	0.02	**−0.00**	0.00	0.00	0.01
pc2	−0.00	−0.00	0.02	**−0.00**	0.00	0.00	0.01
pc3	−0.00	0.00	0.02	**−0.00**	0.00	0.00	0.01

The eQQ Med, Mean, and Max columns provide the corresponding summary statistics of the empirical quantile–quantile function, of Treated vs. Control

covariates that were found to be strongly associated with the $\sqrt{\text{CPD}}$ variable using the IPW method, the PSM method also identifies a significant association between the first two population substructure principal components and $\sqrt{\text{CPD}}$.

To check that the PSM algorithm achieved the desired balance, consider Tables 5 and 6, and notice that for all variables the differences between the two groups after matching (Table 6) are significantly reduced, compared with the differences between the groups when using the original data (Table 5). Note that the education = 0 level is absent from the tables since the secondary response is well-balanced across the two groups in the original data. Another way to visualize the effect of the matching on the distribution is to use side-by-side boxplots. The matching provided the most noticeable improvement in balancing age and PC1 across the two groups, as can be seen in Fig. 3.

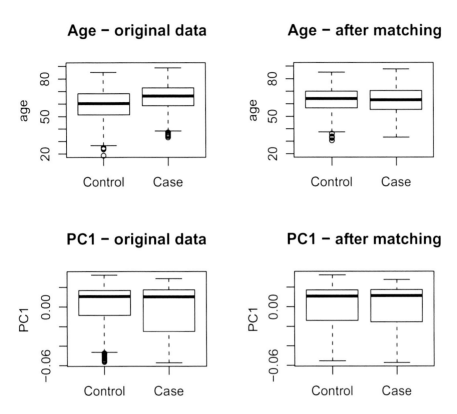

Fig. 3 The distributions of Age and PC1 in the case and control groups, before, and after applying the propensity score matching method

6   Discussion

In this chapter we demonstrated how the analysis of secondary outcomes in case–control studies can be challenging, especially when the cases are characterized by a rare condition. In these situations, extra care must be taken in order to mitigate the selection bias problem that arises because, when the experiment is designed with the primary outcome in mind, the cases are over-sampled with respect to secondary outcomes. We showed two methods, namely IPW and PSM, which can be applied in order to achieve the necessary balance in the data. In both approaches, under certain assumptions the resulting data set 'mimics' a random sampling design with respect to the secondary outcome. Note that this chapter is only meant to present the general problem and describe two possible approaches, but in practice one has to consider other limitations and complications. For example, one underlying assumption is that in the available data, covariates of interest overlap across the two groups. In other words, the range of values of a covariate is the same in both cases and controls. If this assumption does not hold, then these approaches may actually add bias to the estimation. Also, we used complete-case analysis in our demonstration, by deleting any observation which had missing data in any of the variables which were included in our models. Handling missing data presents several challenges in the analysis of secondary outcomes in case–control studies. However, this is beyond the scope of this chapter. Finally, since the result of the secondary outcome analysis often depends on user-specified parameters, it is recommended to perform sensitivity analysis, and to carefully check the assumptions of the secondary outcome model. For example, with PSM the user can choose different logistic regression models to create the propensity scores, then choose from a variety of distance measures to determine similarity between cases and controls, and then choose how many controls to try and match with each case, and how similar the matched pairs should be. Each such configuration of user input has to be validated by using diagnostic plots and tables, as shown here and in much greater detail in the PSM literature.

Acknowledgements The authors wish to thank Dr. David C. Christiani for generously sharing his data. This research was supported in part by the National Institute of Mental Health, Award Number K01MH087219. The content of this paper is solely the responsibility of the authors, and it does not represent the official views of the National Institute of Mental Health or the National Institutes of Health.

References

Abadie, A., Imbens, G.: Large sample properties of matching estimators for average treatment effects. Econometrica **74**(1), 235–267 (2006)

Amos, C.I., Wu, X., Broderick, P., Gorlov, I.P., Gu, J., Eisen, T., Dong, Q., Zhang, Q., Gu, X., Vijayakrishnan, J., Sullivan, K., Matakidou, A., Wang, Y., Mills, G., Doheny, K., Tsai, Y.Y., Chen, W.V., Shete, S., Spitz, M.R., Houlston, R.S.: Genome-wide association scan of tag SNPs identifies a susceptibility locus for lung cancer at 15q25.1. Nat. Genet. **40**(5), 616–622 (2008)

Ghosh, A., Wright, F., Zou, F.: Unified analysis of secondary traits in case-control association studies. J. Am. Stat. Assoc. **108**, 566–576 (2013)

Ho, D.E., Imai, K., King, G., Stuart, E.A.: MatchIt: nonparametric preprocessing for parametric causal inference. J. Stat. Softw. **42**(8), 1–28 (2011). http://www.jstatsoft.org/v42/i08/

Højsgaard, S., Halekoh, U., Yan, J.: The R package geepack for generalized estimating equations. J. Stat. Softw. **15**(2), 1–11 (2005)

Lettre, G., Jackson, A.U., Gieger, C., Schumacher, F.R., Berndt, S.I., Sanna, S., Eyheramendy, S., Voight, B.F., Butler, J.L., Guiducci, C., Illig, T., Hackett, R., Heid, I.M., Jacobs, K.B., Lyssenko, V., Uda, M., Boehnke, M., Chanock, S.J., Groop, L.C., Hu, F.B., Isomaa, B., Kraft, P., Peltonen, L., Salomaa, V., Schlessinger, D., Hunter, D.J., Hayes, R.B., Abecasis, G.R., Wichmann, H.E., Mohlke, K.L., Hirschhorn, J.N.: Identification of ten loci associated with height highlights new biological pathways in human growth. Nat. Genet. **40**(5), 584–591 (2008)

Lin, D.Y., Zeng, D.: Proper analysis of secondary phenotype data in case-control association studies. Genet. Epidemiol. **33**(3), 356–365 (2009)

Monsees, G.M., Tamimi, R.M., Kraft, P.: Genome-wide association scans for secondary traits using case-control samples. Genet. Epidemiol. **33**, 717–728 (2009)

R Core Team: R: A language and environment for statistical computing. R Foundation for Statistical Computing, Vienna, Austria (2014). http://www.R-project.org/

Robins, J., Rotnitzky, A., Zhao, L.: Estimation of regression coefficients when some regressors are not always observed. J. Am. Stat. Assoc. **89**, 198–203 (1994)

Rosenbaum, P., Rubin, D.: The central role of the propensity score in observational studies for causal effects. Biometrika **70**, 41–55 (1983)

Sanna, S., Jackson, A.U., Nagaraja, R., Willer, C.J., Chen, W.M., Bonnycastle, L.L., Shen, H., Timpson, N., Lettre, G., Usala, G., Chines, P.S., Stringham, H.M., Scott, L.J., Dei, M., Lai, S., Albai, G., Crisponi, L., Naitza, S., Doheny, K.F., Pugh, E.W., Ben-Shlomo, Y., Ebrahim, S., Lawlor, D.A., Bergman, R.N., Watanabe, R.M., Uda, M., Tuomilehto, J., Coresh, J., Hirschhorn, J.N., Shuldiner, A.R., Schlessinger, D., Collins, F.S., Davey Smith, G., Boerwinkle, E., Cao, A., Boehnke, M., Abecasis, G.R., Mohlke, K.L.: Common variants in the GDF5-UQCC region are associated with variation in human height. Nat. Genet. **40**(2), 198–203 (2008)

Schifano, E., Li, L., Christiani, D., Lin, X.: Genome-wide association analysis for multiple continuous phenotypes. AJHG **92**(5), 744–759 (2013)

Tchetgen Tchetgen, E.: A general regression framework for a secondary outcome in case-control studies. Biostatistics **15**, 117–128 (2014)

VanderWeele, T.J., Asomaning, K., Tchetgen Tchetgen, E.J., Han, Y., Spitz, M.R., Shete, S., Wu, X., Gaborieau, V., Wang, Y., McLaughlin, J., Hung, R.J., Brennan, P., Amos, C.I., Christiani, D.C., Lin, X.: Genetic variants on 15q25.1, smoking, and lung cancer: an assessment of mediation and interaction. Am. J. Epidemiol. **175**(10), 1013–1020 (2012)

Wei, J., Carrroll, R., Muller, U., Van Keilegon, I., Chatterjee, N.: Locally efficient estimation for homoscedastic regression in the secondary analysis of case-control data. J. Roy. Stat. Soc. Ser. B **75**, 186–206 (2013)

Controlling for Population Density Using Clustering and Data Weighting Techniques When Examining Social Health and Welfare Problems

Lynn A. Agre, N. Andrew Peterson, and James Brady

Abstract Clustering techniques partition the unit of analysis or study subjects into similar groups by a certain variable, thus permitting a model to run on cases with related attributes as a control for sociodemographic differences. Though large-scale national surveys often provide a raw weight variable, when applied without transformation, yields no change in statistical results, thus leading to spurious conclusions about relationships between predictors and outcomes. For example, most research studies using various components of the National Longitudinal Survey on Youth (NLSY) data sets to test hypotheses do not employ a weighting technique or post-stratification procedure to normalize the sample against the population from which it is drawn. Therefore, this chapter will illustrate how an algebraic weight formula introduced by Oh and Scheuren (Weighting adjustment for unit non-response. In: Incomplete Data in Sample Surveys, Chap. 3. Academic Press, New York, 1983), can be used in path analysis to elucidate the relationship between underlying psychosocial mechanisms and health risk behaviors among adolescents in the 1998 NLSY Young Adult cohort. Using the NLSY sample originally surveyed from US population, the association between self-assessed risk perception or risk proneness and how that perception affects the likelihood of an adolescent to engage in substance use and sexual behavior is investigated, separated into clusters by mother's race/ethnicity and educational attainment. To control for oversampling of under represented racial/ethnic groups, mathematically adjusted design weights are then implemented in the calculation of the covariance matrices for each cluster group by race and educational attainment, comparing non-normalized vs. normalized path analysis results. The impact of ignoring weights leading to serious

L.A. Agre (✉)
Department of Statistics and Biostatistics, Rutgers University, 110 Frelinghuysen Road, Hill Center, Busch Campus, New Brunswick, NJ 08854, USA
e-mail: lynn.agre.rutcor@gmail.com; agre@rci.rutgers.edu

N.A. Peterson
School of Social Work, Rutgers University, New Brunswick, NJ, USA

J. Brady
Rutgers University, New Brunswick, NJ, USA

© Springer International Publishing Switzerland 2015
D.-G. Chen, J. Wilson (eds.), *Innovative Statistical Methods for Public Health Data*, ICSA Book Series in Statistics, DOI 10.1007/978-3-319-18536-1_2

bias in parameter estimates, with the underestimation of standards errors will be presented illustrating the distinction between weighted and non-weighted data. As an innovative statistical approach, this application uses a weighted case approach by testing the model on discrete cluster samples of youth by race/ethnicity and mother's educational attainment. Determining public health policy initiatives and objectives requires that the data be representative of the population, ensured by transforming and applying the weight formula to the sample.

Keywords Variance–covariance matrix • Secondary data analysis • Design adjustment • Post-stratification procedure • Transforming raw weights • Oversampling

1 Introduction

Risk proneness and its relationship to depressive symptoms are vital in understanding the underlying processes that determine health risk behaviors among youth, such as alcohol use and sexual behavior. The National Longitudinal Survey on Youth (NLSY) 1998 Young Adult cohort has been selected to illustrate how sensation seeking operates in predicting alcohol use and sexual behavior among adolescents, using a weighted path analysis model. By introducing the weighting technique, particularly with respect to computation of the covariance matrix necessary to execute path analysis, never applied before to these data before in order to normalize against US population, the resulting path model compares the different results when a design effect procedure is applied.

2 Background

The NLSY Young Adult Survey is renowned for over-sampling economically disadvantaged and minority groups and thus is not a nationally representative sample of children. Some components of the questionnaire (i.e., the Center for Epidemiological Studies-Depression (CESD) short form depressive symptom index and other psychosocial, behavioral assessments) are conducted as part of an intensive in-person interview of the respondent conducted by a trained interviewer from the National Opinion Research Center. The largest portion of the survey is self-administered as a confidential questionnaire (regarding risk behavior, teenage sexual behavior, and substance use). Data then need to be weighted against race distribution of the United States, utilizing the raw data weight variable provided for each case record (Hahs-Vaughn and Lomax 2006). In order to normalize the sample against the US population demographics (Hahs-Vaughn and Lomax 2006), an algebraic weight formula is then calculated in SPSS for use with these data, applying the post-stratification algorithm developed by Oh and Scheuren (1983).

From a review of the literature, it appears that most studies using various components of the NLSY Mother–Child cohorts or Young Adult data sets to conduct analyses do not employ the raw data weights, let alone a transformed data weight, in conjunction with an algebraic formula (Crockett et al. 2006; Pachter et al. 2006). Thus, the application of the weighted approach extends the illustration of weighting procedures beyond the econometric and/or demography literature into the broader behavioral and epidemiological sciences (Horowitz and Manski 1998; MaCurdy et al. 1998). The NLSY data weights have been used to examine employment and wage trends, but not the relationship between underlying psychosocial mechanisms and health-related outcomes (MaCurdy et al. 1998). A post-stratification procedure is necessary to reduce bias in standard error estimates (Rubin et al. 1983). This research makes an important contribution by using a weighted case approach in testing the difference between non-weighted vs. weighted models.

Indeed, Lang and Zagorsky (2001) assert that not using weights may intro-duce heteroskedasticity (different variances among the variables). Therefore, it is necessary to examine and compare the standard errors when performing analyses, using a weight formula. Horowitz and Manski (1998) explain the application of the weight formula from Little and Rubin (1987) and Rubin et al. (1983), as applied to econometric analysis. Moreover, MaCurdy et al. (1998) discuss why and how the raw weights in each of the NLSY survey years differ, accounting for the non-response rate and attrition. Since the weights differ in each year and particularly since the calculation of the weight changed in 2002 (Ohio State University and Center for Human Resource Research 2006), MaCurdy et al. (1998) assert that longitudinal analysis using weighted data for multiple wave analysis from the NLSY is not accurate.

Finally, regarding techniques to control for oversampling of certain under represented groups in large population data sets, Stapleton (2002) suggests using design weights in the calculation of the covariance matrices in multi-level and structural equation models. Alternatively, she recommends using the design weight variables as covariates in the hypothesized model. She compares the results of the normalization vs. non-normalization procedures in a structural equation model. Moreover, both Stapleton (2002) and Hahs-Vaughn and Lomax (2006) strongly recommend that ignoring weights leads to serious bias in parameter estimates, with the underestimation of standard errors. Finally, Stapleton et al. (2002) declares "when modeling with effective sample size weights, care must be taken in devel-oping syntax to be submitted to the SEM software program. Using traditional SEM software, the analyst must provide the scaling factor for the between group covariance model (the square root of the common group size)."

3   Method

In a later paper Stapleton (2006) presents an argument for design effect adjusted weighting based on unequal probability selection. Given a probability sample is a proportional selection procedure, then this data collection approach requires post-stratification transformation to adjust for over-sampling of certain under represented racial and ethnic groups. The following proof explains the mathematical rationale for weighting the data, as normalizing the sample against the population from which it is originally drawn.

At the sampling stage, Oh and Scheuren (1983) conceptualize weighting cell estimators in a probability sample representing π_i^{-1} units in the population as

$$t = \sum_i^n Y_i I_i \pi_i^{-1}$$

In this formula, t is the estimator of that group with I as the indicator function or Boolean indicator, i.e. <0,1> in the non-response population where

$$\pi_i = {}^{n_i}\!/_N \; ; \; n_i \text{ is the sample size of } i^{th} \text{ unit and N is the population size,}$$

which is called the Horvitz–Thompson estimator. The t or weight for each observation then is the sum of the all the cases multiplied by the population mean divided by the number of people in that group sampled within the population. The expression below explains that each weight or t is calculated separately for each group sampled in the population, then added to yield a distinct proportion or weight in decimal form for each study subject in the data.

$$t = \left(Y_1 I_1 \; \pi_1^{-1}\right) + \left(Y_2 I_2 \; \pi_2^{-1}\right) + \ldots + \left(Y_n I_n \; \pi_n^{-1}\right)$$

However, the t or weighting cell estimator or raw weight must then be converted to relative weights or mean values, or proportion of that group in the population that was sampled based on race, age, and gender.

$$\bar{y}w = \sum_{i=1}^N w_1 y_i$$

where $w = I \times \pi - 1$

$$\frac{1}{0} = \infty \text{ where } 0 \text{ means no sample selection}$$

So if Ij or population mean is zero then the relative weight is infinity

$$\frac{y_j I_j}{\pi_j = \frac{n_j}{N_j}} \Rightarrow y_j I_j \left(\frac{N_j}{n_j}\right)$$

The result, then, is higher weight or value for that group sample size that is oversampled in order to compensate for under-representation of that particular race or ethnic cluster. With n or 3 groups as in the hypothetical illustration below, nominal weights are calculated based on the average or mean of each group. As an example, for the first group, the weight is equal to 0.1. The second is 0.4 and the third weight is 0.2. The algebraic weight formula, when subsequently applied, yields a revised or transformed sample weight, normalized against the population as follows:

$$w_i = \frac{I_j * \pi_j^{-1}}{\sum_k I_k * \pi_k^{-1}}$$

$$w1 = 0.1; w2 = 0.4; w3 = 0.2$$

Thus, for example when the given raw weight number 1 is equal to 0.1, the transformed weight becomes 0.14.

$$w_i = \frac{0.1}{0.1 + 0.4 + 0.2} = \frac{0.1}{0.7} = \frac{1}{7} = 0.14$$

$$\sum \begin{bmatrix} \pi_1^{-1} & 0.1/0.7 \\ \pi_2^{-1} & 0.4/0.7 \\ \pi_3^{-1} & 0.2/0.7 \end{bmatrix} = 1$$

Since there is unequal selection probability due to cluster sampling of the NLSY, the population mean must be estimated by the weighted mean, because the observations are not independent and are not identically distributed (Stapleton 2002). According to Stapleton (2002, 2006), the unbiased population mean results in unequal inclusion of probabilities, which requires normalization of the raw weights as expressed in the formula below. This is design effect adjustment.

$$\hat{u} = \frac{\sum_{i=1}^{n} y_i}{n} \quad \text{Stapleton}$$

Unbiased estimate population mean refers to selection probability as in cluster design (Steinley and Brusco, 2008), such that the population mean must be estimated by the weighted mean shown as formulas.

$$\hat{u} = \frac{\sum_{i=1}^{n} w_i y_i}{\sum_{i=1}^{n} w_i}$$

$$\frac{w_i n}{\sum w_i} \quad w_i = \text{raw weight}$$

Therefore, sampling variance must be calculated when unequal probabilities are included.

$$\text{var}\,(\widehat{u}) = \frac{\sum_{i=1}^{n} (y_i - \widehat{u})^2}{n\,(n-1)}$$

For equal inclusion probabilities, weights are applied to minimize the variance in the groups with oversampling due to under-representation in a population.

$$\text{var}\,(\widehat{u}) = \frac{\sum_{i=1}^{n} w_i(y_i - \widehat{u})^2}{\sum_{i=1}^{n} w_i \left(\sum_{i=1}^{n} w_i - 1\right)}$$

When the transformed weights in decimals are normalized, the weights total to one. To implement the application of the transformed algebraic weights, the procedure in statistical software entails creating a weighted variance–covariance matrix from the original variables (Stapleton 2002). In SPSS, the variance–covariance matrix is generated with the transformed weight or new weight turned on. The weighted matrix and sample size are then supplied to the SEM software or AMOS for testing the relationship of the paths.

On a programming level, the weighting cell estimator formula is used to transform the raw weights which represent the number of people in that group collected as part of the NLSY 1998 young adult cohort. The first procedure entails selecting "analyze" then clicking on "descriptive statistics" followed by the function "frequency." Using the revised raw sample weight variable provided in the NLSY data set by the Ohio State University, Center for Human Resource Research, the "statistics button" is chosen on the bottom of the draw-down menu window and then "sum." This procedure prints out the sum of the weights of all the cases in these data. A new weight for each variable is then calculated using the following formula:

$$\text{Normalized Weight} = \text{yaw} * n \Big/ \sum$$

yaw = young adult's raw weight variable provided in the NLSY Young Adult
    Data set
n = number of cases in the NLSY Young Adult cohorts 1998
$\sum$ = sum of the raw weights of all cases

An example follows using simple numbers:

	Case#	Weights Weight = Wi
n = 4	1	2
	2	3
	3	1
	4	0.5

Sum of the weight for n = 4 is 6.5
Ratio is 4/6.5

Wi * ratio	
Wi = 2	2*4/6.5 = 1.230769
Wi = 3	3*4/6.5 = 1.846154
Wi = 1	1*4/6.5 = 0.6153846
Wi = 0.5	0.5*4/6.5 = 0.3076923
Total	=4

This normalized weight is then applied to all path analyses executed. While performing analyses, the weight "on" command in SPSS is selected to ensure the variables in the sample are normalized against the US population from which they were originally drawn.

4 Results

4.1 Bivariate

4.1.1 Correlation Table Comparison

All the individual measures in the study were correlated to determine how strongly associated the variables are with each other, yielding a bivariate final sample n of 4,648, as displayed in Table 1. Correlations were also employed to ascertain the relationships among the descriptive as well as scale indicators used in the analyses. Only those correlations that were both significant at $p < 0.05$ or 0.01 and below are discussed. In the correlation Table 1 depicting both weighted and non-weighted Pearson correlation coefficients, some correlations are strengthened with higher values when compared to non-weighted results. Indeed, in some cases, such as alcohol use and age (weighted Pearson correlation coefficient (w.P.c.c. = 0.080) vs. non-weighted Pearson correlation coefficient (n.w.P.c.c. = 0.021)), or sexual risk taking and gender (w.P.c.c. = −0.062 vs. n.w.P.c.c. = 0.005), the association between two weighted variables becomes significant. The correlation values generally remain at the same significance level even when weighted, but some correlation values increase, while a few decrease as indicated in the ensuing paragraphs.

Table 1 Correlations for NLSY 1998 variables used in analysis (n = 4,648): non-weighted vs. weighted (in parentheses)

Variable	1	2	3	4	5	6	7	8	9
1. Age	1.0								
2. Gender Male	0.011 (0.023)	1.0							
3. Race White	−0.103** (−0.076**)	0.033 (0.044**)	1.0						
4. Neighborhood Quality	−0.064** (−0.034*)	0.006 (0.012)	0.247** (0.253**)	1.0					
5. Perceived closeness between parents	−0.120** (−0.140**)	0.010 (−0.003)	0.100** (0.112**)	0.043** (0.079**)	1.0				
6. Depressive symptoms index	−0.001 (−0.005)	−0.169** (−0.188**)	0.020 (0.014)	−0.142** (−0.149**)	0.015 (0.000)	1.0			
7. Risk proneness	−0.123** (−0.104**)	0.088** (0.124**)	0.229** (0.208**)	0.036* (0.011)	0.098** (0.087**)	0.125** (0.121**)	1.0		
8. Alcohol use	0.021 (0.080**)	0.020 (0.033*)	0.141** (0.132**)	0.082** (0.061**)	0.017 (0.040**)	0.013 (0.011)	0.138** (0.153**)	1.0	
9. Sexual risk taking	0.286** (0.295**)	0.005 (−0.062**)	−0.071** (−0.059**)	−0.104** (−0.155**)	−0.112** (−0.149**)	0.112** (0.138**)	0.029 (0.012)	0.105** (0.164**)	1.0

*$p < 0.05$; **$p < 0.01$

Thus, youth's age and white race yielded a weighted Pearson correlation coefficient of -0.076 (vs. n.w.P.c.c. $= -0.103$), with high significance at $p < 0.01$. Neighborhood quality correlated with age at interview date (1998) with a weighted Pearson correlation coefficient of -0.034 (vs. n.w.P.c.c. $= -0.064$) with significance at $p < 0.05$. Perceived parental closeness between the mother and biological father also negatively correlated with youth's age (w.P.c.c. $= -0.140$ vs. n.w.P.c.c. $= -0.120$) and also with risk proneness (w.P.c.c. $= -0.104$ vs. n.w.P.c.c. $= -0.123$) at significance level of $p < 0.01$. Alcohol use (w.P.c.c. $= 0.080$ vs. n.w.P.c.c. $= 0.021$) and sexual risk taking (w.P.c.c. $= 0.295$ vs. n.w.P.c.c. $= 0.286$) were both correlated with age and highly significant at $p < 0.01$.

Male gender produced positive correlations with white race (w.P.c.c. $= 0.044$ vs. n.w.P.c.c. $= 0.033$) and risk proneness (w.P.c.c. $= 0.124$ vs. n.w.P.c.c. $= 0.088$), again significant at $p < 0.01$, and alcohol use (w.P.c.c. $= 0.033$ vs. n.w.P.c.c. $= 0.022$) significant at $p < 0.05$. Male gender negatively correlated with depressive symptoms (w.P.c.c. $= -0.188$ vs. n.w.P.c.c. $= -0.169$, $p < 0.01$) and sexual risk taking (w.P.c.c. $= -0.062$, $p < 0.01$ vs. n.w.P.c.c. $= 0.005$ not significant). White race positively correlated with neighborhood quality (w.P.c.c. $= 0.253$ vs. n.w.P.c.c. $= 0.247$), perceived parental closeness between the mother and biological father (w.P.c.c. $= 0.112$ vs. n.w.P.c.c. $= 0.100$), risk proneness (w.P.c.c. $= 0.208$ vs. n.w.P.c.c. $= 0.229$) and alcohol use (w.P.c.c. $= 0.132$ vs. n.w.P.c.c. $= 0.141$), all significant at $p < 0.01$. However, white race negatively correlated with sexual risk taking (w.P.c.c. $= -0.059$ vs. n.w.P.c.c. $= -0.071$), at $p < 0.01$ significance level. Further, neighborhood quality correlated with perceived parental closeness between the mother and biological father at (w.P.c.c. $= 0.079$ vs. n.w.P.c.c. $= 0.043$) and alcohol use (w.P.c.c. $= 0.061$ vs. n.w.P.c.c. $= 0.082$) also significant at $p < 0.01$. Other negative correlations with neighborhood quality (meaning lower score, worse quality neighborhood) included: depressive symptoms index (w.P.c.c. $= -0.149$ vs. n.w.P.c.c. $= -0.142$) and sexual risk taking (w.P.c.c. $= -0.155$ vs. n.w.P.c.c. $= -0.104$), both highly significant at $p < 0.01$.

The variable perceived parental closeness between mother and biological father (the lower the score, the worse the parenting) also correlated with risk proneness (w.P.c.c. $= 0.087$ vs. n.w.P.c.c. $= 0.098$), alcohol use (w.P.c.c. $= 0.040$ vs. n.w.P.c.c. $= 0.017$, not significant), and sexual risk taking (w.P.c.c. $= -0.149$ vs. n.w.P.c.c. $= -0.112$), all weighted Pearson correlation coefficients significant at $p < 0.01$. Further, depressive symptoms index was associated with risk proneness (w.P.c.c. $= 0.121$ vs. n.w.P.c.c. $= 0.125$), and sexual risk taking (w.P.c.c. $= 0.138$ vs. n.w.P.c.c. $= 0.112$) at significance level of $p < 0.01$. Finally, risk proneness was moderately correlated with alcohol use (w.P.c.c. $= 0.153$ vs. n.w.P.c.c. $= 0.138$), which was also associated with sexual risk taking (w.P.c.c. $= 0.164$ vs. n.w.P.c.c. $= 0.105$) but highly significant at $p < 0.01$.

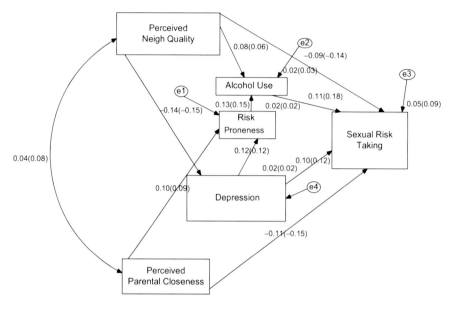

Fig. 1 Non-weighted and weighted path model (weighted values in parentheses)

4.2   Multivariate

4.2.1   Path Comparison

As with the bivariate analysis, the beta coefficients in the path model again change as a consequence of applying weights. Most of the values increase, thereby demonstrating that when the transformed data weights are applied, the association between and among the variables differs from the non-weighted findings. Therefore, as seen in Fig. 1, the weighted path analysis results show that higher neighborhood quality is correlated with higher perceived parental closeness (weighted beta coefficient (w.b.c.) = 0.08 vs. non-weighted beta coefficient (n.w.b.c.) = 0.04). Poorer neighborhood quality is related to higher depression scores (w.b.c. = −0.15 vs. n.w.b.c. = −0.14). Higher neighborhood quality and higher alcohol use are also associated (w.b.c. = 0.06 vs. n.w.b.c. = 0.08) in this model. Poorer neighborhood quality influences higher sexual risk taking (w.b.c. = −0.14 vs. n.w.b.c. = −0.09). Moreover, lower perceived parental closeness between mother and biological father also promotes higher risk proneness (w.b.c. = 0.08 vs. n.w.b.c. = 0.04). Poor perceived parental closeness between mother and biological father is also related to elevated sexual risk taking (w.b.c. = −0.15 vs. n.w.b.c = −0.14). Higher depression scores are associated with increased risk proneness (w.b.c. = 0.12 same as n.w.b.c. = 0.12) and greater sexual risk taking (w.b.c. = 0.12 vs. n.w.b.c. = 0.10). Risk proneness leads to greater alcohol use (w.b.c. = 0.15 vs. n.w.b.c. = 0.13). Finally, greater alcohol use promotes higher sexual risk taking (w.b.c. = 0.18 vs. n.w.b.c. = 0.11).

Table 2 Fit indices for non-weighted vs. weighted model

Measures of fit	Non-weighted 1998 NLSY data (n = 4,648)	Weighted 1998 NLSY data (n = 4,648)
χ^2	15,673 ($p = 0.008$)	6,645 ($p = 0.248$)
CFI	0.981	0.998
AGFI	0.995	0.998
RMSEA	0.021	0.008
TLI	0.942	0.994

Table 3 Indirect, direct, and total comparing non-weighted and weighted effects from path analysis using perceived parental closeness between mother and biological father on sexual risk taking n = 4,648

Variable	Non-weighted			Weighted		
	Total indirect effect	Direct effect	Total effect	Total indirect effect	Direct effect	Total effect
Perceived parental closeness between mother and bio-father	0.001	−0.110	−0.109	0.002	−0.145	−0.143
Neighborhood quality	−0.006	−0.094	−0.100	−0.007	−0.137	−0.144
Depressive symptoms	0.002	0.099	0.101	0.003	0.116	0.119
Risk proneness	0.015	0.000	0.015	0.027	0.000	0.027
Alcohol use	0.000	0.113	0.113	0.000	0.177	0.177

Table 2 presents the fit indices for both the non-weighted vs. weighted path analysis models. The chi-square for both the non-weighted and weighted models is low and not significant at $p < 0.001$, meaning the model has good fit in both cases. However, the weighted chi-square results clearly show a slightly higher chi-square with even less significance at $p < 0.001$. Further, the other fit indices, Comparative Fit Index (CFI), Adjusted Goodness of Fit Index (AGFI), Root Mean Square Error of Approximation (RMSEA) and Tucker Lewis Index (TLI) per Olobatuyi (2006), when comparing the non-weighted to the non-weighted all meet the criteria of between 0.9 and 1. But the weighted model indicates stronger fit with all values closer to the upper threshold than the non-weighted. Thus, the CFI compares the tested model to the null, i.e. no paths between variables. The AGFI measures the amount of variance and covariance in observed and reproduced matrices. The RMSEA is an indicator of parsimony in the model, meaning the simplest and fewest number of variables. Finally, the TLI, using chi-square values of the null vs. the proposed model, reinforces the rigor of this model.

Table 3 describes the direct and indirect effects of all the variables together with perceived parental closeness between mother and biological father and mother and step-father, respectively, used in this path analysis on sexual risk taking dependent variable. Similar findings are reported for both non-weighted and weighted data. Indeed, the detrimental effect of perceived parental closeness on sexual risk taking is evidenced by the negative coefficient value in both models using ratings of the mother and biological father (-0.15 non-weighted vs. weighted -0.03). However, better neighborhood appraisal in the perceived parental closeness between the mother and biological father had a direct effect (0.06) on increased alcohol use. Thus, youth who perceived greater neighborhood quality used more alcohol. However, worse neighborhood quality (-0.14) and lower perceived parental closeness (-0.15) has a direct negative effect on sexual risk taking. Or conversely, teens who perceive a worse environment engage in less sexual activity. Thus, both neighborhood perception and perceived parental closeness have a protective effect on sexual risk taking, which then, in turn, is diminished by risk proneness (0.00) and alcohol use (0.18).

Nevertheless, a paradox arises among indirect effects associated with neighborhood quality. Those youth who rate neighborhood quality as high also report using more alcohol and increased sexual risk taking, which can possibly be attributed to more disposal income. In another indirect effect, lower neighborhood quality operates through higher depression, higher risk proneness, in turn leading to higher alcohol use and higher sexual risk taking (or total effect of -0.144 for biological parents model path analysis, based on four multiplicative paths, then summed together, (per Cohen and Cohen 1983, referring to Fig. 1). The total effects for all variables in the weighted model (Fig. 1) are higher in value than the non-weighted, with the exception of: (1) perceived parental closeness and risk proneness (w.b.c. $= 0.09$ vs. n.w.b.c. $= 0.10$); (2) neighborhood quality and alcohol use (w.b.c $= 0.06$ vs. n.w.b.c. $= 0.08$); and (3) depressive symptoms and risk proneness (both w.b.c. and n.w.b.c. equal to 0.12).

5 Discussion

To date, no published literature documents the weighting technique applied to the variance–covariance matrix used for the path analysis, generated from the NLSY data for this research. The algebraic weight formula is used to transform the raw weights provided in the NLSY Young Adult data set. The raw weights are proportionally calculated based on each case by gender, race, and age. However, the raw weights need to be modified before implemented in the multivariate analysis in order to normalize the sample against the US population. Therefore, the value of each case is now altered to ensure the contribution of those responses within a case are representative of the population distribution in the US. Thus, the weighting technique can now be introduced into future research studies involving the NLSY data sets.

Since the NLSY is a probability cluster sample (Ohio State University and Center for Human Resource Research 2006), which is a selection procedure determined by proportion of a population, a post-stratification procedure is needed to adjust for the study design (Stapleton 2006; Steinley and Brusco 2008). The two standardized path models—one using the non-weighted variance–covariance matrix and the other weighted—reveal slight differences in the path beta coefficient values. While these distinctions are not marked, applying the transformed weight to the variance–covariance matrix does present implications for generalizability and external validity.

Indeed, in path analysis, what happens to the covariance matrix to a degree is data dependent (McDonald 1996). When using mean substitution in a path model, variability and standard error decreases thereby reducing the strength of the correlations and weakening the covariance matrix (Olinsky et al. 2003), as is the case with this example using the NLSY—Young Adult Survey. However, if the missing data is indeed missing at random (MAR), mean substitution is considered the most conservative and therefore the least distorting of the data distribution (Little and Rubin 1987; Shafer and Olsen 1998). Moreover, by applying the algebraic weighting technique shown in this study, the contribution of each variable in the equation is proportionally adjusted to reflect the actual distribution, normalized to reflect the actual population from which the sample is drawn. On a graphical level, the data weighting procedure thus hugs the scatter plot in closer away from the imaginary axes defining the boundaries, tightening the ellipse, yielding a better estimated regression line (Green 1977). Because the underlying notion of causal inferencing is the focus of path analysis (Rothman and Greenland 2005) applying the Rubin (1987) MAR mean substitution is not only required in determining the causal reasoning with large secondary data sets, such as the NLSY, but essential for demonstrating in particular the temporal ordering of the endogenous variables' role in affecting exogenous outcomes (Pearl 2000).

The weighting technique is critical even when the model is applied to primary data. For example, if this model were tested on a sample taken from a geographic area with overrepresentation of a particular ethnicity or race, then the weight formula would need to be applied to ensure generalizability and replicability. Thus, in order to determine policy initiatives and objectives with respect to demonstration projects and/or interventions, the data needs to be representative of the population, standardized against the original distribution ensured by implementing the weight formula.

The effects of individual, family, and neighborhood quality on adolescent substance use and sexual activity are evaluated to explain the relationship of the individual adolescent to the environmental context and how these factors are associated with co-morbid mental and physical health conditions. Understanding the mechanisms, such as how depression, sensation seeking, lack of perceived parental closeness (discord on rules), and poorer neighborhood quality elucidates the link to health risk behaviors in situ. This study makes an important contribution by using a weighted case approach in potentially testing different samples of youth by race/ethnicity. Determining policy initiatives and objectives requires that the data be representative of the population, ensured by applying the weight formula.

References

Cohen, J., Cohen, A.: Applied Multiple Regression/Correlation Analysis for the Behavioral Sciences. Lawrence Erlbaum Associates, Hillsdale (1983)

Crockett, L.J., Raffaelli, M., Shen, Y.-L.: Linking self-regulation and risk proneness to risky sexual behavior: pathways through peer pressure and early substance use. J. Res. Adolesc. **16**, 503–525 (2006)

Green, B.F.: Parameter sensitivity in multivariate methods. J. Multivar. Behav. Res. **12**, 263–287 (1977)

Hahs-Vaughn, D.L., Lomax, R.G.: Utilization of sample weights in single-level structural equation modeling. J. Exp. Educ. **74**, 163–190 (2006)

Horowitz, J.L., Manski, C.F.: Censoring of outcomes and regressors due to survey nonresponse: identification and estimation using weights and imputations. J. Econ. **84**, 37–58 (1998)

Lang, K., Zagorsky, J.L.: Does growing up with a parent absent really hurt? J. Hum. Resour. **36**, 253–273 (2001)

Little, R.J.A., Rubin, D.A.: Statistical Analysis with Missing Data. Wiley, New York (1987)

MaCurdy, T., Mroz, T., Gritz, R.M.: An evaluation of the national longitudinal survey on youth. J. Hum. Resour. **33**, 345–436 (1998)

McDonald, R.P.: Path analysis with composite variables. Multivar. Behav. Res. **31**, 239–270 (1996)

Oh, H.L., Scheuren, F.J.: Weighting adjustment for unit nonresponse. In: Incomplete Data in Sample Surveys, Chap. 3. Academic Press, New York (1983)

Ohio State University, Center for Human Resource Research: NLSY 79 Child & Young Adult Data Users Guide. Ohio State University, Center for Human Resource Research, Columbus (2006). Retrieved from http://www.nlsinfo.org/pub/usersvc/Child-Young-Adult/2004ChildYA-DataUsersGuide.pdf

Olinsky, A., Chen, S., Harlow, L.: The comparative efficacy of imputation methods for missing data in structural equation modeling. Eur. J. Oper. Res. **151**, 53–79 (2003)

Olobatuyi, R.: A User's Guide to Path Analysis. University Press of America, Lanham (2006)

Pachter, L.M., Auinger, P., Palmer, R., Weitzman, M.: Do parenting and home environment, maternal depression, neighborhood and chronic poverty affect child behavioral problems differently in different age groups? Pediatrics **117**, 1329–1338 (2006)

Pearl, J.: Causality: Models, Reasoning and Inference. Cambridge University Press, Cambridge (2000)

Rothman, K.J., Greenland, S.: Causation and causal inference in epidemiology. Am. J. Public Health **95**, S144–S150 (2005)

Rubin, D.B., Olkin, I., Madow, W.G.: Incomplete Data in Sample Surveys. Academic Press, Inc., New York (1983)

Shafer, J.L., Oslen, M.K.: Multiple imputation for multivariate missing-data problems: a data analyst's perspective. Multivar. Behav. Res. **33**, 545–571 (1998)

Stapleton, L.M.: The incorporation of sample weights into multilevel structural equation models. Struct. Equ. Model. **9**, 475–502 (2002)

Stapleton, L.M.: An assessment of practical solutions for structural equation modeling with complex data. Struct. Equ. Model. **13**, 28–58 (2006)

Steinley, D., Brusco, M.J.: A new variable weighting and selection procedure for K-means cluster analysis. Multivar. Behav. Res. **43**, 77–108 (2008)

On the Inference of Partially Correlated Data with Applications to Public Health Issues

Hani M. Samawi and Robert Vogel

Abstract Correlated or matched data is frequently collected under many study designs in applied sciences such as the social, behavioral, economic, biological, medical, epidemiologic, health, public health, and drug developmental sciences in order to have a more efficient design and to control for potential confounding factors in the study. Challenges with respect to availability and cost commonly occur with matching observational or experimental study subjects. Researchers frequently encounter situations where the observed sample consists of a combination of correlated and uncorrelated data due to missing responses. Ignoring cases with missing responses, when analyzing the data, will introduce bias in the inference and reduce the power of the testing procedure. As such, the importance in developing new statistical inference methods to treat partially correlated data and new approaches to model partially correlated data has grown over the past few decades. These methods attempt to account for the special nature of partially correlated data.

In this chapter, we provide several methods to compare two Gaussian distributed means in the two sample location problem under the assumption of partially dependent observations. For categorical data, tests of homogeneity for partially matched-pair data are investigated. Different methods of combining tests of homogeneity based on Pearson chi-square test and McNemar chi-squared test are investigated. Also, we will introduce several nonparametric testing procedures which combine all cases in the study.

H.M. Samawi (✉)
Department of Biostatistics, Jiann-Ping Hsu College of Public Health, Georgia Southern University, Hendricks Hall, Room 1006, Statesboro, GA 30460, USA
e-mail: hsamawi@georgiasouthern.edu

R. Vogel (✉)
Department of Biostatistics, Jiann-Ping Hsu College of Public Health, Georgia Southern University, Hendricks Hall, Room 1013, Statesboro, GA 30460, USA
e-mail: rvogel@georgiasouthern.edu

© Springer International Publishing Switzerland 2015
D.-G. Chen, J. Wilson (eds.), *Innovative Statistical Methods for Public Health Data*,
ICSA Book Series in Statistics, DOI 10.1007/978-3-319-18536-1_3

31

Keywords McNemar test • Pearson chi-square test • Inverse chi-square method • Weighted chi-square test • Tippett method • Partially matched-pair • Case–control and matching studies • T-test • Z-test • Power of the test • *p*-Value of the test • Efficiency • Matched pairs sign test • Sign test • Wilcoxon signed-rank test • Correlated and uncorrelated data

1   Introduction

The importance of statistical inferential methods and modeling approaches to the social, behavioral, economic, biological, medical, epidemiologic, health, public health, and drug developmental sciences has grown exponentially in the last few decades. Many study designs in the aforementioned applied sciences give rise to correlated and partially correlated data due to missing responses. In some instances correlated data arise when subjects are matched to controls because of confounding factors. Other situations arise when subjects are repeatedly measured over time as in repeated measures designs. One assumption to consider is that observations are missing completely at random (MCAR), see, for example, Brunner and Puri (1996) and Brunner et al. (2002). However, Akritas et al. (2002) consider another missing value mechanism, missing at random (MAR). For quantitative responses, statistical methods, including linear and nonlinear models, are established for correlated data. However, for partially correlated data there are concerns which to be addressed due to the complexity of the analysis. In particular, for small sample sizes and when a normality assumption of the underlying populations is not valid.

As an example of partially correlated data for the MCAR design, consider the case where the researcher compares two different treatment regiments for eye redness or allergy and randomly assigns one treatment to each eye for each experimental subject. Some patients may drop out after the first treatment, while other patients may drop out after the second treatment. In this situation, we may have two groups of patients: the first group of patients who received both treatments in each eye, and are considered as paired matched data; and the second group who received only one of the treatments in one of the eyes, and are considered as unmatched data. This study design is illustrated in Table 1.

Moreover, additional examples for partially correlated data can be found in the literature (see, for example, Dimery et al. 1987; Nurnberger et al. 1982; Steere et al. 1985). Several authors have presented various tests considering the problem of estimating the difference of means of a bivariate normal distribution when some observations corresponding to both variables are missing. Under the assumption of bivariate normality and MCAR, Ekbohm (1976) summarized five procedures for testing the equality of two means. Using Monte Carlo results Ekbohm (1976) indicated that the two tests based on a modified maximum likelihood estimator are preferred: one due to Lin and Stivers (1974) when the number of complete pairs is large, and the other proposed in Ekbohm's paper otherwise, provided the variances of the two responses do not differ substantially. When the correlation coefficient

Table 1 Partially matched
study design

Paired subject	Treatment 1	Treatment 2
1	Yes	Yes
2	Yes	Yes
3	Yes	Yes
4	Yes	No
5	Yes	No
6	Yes	No
7	No	Yes
8	No	Yes
9	No	Yes
10	No	Yes

between the two responses is small, two other tests may be used: a test proposed by Ekbohm when the homoscedasticity assumption is not strongly violated, and otherwise a Welch-type statistic suggested by Lin and Stivers (1974) (for further discussion, see Ekbohm 1976).

Alternatively, researchers tend to ignore some of the data—either the correlated or the uncorrelated data depending on the size of each subset. However, in case the missingness not completely at random (MCAR), Looney and Jones (2003) argued that ignoring some of the correlated observations would bias the estimation of the variance of the difference in treatment means and would dramatically affect the performance of the statistical test in terms of controlling type I error rates and statistical power (see Snedecor and Cochran 1980). They propose a corrected z-test method to overcome the challenges created by ignoring some of the correlated observations. However, our preliminary investigation shows that the method of Looney and Jones (2003) pertains to large samples and is not the most powerful test procedure. Furthermore, Rempala and Looney (2006) studied asymptotic properties of a two-sample randomized test for partially dependent data. They indicated that a linear combination of randomized t-tests is asymptotically valid and can be used for non-normal data. However, the large sample permutation tests are difficult to perform and only have some optimal asymptotic properties in the Gaussian family of distributions when the correlation between the paired observations is positive. Other researchers such as Xu and Harrar (2012) and Konietschke et al. (2012) also discuss the problem for continuous variables including the normal distribution by using weighted statistics. However, the procedure suggested by Xu and Harrar (2012) is a functional smoothing to the Looney and Jones (2003) procedure. As such, the Xu and Hara procedure is not a practical alternative for the non-statistician researcher. The procedure suggested by Konietschke et al. (2012) is a nonparametric procedure based on ranking.

The aforementioned methods cannot be used for non-normal and moderate, small sample size data and categorical data. Samawi and Vogel (2011) introduced several weighted tests when the variables of interest are categorical. They showed that their test procedures compete with other tests in the literature. Moreover, there are several attempts to provide nonparametric test procedures under MCAR and MAR designs (for example, see Brunner and Puri 1996; Brunner et al. 2002; Akritas et al. 2002; Im KyungAh 2002; Tang 2007). However, there is still a need for intensive investigation to develop more powerful nonparametric testing procedures for MCAR and MAR designs. Samawi et al. (2014) discussed and proposed some nonparametric testing procedures to handle data when partially correlated data is available without ignoring the cases with missing responses. They introduced more powerful testing procedure which combined all cases in the study. These procedures will be of special importance in meta-analysis where partially correlated data is a concern when combining results of various studies.

2   Tests for Normal Data

Methods that are most commonly used to analyze a combination of correlated and non-correlated when data assumed to be normally distributed data are:

1. Using all data with a t-test for two independent samples assuming no correlation among the observations in the two treatments.
2. Ignoring the paired observations and perform the usual t-test of two independent samples after deleting the correlated data.
3. Ignore the independent observations of treatment 1 and 2 and perform the usual paired t-test on the correlated data.
4. The corrected z-test by Looney and Jones (2003).

To perform the Looney and Jones test, let $\{X_1, X_2, \ldots, X_{n_1}\}$ and $\{Y_1, Y_2, \ldots, Y_{n_2}\}$ denote two independent random samples of subjects receiving either treatment 1 or treatment 2, respectively. Suppose there are n paired subjects in which one member of the pair receives treatment 1 and the other paired member receives treatment 2. Let $\{(U_1, V_1), (U_2, V_2), \ldots, (U_n, V_n)\}$ denote the observed values of the paired (correlated) subjects. Looney and Jones assumed that x- and u-observations come from a common normal parent population and y- and v-observations come from a common normal parent population, which may be different from x and u observations. Let M_1 denote the sample mean for all treatment 1 subjects; that is the mean of all x- and u-values combined, and let M_2 denote the sample mean for all treatment 2 subjects; that is, the mean of all y- and v-values combined. Let S_1^2 denote the sample variance for all treatment 1 subjects and let S_2^2 denote the sample variance for all treatment 2 subjects. The Looney and Jones proposed test statistic is:

$$Z_{Corr} = \frac{M_1 - M_2}{\sqrt{\frac{S_1^2}{(n_1+n)} + \frac{S_2^2}{(n_2+n)} - \frac{2nS_{uv}^2}{(n_1+n)(n_2+n)}}}$$

where S_{uv}^2 is the sample covariance of the paired observations.

Under the null hypothesis, Z_{Corr} has asymptotic $N(0,1)$ distribution. However, this test works only for a large sample size. In case of small sample sizes, the exact distribution is not clear. An approximation to the exact distribution critical values is needed. Bootstrap methods to find the p-value of the test may also work. In addition, under the assumption of a large sample size, this test is not a uniformly powerful test. Its power depends on the correlation between the correlated observations. As an alternative we propose the following test procedure.

2.1 Proposed Weighted Tests by Samawi and Vogel (2014)

As in Looney and Jones (2003), let $\{X_1, X_2, \ldots, X_{n_1}\}$ and $\{Y_1, Y_2, \ldots, Y_{n_2}\}$ denote two independent random samples of subjects receiving either treatment 1 or treatment 2, respectively. Suppose there are n paired subjects in which one member of the pair receives treatment 1 and the other paired member receives treatment 2. Let $\{(U_1, V_1), (U_2, V_2), \ldots, (U_n, V_n)\}$ denote the observed values of the paired subjects. Assume that x- and u-observations come from a common normal parent population $N(\mu_1, \sigma^2)$ and y- and v-observations come from a common normal parent population $N(\mu_2, \sigma^2)$. Let $D_i = U_i - V_i, i = 1, 2, \ldots, n$. D_i is $N\left(\mu_1 - \mu_2, \sigma_D^2\right)$, where $\sigma_D^2 = 2\sigma^2(1 - \rho)$ and ρ is the correlation coefficient between U and V. Let $\overline{X}, \overline{Y}$ and $\overline{D}$ denote the sample means of x-observations, y-observations, and d-observations, respectively. Also, let S_x^2, S_y^2 and S_d^2 denote the sample variances of x-observations, y-observations, and d-observations, respectively. Let $N = n_1+n_2+n$ and $\gamma = \frac{n_1+n_2}{N}$. Samawi and Vogel (2014) proposed the following test procedure for testing the null hypothesis $H_0: \mu_1=\mu_2$, where μ_1 and μ_2 are the respective response means of treatment 1 and treatment 2:

$$T_0 = \sqrt{\gamma}\,\frac{\overline{X} - \overline{Y}}{\sqrt{\frac{S_x^2}{n_1} + \frac{S_y^2}{n_2}}} + \sqrt{1 - \gamma}\,\frac{\overline{D}}{S_d/\sqrt{n}}. \tag{1}$$

When $\gamma=1$, this test reduces to the two-sample t-test. Also, when $\gamma=0$, this test is the matched paired t-test.

Case 1. Large sample sizes will generally mean both a large number of matched paired observations and large number of two independent samples from treatment 1 and treatment 2. By applying Slutsky's Theorem and under the null hypothesis, T_0 has an approximate $N(0,1)$ distribution. The p-value of the test can therefore be directly calculated from the standard normal distribution.

Case 2. Without loss of generality, we will consider that the paired data has small sample size while the independent two-samples from the two treatments have large sample size. To find the distribution of the weighted test, under the null hypothesis, let $T_o = \sqrt{\gamma}X + \sqrt{1 - \gamma}T_k$ where X has $N(0,1)$ and T_k has t-distribution with k degrees of freedom. Then

$$f_{T_0}(t) = \int\limits_{-\infty}^{\infty} \frac{1}{\sqrt{\gamma}} \phi\left(\frac{t - \sqrt{\gamma}x}{\sqrt{1-\gamma}}\right) t_k(x)dx. \tag{2}$$

Nason (2005) in an unpublished report found the distribution of T_o when the degrees of freedom is odd. The distribution provided by Nason (2005) is very complicated and cannot be used directly to find percentiles from this distribution. To find the p-value of T_o you need to use a package published by Nason (2005). Therefore, we provide a simple bootstrap algorithm to find the p-value of test procedure based on the distribution of T_o. A similar approach may be taken when the paired data has large sample size and the independent data has small sample size.

Case 3. Both data sets, the independent samples and the matched paired data, have small sample sizes. Under the null hypothesis T_0 has weighted t-distribution. Let $T_o = \gamma T_{k_1} + (1 - \gamma) T_{k_2}$ where T_{k_1} and T_{k_2} are two independent t-variates with k_1 and k_2 degrees of freedom, respectively. Walker and Saw (1978) derived the distribution of a linear combination of t-variates when all degrees of freedom are odd. In our case, since we have only two t-variates with k_1 and k_2 degrees of freedoms, we need to assume that k_1 and k_2 are odd numbers or we can manipulate the data to have both numbers to be odd. Using Walker and Saw (1978) results, one can find the p-value of the suggested test statistics T_0. However, the Walker and Saw (1978) method still needs an extensive amount of computation. Therefore, a bootstrap algorithm also may be used to find the p-value of T_0.

2.2 New Test Procedure by Samawi and Vogel (2014)

Under the assumption of MCAR, to test the null hypothesis $H_0 : \mu_1 = \mu_2$, they introduced the following notation: $D_i = U_i - V_i, i = 1, 2, \ldots, n$, and $\overline{D} = \dfrac{\sum\limits_{i=1}^{n} D_i}{n}$.
They proposed the following test statistics to test $H_0 : \mu_1 = \mu_2$ as follows:

$$T_{New} = \frac{\overline{D} + (\overline{X} - \overline{Y})}{\sqrt{\theta_1 S_d^2 + \theta_2 S_P^2}}, \tag{3}$$

where $S_d^2 = \dfrac{\sum\limits_{i=1}^{n}(d_i - \overline{d})^2}{n-1}$, $S_P^2 = \dfrac{\sum\limits_{i=1}^{n_1}(X_i - \overline{X})^2 + \sum\limits_{i=1}^{n_2}(Y_i - \overline{Y})^2}{n_1 + n_2 - 2}$, $\theta_1 = \dfrac{1}{n}$ and $\theta_2 = \dfrac{1}{n_1} + \dfrac{1}{n_2}$.

Note that $Var\left(\overline{D} + \overline{X} - \overline{Y}\right) = \theta_1 \sigma_d^2 + \theta_2 \sigma^2$, under the normality assumption and

$$H_0 : \mu_1 = \mu_2, \quad \frac{(n-1)S_d^2}{\sigma_d^2} \xrightarrow{L} \chi_{(n-1)}^2 \quad \text{and} \quad \frac{\sum\limits_{i=1}^{n_1} \left(X_i - \overline{X}\right)^2 + \sum\limits_{i=1}^{n_2} \left(Y_i - \overline{Y}\right)^2}{\sigma^2} \xrightarrow{L} \chi_{(n_1+n_2-2)}^2.$$

Therefore, under the null hypothesis and using Satherwaite's method,

$$T_{New} \xrightarrow{L} t\left(df_s\right); df_s \approx \frac{\left(\theta_1 S_d^2 + \theta_2 S_P^2\right)^2}{\frac{\left(\theta_1 S_d^2\right)^2}{n-1} + \frac{\left(\theta_2 S_P^2\right)^2}{n_1+n_2-2}}. \tag{4}$$

2.3   Bootstrap Method to Estimate the p-Value of T_0 in Case 2 and 3

Uniform bootstrap resampling was introduce by Efron (1979). The uniform resampling for the two independent sample case is discussed by Ibrahim (1991) and Samawi et al. (1996, 1998). We suggest applying uniform bootstrap resampling as a means of obtaining p-values for our test procedure. However, since our test procedure involves t-statistic, there are some conditions discussed by Janssen and Pauls (2003) and Janssen (2005) need to be verified to insure that the test statistic under consideration will have proper convergent rate. They indicated that the bootstrap works if and only if the so-called central limit theorem holds for the test statistics.

   In our case $\{X_1, X_2, \ldots, X_{n_1}\}$ and $\{Y_1, Y_2, \ldots, Y_{n_2}\}$ and $\{(U_1, V_1), (U_2, V_2), \ldots, (U_n, V_n)\}$ are independent samples, thus the bootstrap p-value can be calculated as follows:

1. Use the original sample sets $\{X_1, X_2, \ldots, X_{n_1}\}$ and $\{Y_1, Y_2, \ldots, Y_{n_2}\}$ and $\{(U_1, V_1), (U_2, V_2), \ldots, (U_n, V_n)\}$ to calculate T_0.
2. Let $\{X_1^*, X_2^*, \ldots, X_{n_1}^*\}$ and $\{Y_1^*, Y_2^*, \ldots, Y_{n_2}^*\}$ and $\{(U_1^*, V_1^*), (U_2^*, V_2^*), \ldots, (U_n^*, V_n^*)\}$ be the centered samples by subtracting the sampling means $\overline{X}, \overline{Y}$ and $\left(\overline{U}, \overline{V}\right)$, respectively.
3. With placed probabilities $(\frac{1}{n_1}, \frac{1}{n_2}, \frac{1}{n})$ on the samples in step (2), respectively, generate independently bootstrap samples, namely $\{X_{i1}^{**}, X_{i2}^{**}, \ldots, X_{in_1}^{**}\}$ and $\{Y_{i1}^{**}, Y_{i2}^{**}, \ldots, Y_{in_2}^{**}\}$ and $\{(U_{i1}^{**}, V_{i1}^{**}), (U_{i2}^{**}, V_{i2}^{**}), \ldots, (U_{in}^{**}, V_{in}^{i*})\}$, $i = 1, 2, \ldots, B$.
4. For each $i = 1, 2, \ldots, B$ set of samples in step 3, compute the corresponding bootstrap version of T_0 statistics, namely $T_1^{**}, T_2^{**}, \ldots, T_B^{**}$.
5. The bootstrap p-value is the computed as $P^{**} = \dfrac{\sum\limits_{i=1}^{B} I\left(\left|T_i^{**}\right| \geq |T_0|\right)}{B}$, where

$$I\left(\left|T_i^{**}\right| \geq |T_0|\right) = \begin{cases} 1 & \text{if } \left|T_i^{**}\right| \geq |T_0| \\ 0 & \text{Otherwise.} \end{cases}$$

2.4 Illustration: A Vaginal Pessary Satisfaction Data (Samawi and Vogel 2014)

A vaginal pessary is a removable device placed into the vagina. It is designed to support areas of pelvic organ prolapse. Table 2 contains part of an unpublished study by Dr. Catherine Bagley and Dr. Robert Vogel on the value of estrogen therapy for certain types of patients currently using vaginal pessaries. The data come from a satisfaction survey of women aged 45 or older. The total score is 135 which would be interpreted as complete satisfaction. The data also includes the age of the woman and the number of years she used a pessary (at time of first survey) as well as the date of the second survey.

Table 2 A vaginal pessary satisfaction data (Samawi and Vogel 2014)

Patient	Score1	Score2	Patient	Score1	Score2	Patient	Score1	Score2
1	11	6	22	19	13	43	23	–
2	10	4	23	15	11	44	16	–
3	17	14	24	11	8	45	12	–
4	16	22	25	15	12	46	–	21
5	18	15	26	10	11	47	–	11
6	12	9	27	18	12	48	–	14
7	21	19	28	12	11	49	–	21
8	13	11	29	21	13	50	–	10
9	30	29	30	24	21	51	–	13
10	11	7	31	16	13	52	–	8
11	12	13	32	18	–	53	–	14
12	10	7	33	11	–	54	–	21
13	21	12	34	15	–	55	–	10
14	19	11	35	18	–	56	–	11
15	17	15	36	22	–	57	–	23
16	36	30	37	24	–	59	–	11
17	16	16	38	14	–	60	–	12
18	11	9	39	17	–	61	–	13
19	9	7	40	16	–	62	–	20
20	21	14	41	17	–			
21	13	16	42	24	–			

Table 3 Summary inference

Method	Test	p-Value	Type
Z_{Corr}	4.512	0.00000322	Normal-approximation
T_0	5.529	0.00000000	Bootstrap method
T_{New}	3.435	0.00077690	T-approximation

Table 3 indicates that all of the tests discussed in this paper show strong statistical evidence, that on average, the satisfaction scores are lower on the second survey than on the first survey.

3 Tests for Binary Data

Tests of homogeneity for partially matched-pair data are investigated. Different methods of combining tests of homogeneity based on Pearson chi-square test and McNemar chi-squared test are investigated. Numerical and simulation studies are presented to compare the power of these tests. Data from the National Survey of Children's Health of 2003 (NSCH) is used to illustrate the methods.

For binary data, consider a case–control study used to compare exposure and non-exposure groups to a certain response. In designing a case–control study you may use a matched-pair design, unmatched group design or a combination of both. Table 4 shows the design of matched-pairs case–control study of $T=a+b+c+d$ pairs. Table 5 shows the design of unmatched case–control study of $n = n_{11} + n_{12} + n_{21} + n_{22}$ subjects.

Studies involving matched-pairs are very powerful designs for controlling confounding factors. However, for large cohorts, matched-pairs studies are expensive and consume extra time, making them economically inefficient studies. Other stratification techniques may be used; however, these techniques may compromise the power of the test (see Hennekens and Buring 1987).

One to one matching provides the most statistically efficient design, but more controls per case can provide additional statistical power to the study when attempting to detect an association when it exists. This method is desirable in certain clearly defined circumstances. In this case we will be able to control for general characteristics which are highly correlated with members of a particular group. Hence matching is very useful when case series are small and baseline characteristics are very likely to differ between the studies groups due to chance variability.

Table 4 Design for a matched-pair case–control study

Cases	Control		Total
	Exposed	Non-exposed	
Exposed	a	b	$a+b$
Non-exposed	c	c	$c+d$
Total	$a+c$	$b+d$	$T=a+b+c+d$

Table 5 Design for an unmatched case–control study

	Case	Control	Total
Exposed	$n_{11}(\pi_{1|1})$	$n_{12}(\pi_{2|1})$	n_{1+}
Non-exposed	$n_{21}(\pi_{1|2})$	$n_{22}(\pi_{2|2})$	n_{2+}
Total	n_{+1}	n_{+2}	n

In either case, we propose statistics that will economize resources by enabling an analysis that uses concurrent matched-pair and unmatched studies without the fear of having inadequate sample size. Our proposal involves combining the statistical strengths of matched-pair designs with that of unmatched designs.

3.1   Test of Homogeneity in a Case–Control Study

Testing for no association between exposures and certain response outcomes in a case–control study implies testing for homogeneity of conditional distributions of certain responses given the exposures. Based on Tables 4 and 5, the following hypothesis is tested:

H_0 : no association between the responses of exposed and unexposed groups.

3.2   Existing Methods for Testing the Above Hypotheses for Partially Matched Data

1. The first test of significance of combining more than one table or result was initially proposed by Tippett (1931). He pointed out that $p_1, p_2, \ldots, p_k$ are independent p-values from continuous test statistics, each having a uniform distribution under the null hypothesis. In this case, we reject H_0 at significance level α if $p_{[1]} < 1 - (1 - \alpha)^{1/k}$, where $p_{[1]}$ is the minimum of $p_1, p_2, \ldots, p_k$ (see Hedges and Oklin 1985).
2. Inverse chi-square method. This is the most widely used combination procedure and was proposed by Fisher (1932). Given independent k studies and p-values: $p_1, p_2, \ldots, p_k$, Fisher's procedure uses the product of $p_1, p_2, \ldots, p_k$ to combine the p-values, noting if U has a uniform distribution, then $-2log\ U$ has a chi-square distribution with two degrees of freedom. If H_0 is true then $-2\sum_{i=1}^{k} \log \left(p_i \right)$ is chi-square with 2k degrees of freedom. Therefore, we reject H_0 if $-2\sum_{i=1}^{k} \log \left(p_i \right) > C$, where C is obtained from the upper tail of the chi-square distribution with $2k$ degrees of freedom (see Hedges and Oklin 1985).
3. An incorrect practice is to use the Pearson chi-square test for homogeneity in an unmatched group by converting the matched-pair data in Table 4 to unmatched data in Table 5. Since the two groups of matched and unmatched data are independent, people join the two data sets to one unmatched data set as in Table 6.

Table 6 Combined observations from Tables 4 and 5

	Case	Control	Total
Exposed	$n_{11} + (a + b) = N_{11}$	$n_{12} + (a + c) = N_{12}$	$n_{1+} + (2a + b + c) = N_{1+}$
Non-exposed	$n_{21} + (c + d) = N_{21}$	$n_{22} (b + d) = N_{22}$	$n_{2+} + (b + c + 2d) = N_{2+}$
Total	$n_{+1} + (a + b + c + d) = N_{+1}$	$n_{+2} + (a + b + c + d) = N_{+2}$	$n + 2T = N$

The well-known Pearson chi-square test of homogeneity for 2×2 contingency tables can be used as follows: under the null hypothesis (see Agresti 1990)

$$\chi_1 = \frac{N(N_{11}N_{22} - N_{12}N_{21})^2}{N_{1+}N_{2+}N_{+1}N_{+2}} \; : \; \chi^2_{(1)} \; : Chi - square \text{ distribution with one degree}$$
$$\text{of freedom.}$$
$$(5)$$

If the matched-pair data is small, with only a few pairs of matched data compared to the unmatched data, then investigators tend to ignore the matched-pair portion of the data and test the above hypothesis using a Pearson chi-square test from the design in Table 5 as follows: under the null hypothesis (see Agresti 1990)

$$\chi_2 = \frac{n(n_{11}n_{22} - n_{12}n_{21})^2}{n_{1+}n_{2+}n_{+1}n_{+2}} \; : \; \chi^2_{(1)}. \tag{6}$$

4. If the matched-pair data is large compared to the unmatched data, then investigators tend to ignore the unmatched portion of the data and test the hypothesis of association using the McNemar test from the design in Table 4 as follows: under the null hypothesis (see Agresti 1990)

$$\chi_3 = \frac{(b - c)^2}{b + c} \; : \; \chi^2_{(1)} \tag{7}$$

3.3 Proposed Method of Testing the Above Hypothesis for Partially Matched Data (Samawi and Vogel 2011)

In order to use all information in a study that has both matched-pair data and unmatched data, we propose using a weighted chi-square test of homogeneity. The methods will combine the benefits of using matched-pair data tests with the benefits and strengths of unmatched data test procedures.

1. The proposed test for partially matched-pair data using the design in Tables 7 and 8 is as follows:

$$\chi_w = w\chi_2 + (1 - w)\chi_3, \tag{8}$$

Table 7 Cross tabulation for matched-pairs subjects between Georgia and Washington

| | Insured (GA) | | |
Insured (WA)	No	Yes	Total
No	30	173	203
Yes	256	1,235	1,491
Total	286	1,408	1,694

Table 8 Summary analyses for matched-pairs data

| | McNemar's test | | |
States under study	Statistics	DF	p-Value
GA vs. WA	16.06	1	<0.0001

where $w = \frac{n}{N}$, $N = n + 2T$, n = number of unmatched observation and T = number of pairs and $n = n_1 + n_2$; n_1 = number of cases and n_1 = number of controls.

Under the null hypothesis, if $w = 0.5$, then $2\chi_w \sim \chi^2_{(2)}$. However, when $w \neq 0.5$, an approximation to find the p-value of the χ_w statistic is needed. Therefore, they propose a close approximation to the critical value of χ_w as follows: reject H_0 if $\chi_w > D_\alpha$, where $D_\alpha = e^{0.79 - 1.34w + 1.32w^2 + 0.167\chi^\alpha_{(1)}}$ and $\chi^\alpha_{(1)}$ is the upper α quartile of the chi-square distribution with one degree of freedom. Bootstrap methods can also be employed to find the p-value of the test under the null hypothesis. Our expectation is that the proposed test, χ_w, will outperform other test options with respect to statistical power.

2. A simpler test is a chi-square with two degrees of freedom and is given as follows:

$$\chi_C = \chi_2 + \chi_3. \tag{9}$$

These methods can be extended to $r \times c$ contingency tables for other types of tests of no associations.

3.4 Illustration and Final Results and Conclusions

The data used in this project were obtained from the National Survey of Children' Health of 2003 (NSCH) and contains all US states. Two states, namely Georgia (GA) and Washington (WA) are of our primary concern for the comparison of children insurance disparity. To demonstrate the use of the suggested methods in Sect. 2, we control for two confounding factors, age and gender. Matching is performed on all subjects by age (0–17 years) and gender (male and female) for both states. Georgia is retained as a reference state, and children insurance is the subject of interest. The subsequent section provides summaries of the data analysis based on unmatched, matched-pair, and the combination of unmatched and matched models.

3.4.1 Matched-Pairs Data Analysis

Cross tabulations of insurance and WA State, using Georgia as reference state, are presented in Table 7. A summary of statistical inference using McNemar's test to compare states' children insurance disparities is presented in Table 8.

McNemar's test is used to assess the significance of the difference in insurance disparity between the states of Georgia and Washington controlling for age and gender using the matched-pairs model. There is significant statistical evidence that the children insurance disparity in GA is worse than in WA. Based on the estimated odds ratio, the odds of a child who resides in Georgia not having health insurance are 1.48 more than those living in Washington.

3.4.2 Unmatched Data Analysis (Excluding Matched-Pair Data)

The matched-pairs analysis was based on the part of the data that could be matched. However, the other part of the data is considered unmatched data and the usual Pearson chi-square test is used to test for children's insurance disparity difference between GA and WA States.

The following tables are created from the interviewees who remained unmatched. Pearson's chi-square analysis is therefore conducted to see what kind of information these remaining interviewees will provide. The following tables are derived from this data (Table 9).

Table 10 shows similar conclusion as in Table 8. There is statistical difference in children insurance disparity comparing GA to WA, at level of significance 0.05. Also, based on the estimated odds ratio, the odds of a child residing in Georgia and not having health insurance is 2.1 more than those live in Washington.

3.4.3 Combined Tests of Matched-Pairs and Unmatched Data

Table 11 shows the results of using the suggested methods for combining chi-square tests for partially correlated data.

Table 9 Cross tabulation for unmatched data ignoring the matched paired data

	Insured		
State	No	Yes	Total
GA	25	127	152
WA	20	204	224
Total	45	331	376

Table 10 Summary analysis for unmatched data ignoring the matched-pairs data

States	Statistics	DF	p-Value	Odds ratio	95 % confidence intervals
GA vs. WA	4.86	1	0.0275	2.01	(1.07, 3.76)

Table 11 Suggested tests to combined two independent chi-square tests

Comparison	Weighted chi-square critical value $= 2.99$		Combined chi-square (2 d.f.) p-value		Inverse chi-square Fisher method (4 d.f.) p-value		Tippett method critical value $= 0.025$	
GA vs. WA	9.90	Reject	20.92	<0.0001	26.58	<0.0001	0.000061	Reject

The critical value for the Tippett test is 0.025 and the critical value for the weighted chi-square test is 2.99. The methods that combine tests provide results and conclusion similar to that given in the literature but with greater power. For the situation when we have only marginal significance in one or both types of the data, combining the strength of the two types data (matched-pairs and unmatched data) provides greater power to detect any small difference in conditional probabilities.

In conclusion, choosing the right test for combining the matched and the unmatched data for testing the null hypothesis of homogeneity depends on the impact of weights, and the strength of the association between the case and control groups in both data sets. Our investigation revealed that any of the competing tests: the Combined chi-square, the Inverse chi-square and the Weighted chi-square tests, are recommended since they all show superiority over other tests in most of the cases.

4 Nonparametric Test for Partially Correlated Data

This section discusses and proposes some nonparametric testing procedures to handle data when partially correlated data is available without ignoring the cases with missing responses. We will introduce more powerful testing procedure which combined all cases in the study.

4.1 Combined Sign Tests for Correlated and Uncorrelated Data: Proposed Methods

4.1.1 Sign Test for Correlated Data

Correlated data consists of observations in a bivariate random sample $\{(U_i, V_i), i=1, 2, \ldots, n\}$ where there are n pairs of observations. A comparison is made within each pair (U, V), and the pair is classified as "$+$" if $U > V$, or "$-$" if $U < V$. The underlying populations are assumed to be absolute continuous. Therefore, no ties are assumed. In this paper we assume the MCAR or MAR design and the marginal distributions have the same shape ($F_X(x)$ and $F_Y(y)$) to test the one-sided hypotheses $H_0 : \theta_1 = \theta_2$ and $H_1 : \theta_1 > \theta_2$ where θ_1 is a measure of location (median) of $F_X(x)$ and θ_2 is a measure of location (median) of $F_Y(y)$ (see also

Conover 1999). The matched pairs sign test statistic, denoted by T_1, for testing the above hypotheses, equals the number of "+" pairs:

$$T_1 = \sum_{i=1}^{n} I(U_i > V_i) \tag{10}$$

where $I(U_i > V_i) = \begin{cases} 1 & \text{if } U_i > V_i \\ 0 & \text{otherwise}. \end{cases}$

Alternatively, define $D_i = U_i - V_i, i = 1, 2, \ldots, n$. Then, the null hypothesis (H_o: The median of the differences is zero) can be tested using the sign test. Therefore, the test statistic can be written as: $T_1 = \sum_{i=1}^{n} I(D_i > 0)$. All tied pairs are discarded, and n represents the number of remaining pairs. Depending on whether the alternative hypothesis is one- or two-tailed, and if $n \leq 20$, then use the binomial distribution (i.e., $Bin(n, p = \frac{1}{2})$) for finding the critical region of approximately size α. Under H_o and for $n > 20$, $T_1 \sim N(\frac{n}{2}, \frac{n}{4})$. Therefore, the critical region can be defined based on the normal distribution:

$$Z_1 = \frac{T_1 - (\frac{n}{2})}{\sqrt{\frac{n}{4}}} \xrightarrow{L} N(0, 1). \tag{11}$$

4.1.2 Mann–Whitney Wilcoxon Test for Uncorrelated Data

For uncorrelated data, let $\{X_1, X_2, \ldots, X_{n_1}\}$ and $\{Y_1, Y_2, \ldots, Y_{n_2}\}$ denote two independent simple random samples of subjects exposed to method 1 and method 2, respectively. It can be shown that $H_o : \theta_1 = \theta_2$ is valid for two-independent samples, where θ_1 is a measure of location (median) of $F_X(x)$ and θ_2 is a measure of location (median) of $F_Y(y)$. If the distributions of X and Y have the same shape, then the null hypothesis of interest is $H_0 : \theta_1 - \theta_2 = 0$. Define:

$$T_2 = \sum_{j=1}^{n_1} \sum_{k=1}^{n_2} I(X_j > Y_k), \tag{12}$$

where $I(X_j > Y_k) = \begin{cases} 1 & \text{if } X_j > Y_k \\ 0 & \text{otherwise}. \end{cases}$

Then, T_2 is the Mann–Whitney Wilcoxon two samples test. Therefore, $E(T_2) = \frac{n_1 n_2}{2}$ and $Var(T_2) = \frac{n_1 n_2 (n_1 + n_2 + 1)}{12}$, (for example, see Conover 1999). For large samples and under $H_0 : \theta_1 - \theta_2 = 0$, the critical region can be defined based on the normal distribution (again, see Conover 1999):

$$Z_2 = \frac{T_2 - (\frac{n_1 n_2}{2})}{\sqrt{\frac{n_1 n_2 (n_1 + n_2 + 1)}{12}}} \xrightarrow{L} N(0, 1). \tag{13}$$

4.1.3 Combined Sign Test with Mann–Whitney Wilcoxon Test

Case 1. Small sample sizes For small sample sizes, we propose the following test procedure to combine the sign test for correlated data with the Mann–Whitney Wilcoxon test for uncorrelated data:

(1) Let $T_c = T_1 + T_2$.
(2) Let $0 < \gamma < 1$, then the two sign tests can be combined as follows:
   define $T_\gamma = \gamma T_1 + (1 - \gamma) T_2$.

Using similar notation as that found in Hettmansperger and McKean (2011). We construct the following theorem:

Theorem 1. Given n_1 x' s , n_2 y' s, and n pairs of (u, v) and under H_o, let:
$P_{n_1, n_2}(l) = P_{H_0}(T_2 = l), l = 0, 1, 2, \ldots, n_1 n_2$; and $P_n(i) = P_{H_0}(T_1 = i) = \binom{n}{i}\left(\frac{1}{2}\right)^n, i = 0, 1, 2, \ldots, n$. Then,

(i)

$$P(T_c = t) = \sum_{l+i=t}\sum P_{n_1, n_2}(l) P_n(i), t = 0, 1, 2, \ldots, n_1 n_2 + n; \text{ and} \quad (14)$$

(ii)

$$P(T_\gamma = t) = \sum_{\gamma l + (1-\gamma)i = t}\sum P_{n_1, n_2}(l) P_n(i), \quad (15)$$

where $P_{n_1, n_2}(l) = \frac{n_2}{n_1 + n_2} P_{n_1, n_2-1}(l - n_1) + \frac{n_1}{n_1 + n_2} P_{n_1-1, n_2}(l)$, $P_{n_1, n_2}(l) = \frac{\overline{P}_{n_1, n_2}(l)}{\binom{n_1 + n_1}{n_1}}$, $\overline{P}_{n_1, n_2}(l) = \overline{P}_{n_1, n_2-1}(l - n_1) + \overline{P}_{n_1-1, n_2}(l)$, $\overline{P}_{j,k}(l) = 0$

if $1 < 0, \overline{P}_{j,0}(l)$, and $\overline{P}_{0,k}(l)$ is 1 or 0 as $l = 0$ or $l \neq 0$, respectively.

The proof is a consequence of Theorems 3.2.2 and 3.2.3 in Hettmansperger (1984) and see also Hettmansperger and McKean (2011) Theorem 2.4.3. Examples of these null distributions for selected sample sizes are provided as tables in the Appendix. Furthermore, R codes to calculate the exact discrete distribution of the proposed tests are provided on the following website: http://personal.georgiasouthern.edu/~hsamawi/.

Case 2. Large sample sizes For large sample sizes and under H_o, and let

$$\frac{n}{n+n_1+n_2} \to \gamma \text{ as}$$
$$\{n \to \infty \text{ and large } n_1, n_2 < \infty; \text{ or } n \to \infty \text{ and } n_1 \to \infty \text{ and large } n_2 < \infty;$$
$$\text{or } n, n_1, n_2 \to \infty\}$$

we propose to use:

(i)

$$Z_0 = \frac{T_1 + T_2 - (\frac{q}{2} + \frac{n_1 n_2}{2})}{\sqrt{\frac{q}{4} + \frac{n_1 n_2 (n_1 + n_2 + 1)}{12}}} \overset{L}{\to} N(0, 1); \text{ and} \tag{16}$$

(ii)

$$T_Z = \sqrt{\gamma} Z_1 + \sqrt{1 - \gamma} Z_2 \overset{L}{\to} N(0, 1). \tag{17}$$

4.2 Combined Wilcoxon Signed-Rank Test and Mann–Whitney Wilcoxon Test for Correlated and Uncorrelated Data

4.2.1 Wilcoxon Signed-Rank Test for Correlated Data

If we assume that U and V are exchangeable random variables, then $U - V$ and $V - U$ both have symmetric distributions and the Wilcoxon test is clearly justified. Let $D_i = U_i - V_i, i = 1, 2, \ldots, n$. Under H_0, we may use a Wilcoxon signed-rank test as follows. Let I_i be an indicator for when $|D|_{(i)}$ corresponds to a positive observation, where $|D|_{(1)} < \cdots < |D|_{(n)}$ are the ordered absolute values. Then,

$$T_{WC} = \sum_{i=1}^{n} i I_i = \sum_{i=1}^{n} R_i s(D_i) \tag{18}$$

is the Wilcoxon signed-rank statistic, where R_i is the rank of $|D_i|$ and $I_i = s(D_i)$, where $s(D_i) = 1$ if $D_i > 0$ and 0 otherwise. It has been shown that under the null hypothesis, $E(T_{WC}) = \frac{n(n+1)}{4}$ and $Var(T_{WC}) = \frac{n(n+1)(2n+1)}{24}$. Since D_i has a symmetric distribution under the H_0 assumption, T_{WC} is a linear combination of i.i.d. $Bernoulli(\frac{1}{2})$ random variables. However, for large samples

$$Z_{WC} = \frac{T_{WC} - \frac{n(n+1)}{4}}{\sqrt{\frac{n(n+1)(2n+1)}{24}}} \overset{L}{\to} N(0, 1). \tag{19}$$

Conover (1999) provides an example for such large sample sizes.

4.2.2 Combined Wilcoxon Rank Test with Mann–Whitney Wilcoxon Test

Case 1. Small sample sizes For small sample sizes, we propose the following test procedure to combine the two tests:

(i) Let $T_{cw} = T_{WC} + T_2$ (see Dubnicka et al. 2002).
(ii) Let $0 < \gamma < 1$, then the two sign tests can be combined as follows:
   define $T_{\gamma w} = \gamma T_{WC} + (1 - \gamma) T_2$.

Again, using similar notation as that found in Hettmansperger (1984) and Hettmansperger and McKean (2011), we construct the following theorem:

Theorem 2. Given n_1 x' s , n_2 y' s, and n pairs of (u, v) and under H_0, let

$$P_{n_1, n_2}(l) = P_{H_0}(T_2 = l), l = 0, 1, 2, \ldots, n_1 n_2 \text{ and} \tag{20}$$

$$P_{wn}(b) = P_{H_0}(T_{WC} = b) = \frac{\overline{P}_{wn}(b)}{2^n}, b = 0, 1, 2, \ldots, \frac{n(n+1)}{2}. \tag{21}$$

Then:

(i)

$$P(T_{cw} = t) = \sum_{l+b=t} \sum P_{n_1, n_2}(l) P_{wn}(b), t = 0, 1, 2, \ldots, n_1 n_2 + \frac{n(n+1)}{2};$$

and

(ii)

$$P(T_{\gamma w} = t) = \sum_{\gamma l + (1-\gamma)b = t} \sum P_{n_1, n_2}(l) P_{wn}(b),$$

where $P_{n_1, n_2}(l)$ is the same as that in Theorem 1 and $\overline{P}_n(b) = \overline{P}_{n-1}(b) + \overline{P}_{n-1}(b - n)$, $\overline{P}_0(0) = 1, \overline{P}_0(b) = 0$ and $\overline{P}_n(b) = 0$ for $b < 0$.

The proof is a result of Theorems 3.2.2 and 3.2.3 as well as Exercise 3.7.3 in Hettmansperger (1984). Similarly, examples of these null distributions for selected sample sizes are provided in the Appendix. Additionally, R codes are provided on the following website to calculate the exact discrete distribution of the proposed tests: http://personal.georgiasouthern.edu/~hsamawi/.

Case 2. Large sample sizes For large samples and under H_0, and let

$\frac{n}{n+n_1+n_2} \to \gamma$ as
$\{n \to \infty$ and large $n_1, n_2 < \infty$; or $n \to \infty$ and $n_1 \to \infty$ and large $n_2 < \infty$;
   or $n, n_1, n_2 \to \infty\}$,

we can combine the two tests as follows:

(i)

$$Z_{0D} = \frac{T_{WC} + T_2 - \left(\frac{n(n+1)}{4} + \frac{n_1 n_2}{2}\right)}{\sqrt{\frac{n(n+1)(2n+1)}{24} + \frac{n_1 n_2 (n_1 + n_2 + 1)}{12}}} \xrightarrow{L} N(0,1); \text{ and}$$

(ii)

$$T_Z = \sqrt{\gamma} Z_{WC} + \sqrt{1 - \gamma} Z_2 \xrightarrow{L} N(0,1).$$

4.3   New Test Procedure

Under the assumption of MCAR and in order to test the null hypothesis $H_0 : \theta_1 = \theta_2$, the following notation must be defined: $D_i = U_i - V_i, i = 1, 2, \ldots, n$, and $D_{jk} = X_j - Y_k, j = 1, 2, \ldots, n_1, k = 1, 2, \ldots, n_2$. Let $N = n + n_1 n_2$; $DD_1 = D_1, \ldots, D_n = DD_n; DD_{n+1} = D_{11}, \ldots, D_{n_1 n_2} = DD_N$; and I_m be an indicator when $|DD|_{(m)}$ corresponds to a positive DD observation, where m $= 1, 2, \ldots, N$ and $|DD|_{(1)} < \cdots < |DD|_{(N)}$ are the ordered absolute values. Then,

$$T_{New} = \sum_{m=1}^{N} m I_m = \sum_{m=1}^{N} R_m s(DD_m) \tag{22}$$

is the new signed-rank statistic, where R_m is the rank of $|DD_m|$ and $I_m = s(DD_m)$ is defined above. As in Hettmansperger (1984), Theorem 2.2.1 and Hettmansperger and McKean (2011) Lemma 1.7.1, under the assumption that $\{s(DD_1), \ldots, s(DD_N)\}$ and $\{R_1, \ldots, R_N\}$ are independent we will provide the following results. Using simple probability algebra, we can show that

$$P(s(DD_m) = 1) = P(s(DD_m) = 1, DD_m \in A_1) + P(s(DD_m) = 1, DD_m \in A_2)$$
$$= \frac{1/2}{\binom{N}{n}} + \frac{1/2}{\binom{N}{n_1 n_2}} = \frac{1}{\binom{N}{n}},$$

where $A_1 = \{DD_1, \ldots, DD_n\}$ and $A_2 = \{DD_{n+1}, \ldots, DD_N\}$. The number of permutations of the sequence of N positive and negative signs of DD's is 2^N. Using the convolution of the distribution of Wilcoxon's signed-rank statistic in the Wilcoxon–Mann–Whitney statistic, the null distribution of T_{new} can be written as

$$P(T_{new} = t) = \frac{1}{\binom{N}{n}} \sum_{m=1}^{2^N} P_m(T_{WC} = t_{WC}) P_m(T_2 = t - t_{WC}),$$

$$t = 0, 1, 2, \ldots, \frac{N(N+1)}{2}, \tag{23}$$

where $P_m(T_{WC} = t_{WC})$ and $P_m(T_2 = t - t_{WC})$ and are expressed in Theorem 2 for the mth permutation as $P_m(b) = P_m(T_{WC} = b) = \frac{\overline{P}_m(b)}{2^m}, b = 0, 1, 2, \ldots, \frac{m(m+1)}{2}$ and $\overline{P}_m(b) = \overline{P}_{m-1}(b) + \overline{P}_{m-1}(b - m)$, $\overline{P}_0(0) = 1, \overline{P}_0(b) = 0$ and $\overline{P}_m(b) = 0$ for $b < 0$.

R codes to find (23) by calculating the exact discrete distribution of the proposed test are provided on the following website: http://personal.georgiasouthern.edu/~hsamawi/. Using (22), it is easy to show that the mean and the variance of our proposed test statistic are as follows:

$$E(T_{New}) = \frac{N(N+1)}{2 \cdot \binom{N}{2}}, \tag{24}$$

$$V(T_{New}) = \frac{4N(N+1)(2N+1)\binom{N}{2} - 6N^2(N+1)^2}{24\binom{N}{2}^2}. \tag{25}$$

Note that both the mean and the variance in (24) and (25) are finite and decreasing as N increases, provided that

$\frac{n}{n+n_1+n_2} \to \gamma$ as
$\{n \to \infty$ and large $n_1, n_2 < \infty$; or $n \to \infty$ and $n_1 \to \infty$ and large $n_2 < \infty$; or $n, n_1, n_2 \to \infty\}$.

Under the MCAR design and the null hypothesis, the asymptotic distribution of T_{New} is as follows:

$$Z_{New} = \frac{T_{New} - E(T_{New})}{\sqrt{V(T_{New})}} \xrightarrow{L} N(0, 1). \tag{26}$$

4.4 Illustration Using Genetic Data

Table 12 contains data on eight patients taken from Weidmann et al. (1992). The purpose of this study was to compare the proportions of certain T cell receptor gene families (the Vβ gene families) on tumor infiltrating lymphocytes (TILs) and

Table 12 T cell receptor data (Weidmann et al. 1992)

Patient	VB% TIL	VB% PBL
1	6.7	2.8
2	3.7	3.5
3	4.4	4.1
4	2.3	–
5	4.5	–
6	–	4.0
7	–	14.7
8	–	3.2

Table 13 Results of all suggested tests

Test procedure	Value of the test	p-Value
S_1	11,000	0.5000
S_2	19,000	0.3000
S_3	20,000	0.2103
S_4	5,000	0.1625
S_5	33,000	0.3500
Sign test for matched pairs T_1 (ignoring unmatched data)	3,000	0.1250
Wilcoxon test for matched pairs T_{wc} (ignoring unmatched data)	6,000	0.1250
Mann–Whitney test for two independent samples T_2 (ignoring matched data)	2,000	0.8000
Combined sign with Mann–Whitney tests T_c	5,000	0.5000
Weighted sign with Mann–Whitney tests T_γ, $\gamma = \frac{n}{n+n_1+n_2}$	2,375	0.4000
Combined Wilcoxon with Mann–Whitney tests T_{cw}	8,000	0.2878
Weighted Wilcoxon with Mann–Whitney tests $T_{\gamma w}$	3,500	0.3875
Optimal weighted sign with Mann–Whitney tests $\gamma = \frac{w_i}{2}, w_i = \frac{1}{\sigma_i}$, where σ_i is the standard deviation of the $\sum_{i=1} w_i$ ith test	2,800	0.1500
Optimal weighted Wilcoxon with Mann–Whitney tests	3,840	0.2875
New proposed test (T_{New})	18,000	0.6350

peripheral blood lymphocytes (PBLs) in patients with hepatocellular carcinoma (i.e., matched pairs or block design). Weidmann et al. (1992) expected that more changes would be detected in surface receptors of T lymphocytes in the presence of a tumor. The outcome represented the percentage of T cells of each type showing the Vβ22 receptor. The null hypothesis of equal medians was tested by estimating and comparing the relative proportions of Vβ gene family usage for several patients' TILs and PBLs. However, data are missing for some patients due to factors unrelated to the measurements themselves.

None of the tests provided in Table 13 indicate any statistical significance. Therefore, regardless of the test used, H_0 is not rejected.

Acknowledgements We are grateful to the Center for Child & Adolescent Health for providing us with the 2003 National Survey of Children's Health. Also, we would like to thank the referees and the associate editor for their valuable comments which improved the manuscript.

Appendix

See Tables 14 and 15.

Table 14 Null distribution to T_y, T_c, T_{yw}, and T_{cw} for $n = 2, n_1 = 2, n_2 = 2$ and $\gamma = 0.33$

t_c	$P(T_c = t_c)$	t_y	$P(T_y = t_y)$	t_{cw}	$P(T_{cw} = t_{cw})$	t_{yw}	$P(T_{yw} = t_{yw})$
0	0.041667	0.00	0.041667	0	0.041667	0.00	0.0416665
1	0.125000	0.33	0.083333	1	0.083333	0.33	0.0416665
2	0.208332	0.66	0.041667	2	0.166666	0.66	0.0416665
3	0.249998	0.67	0.041667	3	0.208332	0.67	0.0416665
4	0.208332	1.00	0.083333	4	0.208332	0.99	0.0416665
5	0.125000	1.33	0.041667	5	0.166665	1.00	0.0416665
6	0.041667	1.34	0.083333	6	0.083333	1.33	0.0416665
		1.67	0.166665	7	0.041667	1.34	0.0833325
		2.00	0.083333			1.66	0.0416665
		2.01	0.041667			1.67	0.0833325
		2.34	0.083333			2.00	0.0833325
		2.67	0.041667			2.01	0.0416665
		2.68	0.041667			2.33	0.0833325
		3.01	0.083333			2.34	0.0416665
		3.34	0.041667			2.67	0.0416665
						2.68	0.0416665
						3.00	0.0416665
						3.01	0.0416665
						3.34	0.0416665
						3.67	0.0416665

Table 15 Null distribution to T_γ, T_c, $T_{\gamma w}$, and T_{cw} for $n = 3$, $n_1 = 3$, $n_2 = 2$ and $\gamma = 0.375$

t_c	$P(T_c = t_c)$	t_γ	$P(T_\gamma = t_\gamma)$	$t_{\gamma w}$	$P(T_{\gamma w} = t_{\gamma w})$	t_{cw}	$P(T_{cw} = t_{cw})$
0	0.0125	0.0000	0.01250	0	0.0125	0.0000	0.0125
1	0.0500	0.3750	0.03750	1	0.0250	0.3750	0.0125
2	0.1000	0.6250	0.01250	2	0.0500	0.6250	0.0125
3	0.1500	0.7500	0.03750	3	0.0875	0.7500	0.0125
4	0.1875	1.0000	0.03750	4	0.1125	1.0000	0.0125
5	0.1875	1.1250	0.01250	5	0.1375	1.1250	0.0250
6	0.1500	1.2500	0.0250	6	0.1500	1.2500	0.0250
7	0.1000	1.3750	0.03750	7	0.1375	1.3750	0.0125
8	0.0500	1.6250	0.0750	8	0.1125	1.5000	0.0125
9	0.0125	1.7500	0.01250	9	0.0875	1.6250	0.0250
		1.8750	0.0250	10	0.0500	1.7500	0.0250
		2.0000	0.0750	11	0.0250	1.8750	0.0375
		2.2500	0.0750	12	0.0125	2.0000	0.0250
		2.3750	0.0250			2.1250	0.0125
		2.5000	0.0250			2.2500	0.0375
		2.6250	0.0750			2.3750	0.0500
		2.8750	0.0750			2.5000	0.0375
		3.0000	0.0250			2.6250	0.0250
		3.1250	0.0125			2.7500	0.0250
		3.2500	0.0750			2.8750	0.0375
		3.5000	0.0375			3.0000	0.0500
		3.6250	0.0250			3.1250	0.0375
		3.7500	0.0125			3.2500	0.0250
		3.8750	0.0375			3.3750	0.0250
		4.1250	0.0375			3.5000	0.0375
		4.2500	0.0125			3.6250	0.0500
		4.5000	0.0375			3.7500	0.0375
		4.8750	0.0125			3.8750	0.0125
						4.0000	0.0250
						4.1250	0.0375
						4.2500	0.0250
						4.3750	0.0250
						4.500	0.0125
						4.6250	0.0125
						4.7500	0.0250
						4.8750	0.0250
						5.0000	0.0125
						5.2500	0.0125
						5.3750	0.0125
						5.6250	0.0125
						6.0000	0.0125

References

Agresti, A.: Categorical Data Analysis. Wiley, New York (1990)

Akritas, M.G., Kuha, J., Osgood, D.W.: A nonparametric approach to matched pairs with missing data. Sociol. Methods Res. **30**, 425–457 (2002)

Brunner, E., Puri, M.L.: Nonparametric methods in design and analysis of experiments. In: Ghosh, S., Rao, C.R. (eds.) Handbook of Statistics 13, pp. 631–703. North-Holland/Elsevier, Amsterdam (1996)

Brunner, E., Domhof, S., Langer, F.: Nonparametric Analysis of Longitudinal Data in Factorial Designs. Wiley, New York (2002)

Child and Adolescent Health Measurement Initiative: National Survey of Children with Special Health Care Needs: Indicator Dataset 6. Data Resource Center for Child and Adolescent Health website. Retrieved from: www.childhealthdata.org (2003)

Conover, W.J.: Practical Nonparametric Statistics, 3rd edn. Wiley, New York (1999)

Dimery, I.W., Nishioka, K., Grossie, B., Ota, D.M., Schantz, S.P., Robbins, K.T., Hong, W.K.: Polyamine metabolism in carcinoma of oral cavity compared with adjacent and normal oral mucosa. Am. J. Surg. **154**, 429–433 (1987)

Dubnicka, S.R., Blair, R.C., Hettmansperger, T.P.: Rank-based procedures for mixed paired and two-sample designs. J. Mod. Appl. Stat. Methods **1**(1), 32–41 (2002)

Efron, B.: Bootstrap methods: another look at the jackknife. Ann. Stat. **7**, 1–26 (1979)

Ekbohm, G.: Comparing means in the paired case with missing data on one response. Biometrika **63**(1), 169–172 (1976)

Fisher, R.A.: Statistical Methods for Research Workers, 4th edn. Oliver & Boyd, London (1932)

Hedges, L.V., Oklin, I.: Statistical Methods for Meta-Analysis: Combined Test Procedures. Academic, London (1985)

Hennekens, C.H., Burning, J.E.: Epidemiology in medicine. Boston: Little, Brown (1987)

Hettmansperger, T.P.: Statistical Inference Based on Ranks. Wiley, New York (1984)

Hettmansperger, T.P., McKean, J.W.: Robust Nonparametric Statistical Method, 2nd edn. CRC Press, Taylor & Francis Group, New York (2011)

Ibrahim, H.I.: Evaluating the power of the Mann–Whitney test using the bootstrap method. Commun. Stat. Theory Methods **20**, 2919–2931 (1991)

Im KyungAh: A modified signed rank test to account for missing in small samples with paired data. M.S. Thesis, Department of Biostatistics, Graduate School of Public Health, University of Pittsburgh, Pittsburgh, PA. http://www.worldcat.org/title/modified-signed-rank-test-to-account-for-missing-data-in-small-samples-with-paired-data/oclc/52418573 (2002)

Janssen, A.: Resampling Student's t-type statistics. Ann. Inst. Stat. Math. **57**, 507–529 (2005)

Janssen, A., Pauls, T.: How do bootstrap and permutation tests work? Ann. Stat. **31**, 768–806 (2003)

Konietschke, F., Harrar, S.W., Lange, K., Brunner, E.: Ranking procedures for matched pairs with missing values – asymptotic theory and a small sample approximation. Comput. Stat. Data Anal. **56**, 1090–1102 (2012)

Lin, P., Stivers, L.E.: On difference of means with incomplete data. Biometrika **61**(2), 325–334 (1974)

Looney, S.W., Jones, P.W.: A method for comparing two normal means using combined samples of correlated and uncorrelated data. Stat. Med. **22**, 1601–1610 (2003)

Nason, G.P.: On the sum of t and Gaussian random variables. http://www.maths.bris.ac.uk/~guy/Research/papers/SumTGauss.pdf (2005). Accessed 1 May 2011

Nurnberger, J., Jimerson, D., Allen, J.R., Simmons, S., Gershon, E.: Red cell ouabain-sensitive Na^+-K^+-adenosine triphosphatase: a state marker in affective disorder inversely related to plasma cortisol. Biol. Psychiatry **17**(9), 981–992 (1982)

Rempala, G., Looney, S.: Asymptotic properties of a two-sample randomized test for partially dependent data. J. Stat. Plann. Inference **136**, 68–89 (2006)

Samawi, H.M., Vogel, R.L.: Tests of homogeneity for partially matched-pairs data. Stat. Methodol. **8**, 304–313 (2011)

Samawi, H.M., Vogel, R.L.: Notes on two sample tests for partially correlated (paired) data. J. Appl. Stat. **41**(1), 109–117 (2014)

Samawi, H.M., Woodworth, G.G., Al-Saleh, M.F.: Two-sample importance resampling for the bootstrap. Metron. **LIV**(3–4) (1996)

Samawi, H.M., Woodworth, G.G., Lemke, J.: Power estimation for two-sample tests using importance and antithetic resampling. Biom. J. **40**(3), 341–354 (1998)

Samawi, H.M., Yu, L., Vogel, R.L.: On some nonparametric tests for partially correlated data: proposing a new test. Unpublished manuscript (2014)

Snedecor, G.W., Cochran, W.G.: Statistical Methods, 7th edn. Iowa State University Press, Ames (1980)

Steere, A.C., Green, J., Schoen, R.T., Taylor, E., Hutchinson, G.J., Rahn, D.W., Malawista, S.E.: Successful parenteral penicillin therapy of established Lyme arthritis. N. Engl. J. Med. **312**(14), 8699–8874 (1985)

Tang, X.: New test statistic for comparing medians with incomplete paired data. M.S. Thesis, Department of Biostatistics, Graduate School of Public Health, University of Pittsburgh, Pittsburgh, PA. http://www.google.com/search?hl=en&rlz=1T4ADRA_enUS357US357&q= Tang+X.+%282007%29New+Test+Statistic+for+Comparing+Medians+with+Incomplete+ Paired+Data&btnG=Search&aq=f&aqi=&aql=&oq= (2007)

Tippett, L.H.C.: The Method of Statistics. Williams & Norgate, London (1931)

Walker, G.A., Saw, J.G.: The distribution of linear combinations of t-variables. J. Am. Stat. Assoc. **73**(364), 876–878 (1978)

Weidmann, E., Whiteside, T.L., Giorda, R., Herberman, R.B., Trucco, M.: The T-cell receptor V beta gene usage in tumor-infiltrating lymphocytes and blood of patients with hepatocellular carcinoma. Cancer Res. **52**(21), 5913–5920 (1992)

Xu, J., Harrar, S.W.: Accurate mean comparisons for paired samples with missing data: an application to a smoking-cessation trial. Biom. J. **54**, 281–295 (2012)

Modeling Time-Dependent Covariates in Longitudinal Data Analyses

Trent L. Lalonde

Abstract Often public health data contain variables of interest that change over the course of longitudinal data collection. In this chapter a discussion is presented of analysis options for longitudinal data with time-dependent covariates. Relevant definitions are presented and explained in the context of practical applications, such as different types of time-dependent covariates. The consequences of ignoring the time-dependent nature of variables in models is discussed. Modeling options for time-dependent covariate data are presented in two general classes: subject-specific models and population-averaged models. Specific subject-specific models include random-intercept models and random-slopes models. Decomposition of time-dependent covariates into "within" and "between" components within each subject-specific model are discussed. Specific population-averaged models include the independent GEE model and various forms of the GMM (generalized method of moments) approach, including researcher-determined types of time-dependent covariates along with data-driven selection of moment conditions using the Extended Classification. A practical data example is presented along with example programs for both SAS and R.

1 Introduction and Motivating Examples

The term "longitudinal data" refers to data that involve the collection of the same variables repeatedly over time. Typically the term is used to refer to longitudinal *panel* data, which denotes the case of collecting data repeatedly from the same subjects. This type of data is very common in practice, and allows for researchers to assess trends over time and gives power to typical population comparisons (Zeger and Liang 1992; Diggle et al. 2002; Hedeker and Gibbons 2006; Fitzmaurice et al. 2012). Specific research interests can include comparisons of mean responses at different times; comparisons of mean responses across different populations, accounting for the effects of time; and assessing the impacts of independent

T.L. Lalonde (✉)
Department of Applied Statistics and Research Methods, University of Northern Colorado, Greeley, CO, USA
e-mail: trent.lalonde@unco.edu

© Springer International Publishing Switzerland 2015   57
D.-G. Chen, J. Wilson (eds.), *Innovative Statistical Methods for Public Health Data*,
ICSA Book Series in Statistics, DOI 10.1007/978-3-319-18536-1_4

variables on responses, accounting for the effects of time. Longitudinal models allow these questions to be answered, while accounting for the dependence inherent in repeated observation of the same individuals.

Independent variables in longitudinal studies can be broadly classified into one of two categories: time-independent covariates (TIC), or time-dependent covariates (TDC). The differences between these types of covariates can lead to different research interests, different analysis approaches, and different conclusions.

TIC are independent variables with no within-subject variation, meaning that the value of a TIC does not change for a given individual in a longitudinal study. This type of covariate can be used to make comparisons across populations and to describe different time trends, but does not allow for a dynamic relationship between the TIC and response.

TDC are independent variables that include both within-subject variation and between-subject variation, meaning that the value of a TDC changes for a given individual across time and can also change among different subjects. A TDC can be used to make comparisons across populations, to describe time trends, and also to describe dynamic relationships between the TDC and response. The focus of this chapter will be on appropriate analysis techniques for TDC.

Examples of longitudinal data with TDC arise often and in many disciplines. For example, Phillips et al. (2014) were interested in the associations among marijuana usage, drug craving, and motivation. For "heavy users" of marijuana between the ages of 18 and 30, data were collected three times per day for 14 consecutive days. To model the mean number of times marijuana was used, a longitudinal count model was applied using drug craving and motivation as predictors. Over the course of 14 days, both drug craving and motivation vary both within and between subjects, and therefore should be treated as TDC.

Using the Arizona state inpatient database (SID) for records of hospital visits, Lalonde et al. (2014) modeled the probability of rehospitalization within 30 days of a previous visit. Rehospitalization within this time frame is an important consideration for Medicare funding. Subjects for the study were selected such that each subject in the database had exactly three hospital follow-ups. Using a longitudinal logistic model, predictors of probability of rehospitalization included the number of diagnoses during a hospital visit, the number of procedures performed, and the length of hospital stay. Each of these predictors can vary over the three hospital follow-ups, and therefore should be treated as TDC.

It can be seen that TDC allow for different types of conclusions and relationships than TIC. For example, TDC can be involved in accumulated effects from differing values over time (Fitzmaurice and Laird 1995). It is also clear that certain TDC convey different information than others. For example, variables such as age may change over time, but change predictably. On the other hand, variables such as daily precipitation may change over time but cannot be predicted as age can. In such cases it is important to consider relationships between the TDC and the response across time.

In the following sections, the distinctions among TDC will be explored, including methods of identifying types of TDC. Modeling TDC data using conditional methods is discussed, followed by modeling using marginal methods. The chapter concludes with a data example exemplifying all relevant modeling techniques.

2 Classifying Time-Dependent Covariates

Within a longitudinal study, a TDC can be defined as a variable that involves variation both within subjects and between subjects. The additional variation within subjects is a source of dispersion that must be accounted for in longitudinal models, and can provide insight into dynamic relationships between a TDC and the response.

Various types of TDC can behave differently from each other. Variables such as "time of observation" or "treatment" can change through a study, but these changes are inherently deterministic. While there may be an association between such variables and the response at a given time, the associations should not carry over such that the "treatment" at one time affects the response at a different time. Subject-specific variables such as "systolic blood pressure" or "drug craving" can change over time, although not deterministically. These types of variables are associated with subject characteristics, and as such can often be involved in dynamic "feed-back" relationships with the response. The response at a given time can be affected by the accumulated prior values of such a variable, and correspondingly the value of the response can affect these variables in future observations. Covariates involved in feedback have also been referred to as "time-dependent confounders" (Diggle et al. 2002). Random variables such as "atmospheric pressure" or "unsolicited donations" can change over time, but vary randomly with respect to a system. These types of variables can have accumulated effects on the response, but feedback is unlikely.

It is evident that TDC can be classified according to the nature of the relationship between the TDC and the response. It is important to identify the different types of TDC, as different types of covariates can be associated with different conclusions or different appropriate estimation methods within the same models.

2.1 *Exogeneity*

One of the most common distinctions made of TDC is that of exogeneity (Chamberlain 1982; Amemiya 1985; Diggle et al. 2002). An exogenous variable has a stochastic process that can be determined by factors outside the system under study, and is not influenced by the individual under study. An exogenous TDC can be thought of as a randomly fluctuating covariate that cannot be explained using other variables in the study. It is most important to determine exogeneity with respect to the response. A TDC is said to be exogenous with respect to the response process if that time-dependent variable at one time is conditionally independent of all previous responses.

Formally, let the response for subject i at time t be denoted by Y_{it}, and let x_{it} denote a TDC for subject i at time t. Then $\mathbf{x}$ is exogenous with respect to the response process $\mathbf{Y}$ if

$$f_X\left(x_{it}|Y_{i1},\ldots,Y_{it};x_{i1},\ldots,x_{i(t-1)}\right) = f_X\left(x_{it}|x_{i1},\ldots,x_{i(t-1)}\right), \tag{1}$$

where f_X denotes the density of $\mathbf{x}$. Under the definition of Eq. (1), while x_{it} may be associated with previous covariate values $x_{i1},\ldots,x_{i(t-1)}$, it will not be associated with previous or current responses $Y_{i1},\ldots,Y_{it}$. A consequence of this definition is that the current response Y_{it} will be independent of future covariate values, even if there is an association with prior covariate values,

$$\mathrm{E}\left[Y_{it}|x_{i1},\ldots,x_{iT}\right] = \mathrm{E}\left[Y_{it}|x_{i1},\ldots,x_{i(t-1)}\right]. \tag{2}$$

Exogeneity with respect to the response has important modeling implications. Specifically, the definition implies that the response at any time may depend on prior responses and prior values of the TDC, but will be independent of all other covariate values. There is no feedback cycle of effects between responses and exogenous TDC.

TDC that are not exogenous are referred to as endogenous TDC. An endogenous variable, sometimes called an internal variable, is a variable that is stochastically related to other measured factors in the study. This can also be defined as a variable generated by a process related to the individual under study. In other words, endogenous TDC are associated with an individual effect, and can often be explained by other variables in the study. When the stochastic process of an endogenous TDC can be (at least partially) explained by the response variable, there is said to be feedback between the response and endogenous TDC. This type of relationship should be accounted for in any longitudinal model with TDC.

As discussed by Diggle et al. (2002), exogeneity can be assessed by considering a regression of covariate values x_{it} on both prior covariate values $x_{i1},\ldots,x_{i(t-1)}$ and also prior response values $Y_{i1},\ldots,Y_{i(t-1)}$. If, after controlling for prior covariate values, the current covariate value x_{it} shows an association with past response values, the covariate shows evidence of endogeneity.

2.2 Types of Time-Dependent Covariates

Recent work has focused on further categorization of types of TDC to facilitate interpretations and proper estimation methods for a model. While these additional types can be interpreted generally with respect to the covariate and response, they are defined with respect to an appropriately defined marginal response distribution. Suppose the marginal mean of the response for subject i at time t is denoted by $\mu_{it}(\boldsymbol{\beta})$, where $\boldsymbol{\beta}$ is a vector of mean parameters. This definition may be induced by an appropriately defined generalized linear model. Four types of TDC can be defined using distinctions in the relationships between the rate of change of the mean and raw errors between the response and mean.

Lai and Small (2007) defined three types of TDC, and a fourth type was defined by Lalonde et al. (2014). Each type of TDC is related to the extent of non-exogeneity with respect to the response and can help determine appropriate analysis techniques. A covariate is said to be a Type I TDC if

$$E\left[\frac{\partial \mu_{is}}{\partial \beta_j}(Y_{it} - \mu_{it})\right] = 0 \qquad \forall s, t, \tag{3}$$

where μ_{is} and μ_{it} are evaluated at the true parameter values $\boldsymbol{\beta}$, and j is the index of the TDC in question. The expectation must be satisfied for all combinations of times s and t, suggesting there is no relationship between the TDC and the response at different times. A sufficient condition for a TDC to be Type I is

$$E[Y_{it}|x_{i1}, \ldots, x_{iT}] = E[Y_{it}|x_{it}]. \tag{4}$$

Thus the response is independent of all TDC values at different times. The sufficient requirement of Eq. (4) would seem to be a stronger condition than the exogeneity presented by Eq. (2), in that Eq. (4) requires the response at time t to be independent of all other TDC values, even those prior to t. Variables that involve predictable changes over time, such as age or time of observation, are typically treated as Type I TDCs. A covariate is said to be a Type II TDC if

$$E\left[\frac{\partial \mu_{is}}{\partial \beta_j}(Y_{it} - \mu_{it})\right] = 0 \qquad \forall s \geq t. \tag{5}$$

The expectation must be satisfied when $s \geq t$, but not necessarily when $s < t$, suggesting dependence between the response and covariate. In this case the TDC process is not associated with prior responses, but the response process can be associated with prior TDC values. A sufficient condition for a covariate to be Type II is

$$E[Y_{it}|x_{i1}, \ldots, x_{iT}] = E[Y_{it}|x_{i1}, \ldots, x_{it}].$$

As discussed in Lai and Small (2007), this is similar but not equivalent to exogeneity with respect to the response process. It can be shown that exogeneity is sufficient for a TDC to be of Type II (Chamberlain 1982; Lai and Small 2007). Examples of Type II TDCs include covariates that may have a "lagged" association with the response in that previous TDC values can affect the response, but covariate values will not be affected by previous response values. One example is the covariate "blood pressure medication" as a Type II covariate with the response "blood pressure," as the accumulated effects of medication over time can be expected to have an impact on blood pressure at any time. A covariate is said to be a Type III TDC if

$$E\left[\frac{\partial \mu_{is}}{\partial \beta_j}(Y_{it} - \mu_{it})\right] = 0 \qquad \forall s = t. \tag{6}$$

For Type III TDC, there is no assumption of independence between responses and covariate values at different times. Thus a Type III TDC may involve a feedback cycle between the covariate and response, in which covariate values can be affected by previous response values. One example is the covariate "blood pressure medication" as a Type III covariate with the response "myocardial infarction." While it is expected that medication can impact the probability of MI, an MI event may elicit a change in blood pressure medication. A covariate is said to be a Type IV TDC if

$$E\left[\frac{\partial \mu_{is}}{\partial \beta_j}(Y_{it} - \mu_{it})\right] = 0 \qquad \forall s \leq t. \tag{7}$$

The expectation must be satisfied for $s \leq t$, but not necessarily when $s > t$, suggesting dependence between the response and covariate. For a Type IV TDC, a covariate can be associated with previous response values, but the response is not associated with previous covariate values. A sufficient condition for a covariate to be Type IV is

$$E[Y_{it}|x_{i1}, \ldots, x_{iT}] = E[Y_{it}|x_{it}, \ldots, x_{iT}].$$

Type IV TDC are associated with prior response values, but the response at time t is only associated with the TDC at time t. One example is the covariate "blood pressure" as a Type IV covariate with the response "weight." While there is an association between weight and blood pressure, the direction of the effect seems to be that weight impacts blood pressure, but the reverse is unlikely.

Different types of TDCs are associated with different relationships with the response. It is important to be able to identify different types of TDCs to guide model selection and to provide appropriate interpretations. Lai and Small (2007) proposed selecting the type of TDC by choice of the researcher, but also presented a χ^2 test to compare two different selections of types for TDC. The idea is to construct competing quadratic forms using the expressions from Eqs. (3), (5), (6), and (7) with zero expectation, so that additional expressions from a different selection of a type of TDC can inflate the quadratic form if those additional expressions do not, in fact, have zero expectation. However, this method will only allow for comparisons between possible selections of types of TDC, but will not make the selection for the researcher. The Extended Classification method, described in Sect. 4.3, presents such a process.

3 Subject-Specific Modeling

Longitudinal data models can be thought of as belonging to two classes of estimation: conditional models and marginal models. Conditional models, the focus of this section, are often referred to as mixed models, random effect models, hierarchical models, or mixture models. Conditional models involve specification of a response model, conditional on a random subject effect. This random effect is intended to account for the clustering of responses by subject, and induces "subject-specific" or "cluster-specific" conclusions from the model. Because parameters must condition on the random effect, parameters are interpreted as expected changes for a specific (average) subject and not a comparison between populations. For a discussion of subject-specific and population-averaged models, see Zeger et al. (1988), Neuhaus et al. (1991), and Zeger and Liang (1992).

3.1 Conditional Model Decomposition

Conditional correlated generalized linear models have been covered extensively in the literature (Lee and Nelder 1996; Diggle et al. 2002; Hedeker and Gibbons 2006; Lee et al. 2006; McCulloch et al. 2008; Fitzmaurice et al. 2012). A conditional correlated generalized linear model with random intercept can be written,

Random Component:

$$Y_{it}|u_i \sim \mathcal{D}(\mu(\mathbf{x}_{it}, \mathbf{z}_{it})),$$

$$u_i \sim \mathcal{D}_u(\boldsymbol{\alpha}),$$

Systematic and Link Components:

$$g(\mu(\mathbf{x}_{it}, \mathbf{z}_{it})) = \mathbf{x}_{it}^T \boldsymbol{\beta} + \mathbf{z}_{it}^T \mathbf{v}(\mathbf{u}).$$

In the expression of the random component, $\mathcal{D}$ represents a specific conditional response distribution from the exponential family, and u_i indicates the random subject effect distributed according to $\mathcal{D}_u$ with parameters $\boldsymbol{\alpha}$. In defining conditional models these two distributions are typically completely specified. In the expression of the systematic component, $\mathbf{z}_{it}$ represents a component of the random effects design matrix, and v is a function transforming the random effect to a range on the continuum (Lee and Nelder 1996, 2001). This model is referred to as a "random intercept" model because the random effects are additively included in the systematic component and can be thought of as "errors" associated with the intercept β_0. In a "random-slopes" model, products of random effects with the fixed-effects design matrix components x_{it} can be viewed as "errors" for the fixed-effects parameters β_k, and thus allow the slopes to vary randomly (Lalonde et al. 2013). Random-slopes models are often presented as hierarchical models in which each parameter β_k has an associated linear model with an individual error term and can include predictors.

Here the interpretation of conditional model fixed effects can be made clear. The parameter β_k represents the expected change in the (transformed) mean response for a unit increase in $x_{k,it}$ for an individual subject, holding all other predictors fixed. In other words, if predictor $\mathbf{x}_k$ changes for an individual subject, β_k represents the expected impact on the mean response.

In the presence of TDC, the standard conditional models are often adjusted to allow for both "within" and "between" components of effects associated with TDC (Neuhaus and Kalbfleisch 1998). If a covariate includes both variation within subjects and variation between subjects, it is believed these two distinct sources of variation can be associated with different effects. The term in the model representing each TDC can be decomposed into two terms: one associated with variation within subjects and the other associated with variation between subjects,

$$\beta x_{it} \quad \rightarrow \quad \beta_W(x_{it} - \bar{x}_{i.}) + \beta_B \bar{x}_{i.}.$$

In this expression the parameter β_W represents the expected change in the mean response associated with changes of the TDC within subjects, while the parameter β_B is more of a population-averaged parameter that represents the expected change in the mean response associated with changes of the TDC across subjects.

3.2   An Issue with Estimation

Estimation of parameters in conditional models typically proceeds by using likelihood-based methods (McCullagh and Nelder 1989; Lee et al. 2006). Standard maximum likelihood estimating equations are of the form,

$$\mathbf{S}(\boldsymbol{\beta}) = \sum_{i=1}^{N} \left(\frac{\partial \mu(\boldsymbol{\beta}; \mathbf{x}_i)}{\partial \boldsymbol{\beta}} \right)^T \mathbf{W}_i(\mathbf{Y}_i - \mu(\boldsymbol{\beta}; \mathbf{x}_i)) = \mathbf{0},$$

where the weight matrix $\mathbf{W}_i$ is often taken to be the inverse of the variance–covariance of the marginal response (Diggle et al. 2002). Pepe and Anderson (1994) showed that these estimating equations have zero expectation only if the data meet the assumption,

$$E[Y_{it}|X_{it}] = E[Y_{it}|X_{ij}, j = 1, \ldots, T],   \tag{8}$$

for each TDC. The assumption of Eq. (8) is met trivially for TIC. Notice that exogeneity is not a sufficient condition, as Eq. (2) implies that the response at one time will be independent of an exogenous covariate's values at future times. Equation (8), on the other hand, suggests the response at one time should be independent of covariate values at all other times. When this assumption is satisfied,

$$E\left[S(\boldsymbol{\beta})\right] = E\left[E\left[S(\boldsymbol{\beta})|x_{it}, t = 1, \ldots, T\right]\right]$$

$$= E\left[E\left[\sum_{i=1}^{N}\left(\frac{\partial\mu(\boldsymbol{\beta};\mathbf{x}_i)}{\partial\boldsymbol{\beta}}\right)^{T}\left[\phi\mathbf{V}_i(\lambda(\boldsymbol{\beta};\mathbf{x}_i))\right]^{-1}(\mathbf{Y}_i - \mu(\boldsymbol{\beta};\mathbf{x}_i))|x_{it}, t = 1, \ldots, T\right]\right]$$

$$= E\left[\sum_{i=1}^{N}\left(\frac{\partial\mu(\boldsymbol{\beta};\mathbf{x}_i)}{\partial\boldsymbol{\beta}}\right)^{T}\left[\phi\mathbf{V}_i(\lambda(\boldsymbol{\beta};\mathbf{x}_i))\right]^{-1}E\left[(\mathbf{Y}_i - \mu(\boldsymbol{\beta};\mathbf{x}_i))|x_{it}, t = 1, \ldots, T\right]\right]$$

$$= E\left[\sum_{i=1}^{N}\left(\frac{\partial\mu(\boldsymbol{\beta};\mathbf{x}_i)}{\partial\boldsymbol{\beta}}\right)^{T}\left[\phi\mathbf{V}_i(\lambda(\boldsymbol{\beta};\mathbf{x}_i))\right]^{-1}\times\mathbf{0}\right]$$

$$= \mathbf{0}.$$

In this derivation, the step of removing the derivative term from the inner expectation depends on the assumption of Eq. (8). Depending on the choice of the weight matrix $\mathbf{W}_i$, the estimating equations may require combinations of the first term (the derivative of the systematic component) with the second term (the raw error term) across different times. Specifically, this will be the case for any non-diagonal weight matrix. The assumption presented by Pepe and Anderson (1994) requires that the derivative and raw residual terms are independent at any two time points combined by the weight matrix.

The standard conditional generalized linear models induce a block-diagonal variance–covariance structure for the marginal response, and thus the condition of Eq. (8) must be satisfied if the standard weight matrix is applied. Notice Eq. (8) is a sufficient condition for a covariate to be a Type I TDC. For other types of TDC, the condition is likely not satisfied. If the condition is not satisfied, the likelihood-based estimating equations will not have zero expectation, leading to bias and loss of efficiency in parameter estimates (Pepe and Anderson 1994; Diggle et al. 2002).

4 Population-Averaged Modeling

Unlike the conditional models of Sect. 3, marginal models for longitudinal data do not involve specification of a conditional response distribution using random effects. Instead a marginal model involves specification of the marginal response distribution, or at least moments of the response distribution (McCullagh and Nelder 1989; Hardin and Hilbe 2003; Diggle et al. 2002). This type of model is associated with "population-averaged" interpretations, or standard regression interpretations. Parameters in marginal longitudinal models provide a comparison of the mean response between two populations with different average values of the predictor of interest. While marginal conclusions can be obtained through conditional models, the term "marginal model" will be used to refer to a model specifically intended for marginal expression and interpretations (Lee and Nelder 2004). A marginal correlated generalized linear model can be written,

Random Component:

$$Y_{it} \sim \mathscr{D}\left(\mu(\mathbf{x}_{it}), \phi V(\mu(\mathbf{x}_{it}))\right),$$

Marginal Mean:

$$\ln(\mu(\mathbf{x}_{it})) = \mathbf{x}_{it}^T \boldsymbol{\beta}.$$

For this type of model $\mathscr{D}$ is assumed to be a distribution from the exponential family of distributions, but may not be fully specified within a marginal model. Instead, the mean $\mu(\mathbf{x}_{it})$ and variance $V(\mu(\mathbf{x}_{it}))$ (with possible over dispersion parameter ϕ) are supplied by the researcher. While there are many marginal methods for estimating parameters in a longitudinal generalized linear model, this chapter will focus on two methods: the generalized estimating equations (GEE) and the generalized method of moments (GMM).

4.1 Generalized Estimating Equations

The GEE approach to model fitting has been covered extensively in the literature (Liang and Zeger 1986; Zeger and Liang 1986; Liang et al. 1992; Ziegler 1995; Hardin and Hilbe 2003; Diggle et al. 2002). Briefly, parameter estimates are obtained by solving the equations,

$$\mathbf{S}(\boldsymbol{\beta}) = \sum_{i=1}^{N} \left(\frac{\partial \mu(\boldsymbol{\beta}; \mathbf{x}_i)}{\partial \boldsymbol{\beta}}\right)^T [\phi \mathbf{V}_i(\lambda(\boldsymbol{\beta}; \mathbf{x}_i))]^{-1} (\mathbf{Y}_i - \mu(\boldsymbol{\beta}; \mathbf{x}_i)) = \mathbf{0},$$

where the variance–covariance structure is specified through a working correlation structure $\mathbf{R}_i(\boldsymbol{\alpha})$,

$$\mathbf{V}_i(\lambda(\mathbf{x}_{it})) = \mathbf{A}_i^{1/2} \mathbf{R}_i(\boldsymbol{\alpha}) \mathbf{A}_i^{1/2}.$$

Pepe and Anderson (1994) argued that the structure of the GEE requires satisfaction of the assumption,

$$\mathrm{E}[Y_{it}|X_{it}] = \mathrm{E}[Y_{it}|X_{ij}, j = 1, \ldots, T],$$

so that the GEE will have zero expectation. As with conditional model estimation, this assumption is met trivially for TIC. When the assumption is met, the first term of the GEE can be factored out of the expectation of $\mathbf{S}(\boldsymbol{\beta})$, producing unbiased estimating equations. When the assumption is not met, the GEE will not have zero expectation unless the working correlation structure is selected so that all components of the GEE involve only a single observation time. This is achieved by a diagonal working correlation structure, so Pepe and Anderson (1994) recommended use of the independent working correlation structure in the presence of TDC. However, Fitzmaurice (1995) noted that using the independent working correlation structure when it is not appropriate can lead to substantial losses of efficiency.

Together these results have been taken as instructions to use the independent working correlation structure when applying GEE to longitudinal data with TDC. However, the results of Fitzmaurice (1995) suggest there may be meaningful losses in efficiency depending on the strength of the auto-correlation. Additionally, the approach of applying independent GEE makes no distinction among different types of TDC, or even between exogenous and endogenous covariates. An approach using the GMM addresses these issues.

4.2 Generalized Method of Moments

The GMM is a minimum-quadratic method of estimating parameters (Hansen 1982; Hansen et al. 1996; Hansen 2007). Model parameters $\boldsymbol{\beta}$ can be estimated by minimizing a quadratic form $Q(\boldsymbol{\beta})$ with appropriately chosen components,

$$Q(\boldsymbol{\beta}) = \mathbf{G}^T(\boldsymbol{\beta}; \mathbf{Y}, \mathbf{X})\mathbf{W}^{-1}\mathbf{G}(\boldsymbol{\beta}; \mathbf{Y}, \mathbf{X}),$$

where $\mathbf{G}(\boldsymbol{\beta}; \mathbf{Y}, \mathbf{X})$ is a vector of "moment conditions" with zero expectation and $\mathbf{W}$ is a correspondingly chosen weight matrix. For longitudinal data situations, $\mathbf{G}$ is typically constructed as an average of vectors of "valid moment conditions" for each subject,

$$\mathbf{G}(\boldsymbol{\beta}; \mathbf{Y}, \mathbf{X}) = \frac{1}{N} \sum_{i-1}^{N} \mathbf{g}_i(\boldsymbol{\beta}; \mathbf{Y}, \mathbf{X}).$$

When presenting the GMM, Hansen (1982) argued that the optimal choice for the weight matrix is the inverse of the variance–covariance structure of the subject-level vector of valid moment conditions,

$$\mathbf{W} = \mathrm{Cov}\left(\mathbf{g}_i(\boldsymbol{\beta}; \mathbf{Y}, \mathbf{X})\right).$$

The challenge in applying the GMM is to determine appropriate components of the subject-level vectors of valid moments conditions $\mathbf{g}_i$. In some data applications, the valid moment conditions can involve transformations of the raw residuals using appropriately chosen instrumental variables (Wooldridge 2008). In the situation of longitudinal data with TDC, Lai and Small (2007) proposed defining each element of $\mathbf{g}_i(\boldsymbol{\beta}; \mathbf{Y}, \mathbf{X})$ according to the expected nature of each TDC. Specifically, the expectations associated with Type I, Type II, Type III, and Type IV TDC, Eqs. (3), (5), (6), and (7), respectively, define combinations of times at which components of potential moment conditions will be independent. When components are independent and the expectation of Eqs. (3), (5), (6), and (7) is zero, the argument of the expectation can be treated as one component of the vector of valid conditions,

$$g_{ik}(\boldsymbol{\beta}; \mathbf{Y}, \mathbf{X}) = \left(\frac{\partial \mu_{is}}{\partial \beta_j} \right) (y_{it} - \mu_{it}).$$

The type of TDC will determine which combinations of times form valid moment conditions. For all predictors in the model, the concatenation of all valid moment conditions will form the vector $\mathbf{g}_i$ for each subject. Notice that this method avoids choosing a general weight matrix to apply across all covariates, as with likelihood-based estimation or with the GEE. Instead, the GMM allows expressions to be constructed separately for each TDC, which provides the ability to treat each covariate according to its type. This eliminates a major restriction from both likelihood-based methods and the GEE.

4.3   GMM with Extended Classification

As an alternative to constructing subject vectors of valid moment conditions using researcher-determined types, the Extended Classification process can be used (Lalonde et al. 2014). Through this process, for each TDC the data will be used to determine the specific combinations of times that will construct valid moment conditions for all subjects.

First initial parameter estimates $\hat{\boldsymbol{\beta}}_0$ are obtained using GEE with the independent working correlation structure. Values of both the derivative component and raw residual component of potential moment conditions can be calculated for TDC $\mathbf{x}_j$,

$$\hat{d}_{sj} = \frac{\partial \hat{\boldsymbol{\mu}}_s}{\partial \beta_j},$$

$$\hat{r}_t = \mathbf{y}_t - \hat{\boldsymbol{\mu}}_t,$$

where $\hat{\boldsymbol{\mu}}_t$ represents a vector of predicted mean responses at time t across all subjects, evaluated using $\hat{\boldsymbol{\beta}}_0$. After standardizing both vectors to obtain $\tilde{d}_{sji}$ and $\tilde{r}_{ti}$, the association between these components is then evaluated using Pearson correlation,

$$\hat{\rho}_{sjt} = \frac{\sum (\tilde{d}_{sji} - \bar{\tilde{d}}_{sj})(\tilde{r}_{ti} - \bar{\tilde{r}}_t)}{\sqrt{\sum (\tilde{d}_{sji} - \bar{\tilde{d}}_{sj})^2 \sum (\tilde{r}_{ti} - \bar{\tilde{r}}_t)^2}},$$

and standardized for comparison. Assuming all fourth moments of $\hat{\rho}_{sjt}$ exist and are finite,

$$\rho_{sjt}^* = \frac{\hat{\rho}_{sjt}}{\sqrt{\hat{\mu}_{22}/N}} \sim \mathcal{N}(0,1),$$

where $\hat{\mu}_{22} = (1/N)\sum_i(\tilde{d}_{sji})^2(\tilde{r}_{ti})^2$, and N is the total number of subjects. Significantly correlated components show evidence of non-independence between the derivative and raw residual terms, and therefore the associated product of derivative and raw error should not reasonably have zero expectation and can be omitted as a potential valid moment condition. To account for the large number of hypothesis tests involved in the Extended Classification process, p-values for all correlation tests can be collectively evaluated (Conneely and Boehnke 2007).

The method of Extended Classification removes the potentially subjective decision of the type of each TDC by the researcher and allows the data to determine appropriate valid moment conditions. Extended Classification also allows for more than four discrete types, admitting all possible combinations of times instead of the four cases corresponding to the four types. The Extended Classification process has shown to be effective in determining appropriate types of TDC, with results similar or superior to those of subjectively chosen types (Lalonde et al. 2014).

4.4 Minimization For GMM

To complete GMM estimation it is necessary to minimize the constructed quadratic form $Q(\boldsymbol{\beta})$. Minimization of the quadratic form has been described using three methods: Two-step GMM (TSGMM), iterated GMM (IGMM), and continuously updating GMM (CUGMM) (Hansen et al. 1996).

TSGMM includes separate steps to address the weight matrix and moment conditions. Using initial values $\hat{\boldsymbol{\beta}}_{(0)}$, an estimate of the weight matrix $\hat{\mathbf{W}}_{(0)}$ is obtained and substituted into the quadratic form,

$$Q_{TS}(\boldsymbol{\beta}) = \mathbf{G}^T(\boldsymbol{\beta}; \mathbf{Y}, \mathbf{X})\hat{\mathbf{W}}_{(0)}^{-1}\mathbf{G}(\boldsymbol{\beta}; \mathbf{Y}, \mathbf{X}).$$

The quadratic form is then minimized to obtain final parameter estimates $\hat{\boldsymbol{\beta}}$. The TSGMM process appears to be the most commonly applied method in the literature. The IGMM process involves an iterative repeat of the steps in TSGMM. After the quadratic form Q_{TS} has been minimized to obtain updated parameter estimates $\hat{\boldsymbol{\beta}}_{(1)}$, the estimate of the weight matrix is updated, providing $\hat{\mathbf{W}}_{(1)}$. The process then iterates between updating $\hat{\boldsymbol{\beta}}_{(i)}$ using the quadratic form and updating $\hat{\mathbf{W}}_{(i)}$ using the resulting estimates,

$$\hat{\boldsymbol{\beta}}_{(i+1)} = argmin\left[\mathbf{G}^T(\boldsymbol{\beta}; \mathbf{Y}, \mathbf{X})\hat{\mathbf{W}}_{(i)}^{-1}\mathbf{G}(\boldsymbol{\beta}; \mathbf{Y}, \mathbf{X})\right].$$

Table 1 Cross-classification
of rehospitalization by time

		Time			
		1	2	3	Total
Re-admit	No	231	272	253	756
		46.48 %	54.73 %	50.91 %	
	Yes	266	225	244	735
		53.52 %	45.27 %	49.09 %	

The process completes on sufficient convergence of $\hat{\boldsymbol{\beta}}_{(i)}$. The IGMM process appears to be the least commonly used method in the literature, and is associated with convergence problems (Hansen et al. 1996; Hansen 2007). CUGMM proceeds by treating the weight matrix as a function of the model parameters,

$$Q_{CU}(\boldsymbol{\beta}) = \mathbf{G}^T(\boldsymbol{\beta}; \mathbf{Y}, \mathbf{X})\,(\mathbf{W}(\boldsymbol{\beta}))^{-1}\,\mathbf{G}(\boldsymbol{\beta}; \mathbf{Y}, \mathbf{X}).$$

Estimates are obtained by a single minimization of Q_{CU}.

5 Data Example

In order to exemplify the implementation and interpretation associated with the models discussed in Sects. 3 and 4, an analysis is presented using the Arizona SID (Lalonde et al. 2014).The dataset contains patient information from Arizona hospital discharges for the 3-year period from 2003 through 2005, for individuals admitted to a hospital exactly four times. The dataset includes 1,625 patients with three observations; each observation corresponds to a rehospitalization. It is of interest to model the probability of returning to a hospital within 30 days using the predictors: total number of diagnoses ("Diagnoses"), total number of procedures performed ("Procedures"), length of patient hospitalization ("LOS"), the existence of coronary atherosclerosis ("C.A."), and indicators for time 2 and time 3. Table 1 provides the percentage of the patients who were readmitted to the hospital within 30 days of discharge against the percentages of the patients who were not readmitted for each of their first three hospitalizations.

   All four predictors as well as the two time indicators will be TDC. Results of modeling the probability of rehospitalization within 30 days will be presented using the five models: random-intercept logistic regression with decomposition of TDC (RS); random-slope logistic regression with decomposition of TDC (RS); GEE logistic regression with independent working correlation structure (IGEE); TSGMM logistic regression with the type of each TDC selected by the researcher (GMM-Types); and TSGMM logistic regression using extended classification (GMM-EC). The GMM models will be fit using the TSGMM.

The RI logistic regression model can be written with a decomposition of all TDC, except for the time indicators,

$$\text{logit}(\pi_{it}) = \beta_0 + \sum_{k=1}^{4} (\beta_{kW}(x_{k,it} - \bar{x}_{k,i.}) + \beta_{kB}\bar{x}_{k,i.}) + \beta_{t2}\text{Time2} + \beta_{t3}\text{Time3} + \gamma_{0i},$$

where π_{it} indicates the probability of rehospitalization within 30 days for subject i at time t, and γ_{0i} indicates the random subject effect. The model can be fit using SAS or R with the commands provided in Sect. 7.1.

The RS logistic regression model can be written similarly, including a random slope for the length of stay predictor. This will allow the effect of length of stay on probability of rehospitalization to vary randomly among subjects,

$$\text{logit}(\pi_{it}) = \beta_0 + \sum_{k=1}^{4} (\beta_{kW}(x_{k,it} - \bar{x}_{k,i.}) + \beta_{kB}\bar{x}_{k,i.})$$
$$+ \beta_{t2}\text{Time2} + \beta_{t3}\text{Time3} + \gamma_{0i} + \gamma_{1i}\text{LOS}_{it},$$

where γ_{1i} represents the random variation in the slope for length of stay. The model can be fit using SAS or R with the commands provided in Sect. 7.2.

The IGEE logistic model will be written without the decomposition of TDC, and without random subject effects,

$$\text{logit}(\pi_{it}) = \beta_0 + \sum_{k=1}^{4} \beta_{kW}x_{k,it} + \beta_{t2}\text{Time2} + \beta_{t3}\text{Time3}.$$

This GEE model can be fit with the independent working correlation structure using SAS or R with the commands provided in Sect. 7.3.

The systematic and link components for the GMM-Types model will look identical to that of the IGEE model. For the GMM-Types model, specific types will be assumed for each TDC. Both time indicators will be treated as Type I TDC, as is common for such deterministic variables. Both "length of stay" and "existence of coronary atherosclerosis" will be treated as Type II TDC, as it is reasonable to assume an accumulated effect on the response from these two variables, but it is unlikely that the response at one time will affect future values of these covariates. Both "number of diagnoses" and "number of procedures" will be treated as Type III TDC, as it is reasonable to assume feedback between the probability of rehospitalization within 30 days and these two counts.

For the GMM-EC model there will be no assumptions of specific types of TDC. Instead the extended classification process will be used to select appropriate valid moment conditions to be used in the GMM quadratic form. These GMM methods are not yet available in SAS; R functions written by the author can be requested.

Results of fitting all five models are presented in Table 2. First consider the results of the conditional models. For the model including a random intercept, the variation associated with that intercept (0.1472) is significant, suggesting there is significant individual variation in the baseline probability of rehospitalization within 30 days. For all models the time indicators have significant negative coefficients, which implies the chance of rehospitalization within 30 days is significantly lower for later follow-up visits. This is suggestive of either a patient fatigue effect in which an individual tires of visiting the hospital, or the positive impact of multiple visits on curing an illness.

The decomposed TDC in this model provide interesting interpretations. The "between" components of the TDC provide population-averaged types of conclusions. For example, there is evidence that subjects with higher average length of stay tend to have a higher probability of rehospitalization (0.0736), perhaps an indication of more serious illnesses. The "within" components provide interpretations of individual effects over time. For example, there is evidence that an increase in the number of diagnoses for an individual is associated with a higher probability of rehospitalization (0.0780), perhaps an indication of identifying additional illnesses.

Results for the model including a random-slope for length of stay are similar. Within the RS model, the variation in the length of stay slope (0.0025) is significant, indicating meaningful individual variation in the effect of length of stay on the probability of rehospitalization. The variation in the intercept (0.1512) remains significant. Two changes are evident when compared to the random-intercept model. First, the random-slope model shows a significant positive association with length of stay *within* subjects, suggesting an increase in length of stay over time is associated with a higher probability of rehospitalization within 30 days. Second, the RS model shows a significant positive association with existence of coronary atherosclerosis *between* subjects, suggesting an increase in the probability of rehospitalization within 30 days for subjects who eventually develop coronary atherosclerosis.

Next consider the results of the marginal models. For all three of the models IGEE, GMM-Types, and GMM-EC, the parameter associated with length of stay is positive and significant. This indicates that, when comparing two populations with different average lengths of stay, the population with the higher length of stay has a higher probability of rehospitalization within 30 days. Notice that while all three marginal models show a negative effect for the number of procedures, significance is identified with GMM but not with GEE. This is to be expected, as GMM is intended to improve the efficiency over the conservative IGEE process. Also notice that the signs of significant "between" effects for the conditional models are similar to those of the corresponding effects in the marginal models. This is also to be expected, as "between" effects produce conclusions similar to the population-averaged marginal model conclusions.

Overall fit statistics are provided but may not provide meaningful information for selection between conditional and marginal models. Selecting the most appropriate model is often based on researcher intentions. The IGEE model is a safe choice,

Table 2 Conditional and marginal logistic regression models

Parameter estimates and significance

	RI—within	RI—between	RS—within	RS—between	IGEE	GMM-types	GMM-EC
Diagnoses	0.0780***	0.0444	0.0686**	0.0362	0.0648***	0.0613***	0.0573***
Procedures	0.0188	−0.0824**	0.0092	−0.0915**	−0.0306	−0.0458*	−0.0366•
LOS	0.0008	0.0736***	0.0200*	0.0952***	0.0344***	0.0530***	0.0497***
C.A.	−0.2607*	0.2223	−0.2646*	0.3050*	−0.1143	−0.0536	−0.0802
Time 2	−0.3730***		−0.4061***		−0.3876***	−0.4004***	−0.3933***
Time 3	−0.2130**		−0.2357**		−0.2412***	−0.2417***	−0.2633***
Intercept	0.1472**		0.1512•				
Slope	—		0.0025*				
Gen χ^2/DF	0.98		0.96				
QIC					6648.52		
QICu					6646.56		

0 *** 0.001 ** 0.01 * 0.05 • 0.10

but generally lacks the power of the GMM models. The conditional models are an appropriate choice when subject-specific designs and conclusions are of interest, but also impose the assumption of a block-diagonal marginal variance–covariance structure.

The most powerful and appropriate choice appears to be the GMM method that avoids the necessary condition of Eq. (8) presented by Pepe and Anderson (1994), and allows for TDC to be treated differently from each other. In this sense the Extended Classification method provides the most flexibility, as moment conditions are selected individually based on empirical evidence from the dataset. In this data example the results of both the GMM-Types and GMM-EC models are quite similar, yielding the same signs of parameter estimates and similar significance levels, which suggests the researcher-selected types of covariates are probably appropriate according to the dataset.

6 Discussion

TDC occur commonly in practice, as data collected for longitudinal studies often change over time. There are numerous ways to classify TDC. The most common type of classification is as exogenous versus endogenous covariates. Exogenous covariates vary according to factors external to the system under consideration, while endogenous covariates show association with other recorded variables. It is most important to identify exogeneity with respect to the response variable.

TDC more recently have been classified according to four "types" that reflect the nature of the association between the TDC and the response. While these definitions are related to exogeneity, they do not represent the same characteristics. Instead, the different types of TDC reflect different levels of association between covariates and responses at different times, with the most substantial relationship a "feedback" loop between covariates and response at different times.

Existing methods for modeling longitudinal data with TDC can be split into two classes: conditional models and marginal models. Conditional models incorporate random effects into the systematic component of the model to account for the autocorrelation in responses. To accommodate TDC, individual regression terms can be decomposed into contributions from variation "within" subjects and variation "between" subjects. When maximum-likelihood-type methods are applied to estimate parameters in conditional models, there is an implicit assumption of independence between the response at one time and covariate values at other times. If this assumption is not met, the likelihood estimating equations will not have zero expectation because of off-diagonal components of the response variance–covariance structure, which can bias parameter estimates.

Marginal models, on the other hand, define a marginal response (quasi-) distribution through specification of a marginal mean and a marginal variance–covariance structure. The most commonly used such method is the GEE. To accommodate TDC, it has been recommended that the independent working correlation structure is applied when using GEE. This recommendation is made to avoid satisfying a necessary condition for the GEE to have zero expected value, as individual estimating equations that combine components at different times may not have zero expectation due to dependence between responses and covariates at different times. However, the use of independent GEE can lead to meaningful losses in efficiency if the autocorrelation is substantial.

An alternative to both conditional models and GEE estimation is the use of the GMM. The GMM can be used to treat each TDC differently, depending on the type of covariate, and to avoid issues with estimating equations constructed from non-independent components. The GMM can be applied by allowing the researcher to identify the type of each TDC, or the Extended Classification can be used to allow the data to determine the nature of the relationship between each TDC and the response. In the future, the GMM with Extended Classification should be improved and utilized as a standard method for analysis of longitudinal data with TDC.

7 Example SAS and R Commands

7.1 Random-Intercept Models

The random-intercept (RI) model discussed in Section LABEL can be fit using the following SAS commands.

```
/* PROC GLIMMIX DOES NOT REQUIRE INITIAL VALUES */
PROC GLIMMIX DATA=ASID_DATA;
    CLASS subject_id;
    MODEL readmission(event = '1') = diagnoses_w diagnoses_b
                            procedures_w procedures_b
                            LOS_w LOS_b
                            CA_w CA_b
                            time2 time3
                            / DIST=BINARY LINK=LOGIT
                                DDFM=BW SOLUTION;
    RANDOM INTERCEPT/ subject=subject_id;
RUN;

/* PROC NLMIXED REQUIRES INITIAL VALUES:USE INDEPENDENT GEE */
PROC NLMIXED DATA=ASID_DATA QPOINTS=30;
    PARMS beta0= beta1= beta2= beta3= beta4= beta5=
                beta6= beta7= beta8= beta9= beta10=;
    eta = u + beta0 + beta1*diagnoses_w
                + beta2*diagnoses_b
                + beta3*procedures_w
                + beta4*procedures_b
                + beta5*LOS_w + beta6*LOS_b
                + beta7*CA_w + beta8*CA_b
```

```
                        + beta9*time2 + beta10*time3;
    exp_eta = exp(eta);
    pi = ((exp_eta)/(1+exp_eta));
    MODEL readmission ~ BINARY(pi);
    RANDOM u ~ NORMAL(0, sigmau*sigmau)SUBJECT=subject_id;
RUN;
```

Alternatively, the model can be fit using R with the following commands.

```
install.packages("lme4")
library(lme4)
# USE start=c(diagnoses_w=, ... ) OPTION TO SPECIFY
    INITIAL VALUES #
# USE INDEPENDENT GEE FOR INITIAL VALUES #
R_Int = glmer(readmission ~ diagnoses_w+diagnoses_b
            +procedures_w+procedures_b+LOS_w+LOS_b
              +CA_w+CA_b
            +time2+time3 + (1|subject_id),family=binomial,
            REML=FALSE,data=ASID_DATA)
summary(R_Int)
```

7.2   Random-Slope Models

The random-slope (RS) model discussed in Section LABEL can be fit using the following SAS commands.

```
/* PROC GLIMMIX DOES NOT REQUIRE INITIAL VALUES */
PROC GLIMMIX DATA=ASID_DATA;
    CLASS subject_id;
    MODEL readmission(event = '1') = diagnoses_w diagnoses_b
                                procedures_w procedures_b
                                LOS_w LOS_b
                                CA_w CA_b
                                time2 time3
                                / DIST=BINARY LINK=LOGIT
                                    DDFM=BW SOLUTION;
    RANDOM INTERCEPT LOS / subject=subject_id;
run;

/* PROC NLMIXED REQUIRES INITIAL VALUES:
    USE INDEPENDENT GEE */
PROC NLMIXED DATA=ASID_DATA QPOINTS=30;
    PARMS beta0= beta1= beta2= beta3= beta4= beta5=
                beta6= beta7= beta8= beta9= beta10=;
    eta = u + beta0 + beta1*diagnoses_w + beta2*diagnoses_b
                + beta3*procedures_w + beta4*procedures_b
                + beta5*LOS_w + beta6*LOS_b
```

```
                    + beta7*CA_w + beta8*CA_b
                    + beta9*time2 + beta10*time3
                    + rb1*LOS;
    exp_eta = exp(eta);
    pi = ((exp_eta)/(1+exp_eta));
    MODEL readmission ~ BINARY(pi);
    RANDOM u rb1 ~ NORMAL([0, 0], [s2u, 0, s2f])
    SUBJECT=subject_id;
RUN;
```

Alternatively, the model can be fit using R with the following commands.

```
install.packages("lme4")
library(lme4)
# USE start=c(diagnoses_w=, ... ) OPTION TO SPECIFY
    INITIAL VALUES #
# USE INDEPENDENT GEE FOR INITIAL VALUES #
R_Slopes = glmer(readmission ~ diagnoses_w+diagnoses_b
             +procedures_w+procedures_b+LOS_w+LOS_b+CA_w+CA_b
             +time2+time3 + (1|subject_id)+(0+LOS|subject_id),
             family=binomial, REML=FALSE,
             start=c(diagnoses_w=, . . .),data=ASID_DATA)
summary(R_Int)
```

7.3   Independent GEE

```
PROC GENMOD DATA=ASID_DATA;
    CLASS subject_id;
    MODEL readmission = diagnoses procedures LOS CA
                        time2 time3
                          / DIST=BINOMIAL LINK=LOGIT;
    REPEATED SUBJECT = id / TYPE=IND;
RUN;
```

Alternatively, the model can be fit using R with the following commands.

```
install.packages("geepack")
library(geepack)
Ind_GEE = geeglm(readmission ~ diagnoses+procedures+LOS+CA
                   +time2+time3, family=binomial,
                   id=subject_id,corstr="independence",
                   data=ASID_DATA)
summary(Ind_GEE)
```

References

Amemiya, T.: Advanced Econometrics. Harvard University Press, Cambridge (1985)

Chamberlain, G.: The general equivalence of granger and sims causality. Econometrica **50**, 569–582 (1982)

Conneely, K.N., Boehnke, M.: So many correlated tests, so little time! rapid adjustment of p-values for multiple correlated tests. Am. J. Hum. Genet. **81**, 1158–1168 (2007)

Diggle, P.J., Heagerty, P., Liang, K.Y., Zeger, S.L.: Analysis of Longitudinal Data, 2nd edn. Oxford University Press, Oxford (2002)

Fitzmaurice, G.M.: A caveat concerning independence estimating equations with multiple multivariate binary data. Biometrics **51**, 309–317 (1995)

Fitzmaurice, G.M., Laird, N.M.: Regression models for a bivariate discrete and continuous outcome with clustering. J. Am. Stat. Assoc. **90**(431), 845–852 (1995)

Fitzmaurice, G.M., Laird, N.M., Ware, J.H.: Applied Longitudinal Analysis, 2nd edn. Wiley, Hoboken (2012)

Hansen, L.P.: Large sample properties of generalized method of moments estimators. Econometrica **50**(4), 1029–1054 (1982)

Hansen, L.P.: Generalized Method of Moments Estimation, pp. 1–14. Department of Economics, University of Chicago, Chicago (2007)

Hansen, L.P., Heaton, J., Yaron, A.: Finite-sample properties of some alternative gmm estimators. J. Bus. Econ. Stat. **14**(3), 262–280 (1996)

Hardin, J.W., Hilbe, J.M.: Generalized Estimating Equations. Chapman & Hall, New York (2003)

Hedeker, D., Gibbons, R.D.: Longitudinal Data Analysis. Wiley-Interscience, Hoboken (2006)

Lai, T.L., Small, D.: Marginal regression analysis of longitudinal data with time-dependent covariates: a generalized method-of-moments approach. J. Roy. Stat. Soc. Ser. B **69**(1), 79–99 (2007)

Lalonde, T.L., Nguyen, A.Q., Yin, J., Irimate, K., Wilson, J.R.: Modeling correlated binary outcomes with time-dependent covariates. J. Data Sci. **11**, 715–738 (2013)

Lalonde, T.L., Wilson, J.R., Yin, J.: Gmm logistic regression models for longitudinal data with time dependent covariates and extended classifications. Stat. Med. **33**, 4756–4769 (2014)

Lee, Y., Nelder, J.A.: Hierarchical generalized linear models. J. Roy. Stat. Soc. Ser. B (Methodological) **58**(4), 619–678 (1996)

Lee, Y., Nelder, J.A.: Hierarchical generalised linear models: a synthesis of generalised linear models, random-effect models and structured dispersions. Biometrika **88**(4), 987–1006 (2001)

Lee, Y., Nelder, J.A.: Conditional and marginal models: another view. Stat. Sci. **19**(2), 219–228 (2004)

Lee, Y., Nelder, J.A., Pawitan, Y.: Generalized Linear Models with Random Effects, 1st edn. Chapman & Hall/CRC, Boca Raton (2006)

Liang, K.Y., Zeger, S.L.: Longitudinal data analysis using generalized linear models. Biometrika **73**, 13–22 (1986)

Liang, K.Y., Zeger, S.L., Qaqish, B.: Multivariate regression analyses for categorical data. J. Roy. Stat. Soc. Ser. B **54**(1), 3–40 (1992)

McCullagh, P., Nelder, J.A.: Generalized Linear Models, 2nd edn. Chapman & Hall, London (1989)

McCulloch, C.E., Searle, S.R., Neuhaus, J.M.: Generalized, Linear, and Mixed Models, 2nd edn. Wiley Series in Probability and Statistics. Wiley, Hoboken (2008)

Neuhaus, J.M., Kalbfleisch, J.D.: Between- and within-cluster covariate effects in the analysis of clustered data. Biometrics **54**, 638–645 (1998)

Neuhaus, J.M., Kalbfleisch, J.D., Hauck, W.W.: A comparison of cluster-specific and population-averaged approaches for analyzing correlated binary data. Int. Stat. Rev. **59**(1), 25–35 (1991)

Pepe, M.S., Anderson, G.L.: A cautionary note on inference for marginal regression models with longitudinal data and general correlated response data. Commun. Stat. Simul. Comput. **23**, 939–951 (1994)

Phillips, M.M., Phillips, K.T., Lalonde, T.L., Dykema, K.R.: Feasibility of text messaging for ecologocial momentary assessment of marijuana use in college students. Psychol. Assess. **26**(3), 947–957 (2014)

Wooldridge, J.M.: Introductory Econometrics: A Modern Approach, 4th edn. Cengage Learning, South Melbourne (2008)

Zeger, S.L., Liang, K.Y.: Longitudinal data analysis for discrete and continuous outcomes. Biometrics **42**, 121–130 (1986)

Zeger, S.L., Liang, K.Y.: An overview of methods for the analysis of longitudinal data. Stat. Med. **11**(14–15), 1825–1839 (1992)

Zeger, S.L., Liang, K.Y., Albert, P.S.: Models for longitudinal data: a generalized estimating equation approach. Biometrics **44**(4), 1049–1060 (1988)

Ziegler, A.: The different parametrizations of the gee1 and gee2. In: Seeber, G.U.H., et al. (eds.) Statistical Modelling, pp. 315–324. Springer, New York (1995)

Solving Probabilistic Discrete Event Systems with Moore–Penrose Generalized Inverse Matrix Method to Extract Longitudinal Characteristics from Cross-Sectional Survey Data

Ding-Geng (Din) Chen, Xinguang (Jim) Chen, and Feng Lin

Abstract A novel probabilistic discrete event systems (PDES) model was established by the research group of Chen and Lin to quantify smoking behavior progression across multiple stages with cross-sectional survey data. Despite the success of the research, this PDES model requires extra some exogenous equations to be obtained and solved. However, exogenous equations are often difficult if not impossible to obtain. Even if additional exogenous equations are obtained, data used to generate such equations are often error-prone. We have found that Moore–Penrose (M–P) generalized inverse matrix theory can provide a powerful approach to solve an admissible linear-equation system when the inverse of the coefficient matrix does not exist. In this chapter, we report our work to systemize the PDES modeling in characterizing health risk behaviors with multiple progression stages. By applying the M–P theory, our research demonstrates that the PDES model can be solved without additional exogenous equations. Furthermore, the estimated results with this new approach are scientifically stronger than the original method. For practical application, we demonstrate the M–P Approach using the open-source R software with real data from 2000 National Survey of Drug Use and Health. The removal of the need of extra data enhances the feasibility of this novel and powerful PDES method in investigating human behaviors, particularly, health related behaviors for disease prevention and health promotion.

D.-G. Chen (✉)
School of Social Work, University of North Carolina, Chapel Hill, NC 27599, USA
e-mail: dinchen@email.unc.edu

X. (Jim) Chen
Department of Epidemiology, University of Florida, 2004 Mowry Road, CTRB #4228, Gainesville, FL 32610, USA
e-mail: jimax.chen@ufl.edu

F. Lin
Department of Electrical and Computer Engineering, Electric-drive Vehicle Engineering, Wayne State University, Detroit, MI 48202, USA
e-mail: flin@ece.eng.wayne.edu

© Springer International Publishing Switzerland 2015
D.-G. Chen, J. Wilson (eds.), *Innovative Statistical Methods for Public Health Data*, ICSA Book Series in Statistics, DOI 10.1007/978-3-319-18536-1_5

Keywords Discrete event systems • Matrix inverse • Moore–Penrose generalized inverse matrix • Cross-sectional survey • Longitudinal transition probability

1 Background

To extract and model the longitudinal properties of a behavioral system with multiple stages of progression, such as cigarette smoking with cross-sectional survey data, Chen, Lin, and colleagues (Chen and Lin 2012; Chen et al. 2010; Lin and Chen 2010) established a method based on the probabilistic discrete event systems (PDES) theory originally developed for systems engineering and manufacturing. They first conceptualized the continuous development process of a behavior (such as cigarette smoking) as a PDES with multiple progression stages (also known as states). These states describe the process of behavioral progression with the transitions from one stage to another. This model has been successfully used in describing the dynamics of cigarette smoking behavior (Chen and Lin 2012; Chen et al. 2010) and responses to smoking prevention intervention among adolescents in the United States (Chen et al. 2012). The authors also developed methods to estimate transitional probabilities in the PDES models from cross-sectional survey data for smoking behavior. An innovation of this method is that despite that no individual respondents are followed up in a cross-sectional survey; data collected through cross-sectional surveys do contain longitudinal information to quantify behavior progression. The challenge is how to extract the information from the data in order to estimate the transitional probabilities. PDES is one such method.

Intuitively, this can be demonstrated by relating data from a cross-sectional survey with data from a longitudinal survey as shown in Fig. 1. Suppose that we randomly select a sample of subjects 10 years old in 2001 and follow them annually

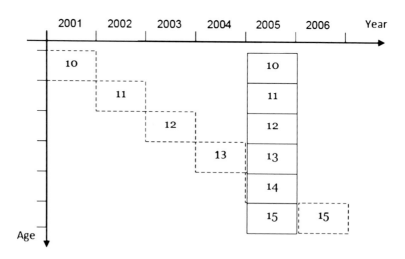

Fig. 1 Relate longitudinal design with cross-sectional design

up to 2006. By the end of the last follow-up, we will have longitudinal data for this birth cohort by years from 2001 to 2006, corresponding to the age groups from 10 to 15 (the dashed-lined boxes in the figure). Transitional probabilities that describe the progression of the smoking behavior (e.g., from nerve user to experimenters, to regular user, etc.) during 1 year period can then be estimated directly by dividing the number of new users identified during the 1-year follow-up and the total number of at-risk subjects at the beginning of each period.

In contrast to the longitudinal data, if one-wave cross-sectional survey was conducted with a random sample of individual subjects 10–15 years old in 2005, we would have data by age for subjects also 10–15 years old (the solid-lined boxes, Fig. 1) as compared to the longitudinal data collected from 2001 to 2006. If we add up the number of various types of smokers by age, the differences in the numbers of these smokers between any two consecutive age groups from the cross-sectional data are analogous to the differences in the numbers of smokers in a birth cohort in any two consecutive years from the longitudinal survey in the same age range. In another word, cross-sectional data do contain longitudinal information.

Besides the fact that cross-sectional surveys are less costly to collect, and hence much more survey data are available, cross-sectional data have advantages over longitudinal data in the following aspects. (1) Selection biases due to attrition: attrition or loss of follow-up is a common and significant concern with survey data collected through a longitudinal design. Data from social behavior research indicate that participants who missed the follow-up are more likely to be smokers (or other drug users). This selective attrition will threaten the validity of longitudinal data. (2) Inaccuracy of survey time: for an ideal longitudinal survey, each wave of data collection should be completed at one time point (e.g., January 1, 2005 for wave 1 and January 1, 2006 for wave 2). However, a good survey usually involves a population with large numbers of participants. Collecting data from such large samples cannot be completed within 1 or 2 days, resulting in time errors in measuring behavior progression even with advanced methodologies. For example, a participant may be surveyed once on January 1, 2005 and then again on March 1, 2006, instead of January 1, 2006. This will cause a time error. (3) Hawthorne (survey) effect: repeatedly asking the same subjects the same questions over time may result in biased data. (4) Recall biases: to obtain data on behavior dynamics, a longitudinal survey may ask each participant to recall in great detail on his or her behavior in the past (e.g., exact date of smoking onset, exact age when voluntarily stopped smoking after experimentation); this may result in erroneous data due to memory loss. (5) Age range of the subjects in a longitudinal sample shifts up as the subjects are followed up over time, affecting the usefulness of such data. (6) Time required: longitudinal survey takes several years to complete, while cross-sectional survey can be done in a relatively short period of time.

Despite the success, the established PDES method has a limitation: the model cannot be determined without extra exogenous equations. Furthermore, such equations are often impractical to obtain and even if an equation is derived, the data supporting the construction of the equation may be error prone. To overcome the limitation of the PDES modeling, we propose to use the Moore–Penrose (M–P)

inverse matrix method that can solve the established PDES model without exogenous equation(s) to create a full-ranked coefficient matrix. The Moore–Penrose
(M–P) generalized inverse matrix theory (Moore and Barnard 1935; Penrose 1955)
is a powerful tool to solve a linear equation system that cannot be solved by using
the classical inverse of the coefficient matrix. Although M–P matrix theory has been
used to solve challenging problems in operation research, signal process, system
controls, and various other fields (Campbel and Meyer 1979; Ying and Jia 2009;
Nashed 1976; Cline 1979), to date this method has not been used in human behavior
research. In this chapter, we demonstrate the applicability of this M–P Approach
with PDES modeling in characterizing the health risk behavior of an adolescent
population. The application of the M–P inverse matrix based methodology (or M–P
Approach for short) will increase the efficiency and utility of PDES modeling in
investigating many dynamics of human behavior. To facilitate the use of the M–P
Approach, an R program with examples and data are provided in Appendix for
interested readers to apply their own research data.

2   A Review of the PDES for Smoking Behavior

We give a brief review in this section on PDES model and detailed descriptions for
this PDES can be found from Lin and Chen (2010) and Chen and Lin (2012). We
make use of the notations in Lin and Chen (2010) to describe the PDES model.
According to Lin and Chen (2010), in estimating the transitional probability with
cross-sectional survey data to model smoking multi-stage progression (Fig. 2), five
behavioral states/stages are defined to construct a PDES as follows:

- NS—never-smoker, a person who has never smoked by the time of the survey.
- EX—experimenter, a person who smokes but not on a regular basis after
  initiation.

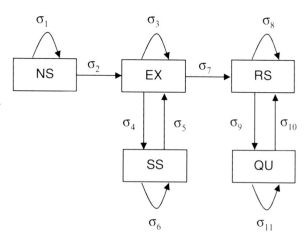

Fig. 2 Probabilistic discrete event system model of the smoking behavior. States are: *NS* never smoker, *EX* experimenter, *SS* self stopper, *RS* regular smoker, and *QU* quitter. σ_i's are events and corresponding probabilities of transitions among states

- SS—self stopper, an ex-experimenter who stopped smoking for at least 12 months.
- RS—regular smoker, a smoker who smokes on a daily or regular basis.
- QU—quitter, a regular smoker who stopped smoking for at least 12 months.

The smoking dynamics as shown in Fig. 2 can be described using the PDES model:

$$G = (Q, \Sigma, \delta, q_o) \tag{1}$$

In the figure Q is the set of discrete states. In this smoking behavior model of Fig. 2, $Q = \{NS, EX, SS, RS, QU\}$. $\sum$ is the set of events. In Fig. 2, $\Sigma = \{\sigma_1, \sigma_2, \ldots \sigma_{11}\}$, where each σ_i is an event describing the transition among the multiple smoking behaviors. For example σ_2 is the event of starting smoking. $\delta : Q \times \Sigma \rightarrow Q$ is the transitional function describing what event can occur at which state and the resulting new states. For example, in Fig. 2, $\delta (NS, \sigma_2) = EX$. q_o is the initial state. For the smoking behavior model in Fig. 2, $q_o = NS$. With slight abuse of notation, we also use q to denote the probability of the system being at state q and use σ_i to denote the probability of σ_i occurring. Therefore, NS also denotes the probability of being a never-smoker and σ_2 also denotes the probability of starting smoking. If it is important to specify the age, then we will use a to denote age. For example, $\sigma_2(a)$ denotes the event or the probability of starting smoking at age a.

Based on the PDES model shown in Fig. 2, the following equation set can be defined conceptually:

$$NS (a + 1) = NS(a) - NS(a)\sigma_2(a) \tag{2}$$

$$EX (a + 1) = EX(a) + NS(a)\sigma_2(a) + SS(a)\sigma_5(a) - EX(a)\sigma_4(a) - EX(a)\sigma_7(a) \tag{3}$$

$$SS (a + 1) = SS(a) + EX(a)\sigma_4(a) - SS(a)\sigma_5(a) \tag{4}$$

$$RS (a + 1) = RS(a) + EX(a)\sigma_7(a) + QU(a)\sigma_{10}(a) - RS(a)\sigma_9(a) \tag{5}$$

$$QU (a + 1) = QU(a) + RS(a)\sigma_9(a) - QU(a)\sigma_{10}(a) \tag{6}$$

For example, Eq. (2) states that the percentage of people who are never-smoker at age $a + 1$ is equal to the percentage of people who are never-smoker at age a, subtracted from the percentage of people who are never-smoker at age a, times the percentage of never-smokers who start smoking at age a. Similar explanations can be given for the other equations. Furthermore, we have the following additional equations with respect to Fig. 2.

$$\sigma_1(a) + \sigma_2(a) = 1 \tag{7}$$

$$\sigma_3(a) + \sigma_4(a) + \sigma_7(a) = 1 \tag{8}$$

$$\sigma_5(a) + \sigma_6(a) = 1 \tag{9}$$

$$\sigma_8(a) + \sigma_9(a) = 1 \tag{10}$$

$$\sigma_{10}(a) + \sigma_{11}(a) = 1 \tag{11}$$

The above ten equations from Eqs. (2) to (11) can be casted into the matrix format:

$$
\begin{bmatrix}
0 & -NS(a) & 0 & 0 & 0 & 0 & 0 & 0 & 0 & 0 & 0 \\
0 & NS(a) & 0 & -EX(a) & SS(a) & 0 & -EX(a) & 0 & 0 & 0 & 0 \\
0 & 0 & 0 & EX(a) & -SS(a) & 0 & 0 & 0 & 0 & 0 & 0 \\
0 & 0 & 0 & 0 & 0 & 0 & EX(a) & 0 & -RS(a) & QU(a) & 0 \\
0 & 0 & 0 & 0 & 0 & 0 & 0 & 0 & RS(a) & -QU(a) & 0 \\
1 & 1 & 0 & 0 & 0 & 0 & 0 & 0 & 0 & 0 & 0 \\
0 & 0 & 1 & 1 & 0 & 0 & 1 & 0 & 0 & 0 & 0 \\
0 & 0 & 0 & 0 & 1 & 1 & 0 & 0 & 0 & 0 & 0 \\
0 & 0 & 0 & 0 & 0 & 0 & 0 & 1 & 1 & 0 & 0 \\
0 & 0 & 0 & 0 & 0 & 0 & 0 & 0 & 0 & 1 & 1
\end{bmatrix}
\begin{bmatrix}
\sigma_1(a) \\ \sigma_2(a) \\ \sigma_3(a) \\ \sigma_4(a) \\ \sigma_5(a) \\ \sigma_6(a) \\ \sigma_7(a) \\ \sigma_8(a) \\ \sigma_9(a) \\ \sigma_{10}(a) \\ \sigma_{11}(a)
\end{bmatrix}
$$

$$
=
\begin{bmatrix}
NS(a+1) - NS(a) \\
EX(a+1) - EX(a) \\
SS(a+1) - SS(a) \\
RS(a+1) - RS(a) \\
QU(a+1) - QU(a) \\
1 \\
1 \\
1 \\
1 \\
1
\end{bmatrix}.
\tag{12}
$$

Equation (12) is denoted by $A\sigma = b$ where A is the coefficient matrix, the bolded σ is the solution vector and vector b denotes the right-side of Eq. (12).

It can be shown that $rank(A) = 9$. Therefore, among the 10 equations, only 9 are independent. However there are 11 transitional probabilities, $\sigma_1(a), \sigma_2(a), \ldots, \sigma_{11}(a)$ to be estimated. Therefore the PDES equation set (12) cannot be solved uniquely as indicated in Lin and Chen (2010). This situation will restrict the application of this novel approach in research and practice.

To solve this challenge, Lin and Chen (2010) sought to derive two more independent equations by squeezing the survey data to define two additional progression stages (1) $\overline{SS}$, old self-stoppers (e.g., those who stopped smoking 1 year ago) and (2) $\overline{QU}$, old quitters (e.g., those who quit smoking 1 year ago). With data for these two types of newly defined smokers, two more independent equations $\overline{SS}(a+1) = SS(a)\sigma_6(a)$ and $\overline{QU}(a+1) = QU(a)\sigma_{11}(a)$ are derived to ensure the equation set (12) has a unique solution. However, the introduction of the two types of smokers $\overline{SS}$ and $\overline{QU}$ may have also brought in more errors from the data because two types of smokers must be derived from recalled data 1 year earlier than other data. If this is the case, errors introduced through these two newly defined smokers will affect the estimated transitional probabilities that are related to self-stoppers and quitters, including σ_3, σ_4, σ_5, σ_6, σ_{10}, and σ_{11} (refer to Fig. 2). When searching for methods that can help to solve Eq. (12) without depending on the two additional equations, we found that the generalized inverse matrix approach can be applied here successfully. It is this "M–P Approach" that makes the impossible PDES model possible.

3   Generalized-Inverse Matrix for PDES

In matrix theory, the generalized-inverse of a matrix A with dimension $m \times n$ (i.e., m rows with m equations and n columns with n variables) is defined as: $AA^-A = A$ where A^{-1} is called the generalized-inverse of A. The purpose of introducing a generalized-inverse for a matrix is to have a general solution $\sigma = A^-b$ for any linear system $A\sigma = b$ (corresponding to the PDES described in Eq. 12) regardless of the existence of the inverse of coefficient matrix A. With this extension, if A is invertible, i.e. A^{-1} exists, the linear system $A\sigma = b$ would be equivalent to the classical solution $\sigma = A^{-1}b$ as commonly known in any elementary linear algebra course. From the definition of the generalized inverse matrix, it can be seen that $A^- = A^{-1}$ if A is a full-rank matrix, that is, rank $(A) = m = n$. Obviously as described earlier, the matrix A for the PDES system (Eq. 12) is not a full-rank matrix $(m < n)$, in another word, the system is complete but the observed data to solve the system is incomplete. Therefore a system without fully observed data like the PDES model cannot be solved using the classic matrix approach. With the introduction of the generalized-inverse matrix approach, we will show that for any matrix equation $A\sigma = b$, including the PDES described in Eq. (12):

(a) $\sigma = A^-b$ is a solution to $A\sigma = b$
(b) The general solution to the PDES matrix equation of $A\sigma = b$ can be expressed in $\sigma = A^-b + (I - A^-A)z$ where A^- is any fixed generalized-inverse of A, while z represents an arbitrary vector.

Therefore, the generalized-inverse A^- is not unique which is equivalent to say that the PDES equation system (12) cannot be solved uniquely as indicated in Lin and Chen (2010). To practically solve this challenge, Lin and Chen (2010) sought to derive two exogenous equations in order to solve for 11 parameters. However, the data used to construct those exogenous equations are hard to obtain and error-prone.

Inspired by the general inverse matrix theory, particularly the work by Moore and Barnard (1935) and Penrose 1955, we introduced a mathematical approach to this problem: the M–P Approach.

In his famous paper, Moore and Barnard (1935) proposed four conditions to the generalized-inverse A^- defined above. They are as follows:

(1)

$$AA^-A = A \tag{13}$$

The original definition of generalized-inverse matrix is to allow any admissible linear system $A\sigma = b$ to be solved easily by matrix representation regardless of the existence of the inverse of coefficient matrix. Extending the classical inverse matrix definition, $AA^{-1} = I$ with the identity matrix I, which is equivalent to $AA^{-1}A = (AA^{-1})A = IA = A$, AA^- is relaxed and no longer needs to be an identity matrix. With this extension, the only requirement is that AA^- will map all column vectors of A to the same column vectors, respectively.

(2)

$$A^-AA^- = A^- \tag{14}$$

The second condition makes A^- a generalized reflexive inverse of A. Similar to the original definition of a generalized-inverse matrix, this added condition is to guarantee that the classical inverse matrix definition of $A^{-1}A = I$ can still hold from this generalized-inverse so that $A^{-1}AA^{-1} = A^{-1}$ when the inverse exists. With this condition A^-A does not need to be an identity matrix, but to map all column vectors of A^- to the same column vectors, respectively.

(3)

$$(AA^-)' = AA^- \tag{15}$$

The third condition requires the transpose of AA^- to be itself. It indicates that AA^- is a Hermitian matrix. This is intuitively true that when A is invertible, $AA^- = AA^{-1} = I$ and the transpose of identity matrix I is itself

(4)

$$(A^-A)' = A^-A \tag{16}$$

The fourth condition is similar to the third condition. It indicates that A^-A is a Hermitian matrix with an intuitive explanation similar to the third condition.

Moore's extended definition did not receive any attention in the mathematics field for 20 years until Penrose 1955 proved the uniqueness of Moore's definition. Since Penrose's work, this definition has been named as Moore–Penrose generalized-inverse and is typically denoted as A^+. The Moore–Penrose generalized inverse has several mathematical properties, and the most relevant one to PDES is that the solution of $\sigma = A^+ b$ is unique as well as being the minimum-norm (i.e., minimum length) solution to the PDES model among all the solutions in $\sigma = A^- b$. It provides a mathematical approach to overcome the challenge in solving a PDES model with a non-full rank coefficient matrix.

4   Demonstration with the MASS Package in R

To demonstrate the M–P Approach in solving the PDES model, a linear equation system without full rank, we make use of the R library "MASS" (Venables and Ripley 2002). This package includes a function named "*ginv.*" It is devised specifically to calculate the Moore–Penrose generalized-inverse of a matrix. We used this function to calculate the Moore–Penrose generalized-inverse of the coefficient matrix A in the PDES smoking behavior model described in Eq. (12).

As presented in Lin and Chen (2010), smoking data from 2000 National Survey on Drug Use and Health (NSDUH) are compiled for US adolescents and young adults aged 15–21 (Table 1). According to the PDES, the state probability for each of the seven types of smokers by single year of age was calculated with the NSDUH data (Table 1). The state probabilities were estimated as the percentages of subjects in various behavioral states. Since the five smoking stages (i.e., NS, EX, SS, RS, QU) are all defined on the current year, the sum of them were one (i.e., 100 %) where $\overline{SS}$ and $\overline{QU}$ were defined as the participants who self-stopped smoking and quit 1 year before.

With data for the first five types of smokers in Table 1, we estimated the transition probabilities with the M–P Approach. The results are shown in Table 2.

For validation and comparison purpose, we also compute the transitional probabilities using data for all seven types of smokers and the original PDES method by Lin and Chen (2010) using R (Codes are included also in Appendix). The results from Table 3 were almost identical to those reported in the original study by Lin and Chen (2010).

As expected, by comparing the results in Table 2 with those in Table 3, for the five transitional probabilities (e.g., $\sigma_1, \sigma_2, \sigma_7, \sigma_8, \sigma_9$) that are not directly affected by the two additionally defined stages $\overline{SS}$ or old self-stoppers and $\overline{QU}$ or old quitters,

Table 1 Percentages of people in 2000 NSDUH smoking data (state probabilities)

Age	NS	EX	SS	RS	QU	$\overline{SS}$	$\overline{QU}$
15	63.65	12.81	14.74	7.84	0.66	8.61	0.42
16	53.10	15.57	17.69	12.45	0.88	12.36	0.40
17	46.95	16.56	17.00	17.99	1.18	12.83	0.54
18	41.20	16.11	16.40	24.46	1.64	11.24	0.87
19	35.55	15.89	15.89	30.50	2.08	11.83	1.34
20	31.75	15.09	16.05	34.69	2.36	12.29	1.51
21	30.35	13.69	17.20	35.77	2.94	13.05	1.73

Table 2 Transitional probabilities of the PDES smoking model from "M–P Approach"

Age	σ_1	σ_2	σ_3	σ_4	σ_5	σ_6	σ_7	σ_8	σ_9	σ_{10}	σ_{11}
15	0.83	0.17	0.10	0.52	0.26	0.74	0.38	0.93	0.07	0.54	0.46
16	0.88	0.12	0.22	0.40	0.40	0.60	0.38	0.94	0.06	0.53	0.47
17	0.88	0.12	0.20	0.38	0.41	0.59	0.42	0.94	0.06	0.53	0.47
18	0.86	0.14	0.21	0.39	0.41	0.59	0.40	0.95	0.05	0.53	0.47
19	0.89	0.11	0.28	0.43	0.43	0.57	0.28	0.95	0.05	0.53	0.47
20	0.96	0.04	0.37	0.52	0.42	0.58	0.11	0.95	0.05	0.53	0.47

Table 3 Replication of the transitional probabilities of the PDES smoking model derived with the original method by Lin and Chen and data from the 2000 NSDUH but computed using R

Age	σ_1	σ_2	σ_3	σ_4	σ_5	σ_6	σ_7	σ_8	σ_9	σ_{10}	σ_{11}
15	0.83	0.17	0.21	0.42	0.16	0.84	0.38	0.94	0.06	0.39	0.61
16	0.88	0.12	0.36	0.27	0.27	0.73	0.38	0.95	0.05	0.39	0.61
17	0.88	0.12	0.28	0.31	0.34	0.66	0.41	0.96	0.04	0.26	0.74
18	0.86	0.14	0.35	0.25	0.28	0.72	0.40	0.97	0.03	0.18	0.82
19	0.89	0.11	0.48	0.24	0.23	0.77	0.28	0.97	0.03	0.27	0.73
20	0.96	0.04	0.62	0.28	0.19	0.81	0.11	0.97	0.03	0.27	0.73

Note: The results calculated using R in this study are almost identical to those reported in the original study reported by Lin and Chen (2010) with a few minor discrepancies

the results from the "M–P Approach" are almost identical to those from the original method. On the contrary, however, the other six estimated probabilities (σ_3, σ_4, σ_5, σ_6, σ_{10}, σ_{11}) have noticeable differences between the two methods. For example, compared with the original estimates by Lin and Chen (2010), σ_{10} (the transitional probability to relapse to smoke again) with the "M–P Approach" are higher and σ_{11} (the transitional probability of remaining as quitters) are lower; furthermore, these two probabilities show little variations across ages compared to the originally reported results.

To our understanding, the results from the "M–P Approach" are more valid for a number of reasons. (1) The M–P Approach did not use additional data from which more errors could be introduced. (2) More importantly, the results from the M–P Approach scientifically make more sense than those estimated with the original method. Using σ_{10} and σ_{11} as examples, biologically, it has been documented that it is much harder for adolescent smokers who quit and remain as quitters than to relapse and smoke again (Turner et al. 2005; Kralikova et al. 2013; Reddy et al. 2003). Consistent with this finding, the estimated σ_{10} (quitters relapse to regular smokers) was higher and σ_{11} (quitters remain as quitters) was lower with the new method than those with the original method. The results from the "M–P Approach" more accurately characterize these two steps of smoking behavior progression. Furthermore, the likelihood to relapse or to remain as quitter is largely determined by levels of addiction to nicotine, rather than chronological age (Panlilio et al. 2012;

Carmody 1992; Drenan and Lester 2012; Govind et al. 2009; De Biasi and Salas 2008). Consistent with this evidence, the estimated σ_{10} and σ_{11} with the "M–P Approach" varied much less along with age than those estimated with the original method. Similar evidence, supporting a high validity of the "M–P Approach," is the difference in the estimated σ_6 (self-stoppers remaining as self-stoppers) between the two methods. The probability estimated through the "M–P Approach" showed a declining trend with age, reflecting the dominant influence of peers and society rather than nicotine dependence (Turner et al. 2005; Lim et al. 2012; Castrucci and Gerlach 2005). However, no clear age trend was observed in the same probability σ_6 estimated using the original method by Lin and Chen (2010).

5   Discussion and Conclusions

The Moore–Penrose generalized-inverse matrix theory has significant applications in many fields, including multivariate analysis, operation research, neural network analysis, pattern recognition, system control, and graphics processing. However, to our knowledge, this is the first time that this "M–P Approach" is used in solving a PDES model to describe smoking behavior progression in an adolescent population. Our study fills a methodology gap in PDES modeling. With the introduction of the "M–P Approach," we illustrated its application with the same data reported in the original study (Lin and Chen 2010) with the R software. Results from the analysis using the "M–P Approach", although using less data, are scientifically stronger than the results from the original analysis.

Findings of this study provide evidence that the "M–P Approach" can be used to solve a PDES model constructed to characterize complex health behaviors even if the coefficient matrix does not have full rank in this real world application. Behavioral modeling, like in many other systems research fields, has frequently been challenged because of the lack of "fully" observed data to quantitatively characterize a system, even when the system is constructed based on scientific theory or data. The success of this study implies that the introduction of the "M–P Approach" will greatly facilitate system modeling of various human behaviors beyond PDES approach and cigarette smoking. This method also reduces the need for extra exogenous data.

According to the "M–P Approach," as long as a model is "true" (e.g., as long as it has a solution), it should be solvable even the true system is partially observable. In our study, since the PDES smoking model has been proved to be true through previous analysis, we conclude that the "M–P Approach" works. This success is not by chance. Similar to a system with extra observed data (e.g., multiple regression with the number of equations greater than the number of unknowns) that can be solved using the "M–P Approach" (e.g., the least square approach is in theory an "M–P Approach"), a system with the number of unknowns greater than the number of independent equations (e.g., partially observed data) can also be solved based on the minimum-norm approach with M–P inverse matrix.

Acknowledgements This research is supported in part by National Science Foundation (Award #: ECS-0624828, PI: Lin), National Institute of Health (Award #: 1R01DA022730-01A2, PI: ChenX) and the Eunice Kennedy Shriver National Institute of Child Health and Human Development (NICHD, R01HD075635, PIs: ChenX and Chen D).

Appendix: R Program for Implementation of PDES

The following R program is step-by-step illustration to the original PDES calculations in Lin and Chen (2010) and the new PDES with generalized-inverse matrix theory.

```
### Step 1: Read in the data from Table 1 from Lin and Chen (2010)
dat = read.csv("smokedata.csv", header = T)
```

```
###Step 2: Verify the PDES calculation in Table 2 in Lin and Chen (2010)
#Step 2.1. R function to calculate the transition probabilities
PDES.Prob = function(a){
# get the coefficient matrix in equation 2
r1 = c(0,-dat$NS[a],0, 0, 0, 0, 0, 0,0,0,0)
r2 = c(0,dat$NS[a],0,-dat$EX[a],dat$SS[a],0,-dat$EX[a],0,0,0,0)
r3 = c(0,0,0,dat$EX[a],-dat$SS[a],0,0,0,0,0,0)
r4 = c(0,0,0,0,0,0,dat$EX[a],0,-dat$RS[a],dat$QU[a],0)
r5 = c(1,1,0,0,0,0,0,0,0,0,0)
r6 = c(0,0,1,1,0,0,1,0,0,0,0)
r7 = c(0,0,0,0,1,1,0,0,0,0,0)
r8 = c(0,0,0,0,0,0,0,1,1,0,0)
r9 = c(0,0,0,0,0,0,0,0,0,1,1)
r10 = c(0,0,0,0,0,dat$SS[a],0,0,0,0,0)
r11 = c(0,0,0,0,0,0,0,0,0,0,dat$QU[a])
out = rbind(r1,r2,r3,r4,r5,r6,r7,r8,r9,r10,r11)
coef.mat = solve(out)
# get the right-side vector
vec = c(dat$NS[a + 1]-dat$NS[a],dat$EX[a + 1]-dat$EX[a],dat$SS[a + 1]-dat$SS
    [a],dat$RS[a + 1]dat$RS[a],1,1,1,1,1,dat$OSS[a + 1],dat$OQU[a + 1])
t(coef.mat%*%matrixvec, ncol = 1))
} # end of "PDES.Prob"
# Step 2.2: Calculation to produce Table 2
tab2 = rbind(PDES.Prob(1), PDES.Prob(2), PDES.Prob(3), PDES.Prob(4),
                PDES.Prob(5),PDES.Prob(6))
colnames(tab2) = paste("sig",1:11,sep = "")
rownames(tab2) = dat$Age[-7]
print(tab2) # to get the Table 2 from Lin and Chen (2010):
```

```
### Step 3: PDES with Generalized-Inverse on Equation (2.12)
#Step 3.1. Function to calculate the transition probabilities
```

```
library(MASS)
newPDES = function(a){
# get the coefficient matrix in equation 1 (10 equations)
r1 = c(0,-dat$NS[a],0,0,0,0,0,0,0,0)
r2 = c(0,dat$NS[a],0,-dat$EX[a],dat$SS[a],0,-dat$EX[a],0,0,0,0)
r3 = c(0,0,0,dat$EX[a],-dat$SS[a],0,0,0,0,0)
r4 = c(0,0,0,0,0,0,dat$EX[a],0,-dat$RS[a],dat$QU[a],0)
r5 = c(0,0,0,0,0,0,0,0, dat$RS[a],-dat$QU[a],0)
r6 = c(1,1,0,0,0,0,0,0,0,0,0)
r7 = c(0,0,1,1,0,0,1,0,0,0,0)
r8 = c(0,0,0,0,1,1,0,0,0,0,0)
r9 = c(0,0,0,0,0,0,0,1,1,0,0)
r10 = c(0,0,0,0,0,0,0,0,0,1,1)
out = rbind(r1,r2,r3,r4,r5,r6,r7,r8,r9, r10)
# get the right-side vector
vec = c(dat$NS[a + 1]-dat$NS[a],dat$EX[a + 1]-dat$EX[a],dat$SS[a + 1]-dat$SS
    [a],dat$RS[a + 1]-dat$RS[a],dat$QU[a + 1]-dat$QU[a], 1,1,1,1,1)
t(ginv(out)%*%matrix(vec, ncol = 1))
} # end of "newPDES"
# Step 3.2. Calculations to generate Table 1 in the current paper
newtab2 = rbind(newPDES(1),newPDES(2),newPDES(3),newPDES(4),newPDES
    (5),newPDES(6))
colnames(newtab2) = paste("sig",1:11,sep = "")
rownames(newtab2) = dat$Age[-7]
print(newtab2) # Output as seen in Table 2 in the current paper
```

References

Campbel, S.L., Meyer, C.D.J.: Generalized Inverses of Linear Transformations. Pitman, London (1979)

Carmody, T.P.: Preventing relapse in the treatment of nicotine addiction: current issues and future directions. J. Psychoactive Drugs **24**(2), 131–158 (1992)

Castrucci, B.C., Gerlach, K.K.: The association between adolescent smokers' desire and intentions to quit smoking and their views of parents' attitudes and opinions about smoking. Matern. Child Health J. **9**(4), 377–384 (2005)

Chen, X., Lin, F.: Estimating transitional probabilities with cross-sectional data to assess smoking behavior progression: a validation analysis. J. Biom. Biostat. **2012**, S1-004 (2012)

Chen, X., Lin, F., Zhang, X.: Validity of PDES method in extracting longitudinal information from cross-sectional data: an example of adolescent smoking progression. Am. J. Epidemiol. **171**, S141 (2010)

Chen, X.G., Ren, Y., Lin, F., MacDonell, K., Jiang, Y.: Exposure to school and community based prevention programs and reductions in cigarette smoking among adolescents in the United States, 2000–08. Eval. Program Plann. **35**(3), 321–328 (2012)

Cline, R.E.: Elements of the Theory of Generalized Inverses for Matrices. Modules and Monographs in Undergraduate Mathematics and its Application Project. Education Development Center, Inc., Knoxville (1979)

De Biasi, M., Salas, R.: Influence of neuronal nicotinic receptors over nicotine addiction and withdrawal. Exp. Biol. Med. (Maywood) **233**(8), 917–929 (2008)

Drenan, R.M., Lester, H.A.: Insights into the neurobiology of the nicotinic cholinergic system and nicotine addiction from mice expressing nicotinic receptors harboring gain-of-function mutations. Pharmacol. Rev. **64**(4), 869–879 (2012)

Govind, A.P., Vezina, P., Green, W.N.: Nicotine-induced upregulation of nicotinic receptors: underlying mechanisms and relevance to nicotine addiction. Biochem. Pharmacol. **78**(7), 756–765 (2009)

Kralikova, E., et al.: Czech adolescent smokers: unhappy to smoke but unable to quit. Int. J. Tuberc. Lung Dis. **17**(6), 842–846 (2013)

Lim, M.K., et al.: Role of quit supporters and other factors associated with smoking abstinence in adolescent smokers: a prospective study on quitline users in the Republic of Korea. Addict. Behav. **37**(3), 342–345 (2012)

Lin, F., Chen, X.: Estimation of transitional probabilities of discrete event systems from cross-sectional survey and its application in tobacco control. Inf. Sci. (Ny) **180**(3), 432–440 (2010)

Moore, E.H., Barnard, R.W.: General Analysis, Parts I. The American Philosophical Society, Philadelphia (1935)

Nashed, M.Z.: Generalized Inverses and Applications. Academic, New York (1976)

Panlilio, L.V., et al.: Novel use of a lipid-lowering fibrate medication to prevent nicotine reward and relapse: preclinical findings. Neuropsychopharmacology **37**(8), 1838–1847 (2012)

Penrose, R.: A Generalized Inverse for Matrices, vol. 51. Proceedings of the Cambridge Philosophical Society (1955)

Reddy, S.R., Burns, J.J., Perkins, K.C.: Tapering: an alternative for adolescent smokers unwilling or unable to quit. Pediatr. Res. **53**(4), 213a–214a (2003)

Turner, L.R., Veldhuis, C.B., Mermelstein, R.: Adolescent smoking: are infrequent and occasional smokers ready to quit? Subst. Use Misuse **40**(8), 1127–1137 (2005)

Venables, W.N., Ripley, B.D.: Modern Applied Statistics with S, 4th edn. Springer, New York (2002)

Ying, Z., Jia, S.H.: Moore–Penrose generalized inverse matrix and solution of linear equation group. Math. Pract. Theory **39**(9), 239–244 (2009)

Part II
Modelling Incomplete or Missing Data

On the Effects of Structural Zeros in Regression Models

Hua He, Wenjuan Wang, Ding-Geng (Din) Chen, and Wan Tang

Abstract Count variables are commonly used in public health research. However, the count variables often do not precisely capture differences among subjects in a study population of interest. For example, drinking outcomes such as the number of days of any alcohol drinking (DAD) over a period of time are often used to assess alcohol use in alcohol studies. A DAD value of 0 for a subject could mean that the subject was continually abstinent from drinking such as lifetime abstainers or that the subject was alcoholic, but happened not to use any alcohol during the period of time considered. In statistical analysis, zeros of the first kind are referred to as structural zeros, to distinguish them from the second type, sampling zeros. As the example indicates, the structural and sampling zeros represent two groups of subjects with quite different psychosocial outcomes. Although many recent studies have begun to explicitly account for the differences between the two types of zeros in modeling drinking variables as responses, none have acknowledged the implications of the different types of zeros when such drinking variables are used as predictors. This chapter is an updated version of He et al. (J Data Sci 12(3), 2014), where we first attempted to tackle the issue and illustrate the importance of disentangling the structural and sampling zeros in alcohol research using simulated as well as real study data.

1 Introduction

Count data with structural zeros is a common phenomenon in public health research and it is important, both conceptually and methodologically, to pay special attention to structural zeros in such count variables. Structural zeros refer to zero responses

H. He (✉) • W. Wang • W. Tang
Department of Biostatistics and Computational Biology, University of Rochester
Medical Center, 265 Crittenden Blvd., Box 630, Rochester, NY 14642, USA
e-mail: hua_he@urmc.rochester.edu; amywshawn@gmail.com; wan_tang@urmc.rochester.edu

D.-G. Chen
School of Social Work, University of North Carolina, Chapel Hill, NC 27599, USA
e-mail: dinchen@email.unc.edu

© Springer International Publishing Switzerland 2015
D.-G. Chen, J. Wilson (eds.), *Innovative Statistical Methods for Public Health Data*,
ICSA Book Series in Statistics, DOI 10.1007/978-3-319-18536-1_6

by those subjects whose count responses will always be zero, in contrast to random (or sampling) zeros that occur in subjects whose count responses can be greater than zero, but appear to be zero due to sampling variability. For example, the number of days of alcohol drinking (DAD) is commonly used to measure alcohol consumptions in alcohol research. Subjects who were always, or become, continually abstinent from drinking during a given time period yield structural zeros and form a non-risk group of individuals in such drinking outcomes, while the remaining subjects constitute the at-risk group. In HIV/AIDS research, the number of sexual partners is often used as a risk factor for HIV/AIDS; subjects with lifetime celibacy yield structural zeros and then consist of the non-risk group for HIV/AIDS, while subjects who happened to have no sex during the study time have random zeros and are part of an at-risk group for HIV/AIDS. Such a partition of the study population is not only supported by the excessive number of zeros observed in the distributions of count responses such as alcohol consumptions from many epidemiologic studies focusing on alcohol and related substance use, but also conceptually needed to serve as a basis for causal inference, as the two groups of subjects can have quite different psychosocial outcomes. In fact, the issue of structural zeros has been well acknowledged (Horton et al. 1999; Pardini et al. 2007; Neal et al. 2005; Hagger-Johnson et al. 2011; Connor et al. 2011; Buu et al. 2011; Fernandez et al. 2011; Cranford et al. 2010; Hildebrandt et al. 2010; Hernandez-Avila et al. 2006) and it has been an active research topic for over a decade. However, nearly all of the studies focus on the cases when the count variables are treated as response (outcome) variables, by using mixture modeling approaches such as zero-inflated Poisson (ZIP) models (Hall 2000; Hall and Zhang 2004; Yu et al. 2012; Tang et al. 2012) to model both the count outcome for at-risk group and the structural zeros for non-risk group. However, it is also important to study the issue of structural zeros when such count variables are serving as predictors.

For instance, DAD is often used as a predictor to study the effects of alcohol use on other psychosocial outcomes such as depression. Common approaches are to treat the DAD as continuous predictor or dichotomize it as a binary predictor (zeros vs. non-zeros, i.e., positive outcomes). Both approaches cannot distinguish the differential effects of structural zeros from their random counterparts. Compared to the dichotomized version of the count variable, the continuous DAD predictor allows one to study the dose effects of alcohol use, but it cannot model the differential effects between structural and random zeros on the outcome, nor can it result in valid inference on other components of the models. This practice is often adopted for modeling convenience, but in many studies it does not reflect the true associations of variables involved. Hence it is essential to model the difference between the structural and random zeros.

In this chapter, we use simulated studies as well as real study data to illustrate the importance of modeling the differential effects of structural zeros when a count variable is used as a predictor. In Sect. 2, we present some background for the structural zeros issue in regression models with such count variables as predictors. We then propose models to assess the differential effects of structural zeros in Sect. 3, and compare the proposed models with conventional models where the effects of structural and random zeros are not delineated in terms of possible biases that may result and the impact on power using simulation studies in Sect. 4. The results from a real data example are presented in Sect. 5, and the chapter is concluded with a discussion in Sect. 6. Much of the material in this chapter was previously presented in He et al. (2014).

2 Background

Count variables in public health, especially in behavioral research, often measure the severity of some kind of behavior such as alcohol use and often contain excessive zeroes, referred to as structural zeroes. The presence of structural zeroes has long been acknowledged as a serious problem for data analysis (Clifford Cohen 1965; Johnson and Kotz 1969; Lachenbruch 2001). In practice, such count variables are treated in a variety of ways when they are analyzed as the response variables. For example, in alcohol studies the DAD has been transformed to percentages as in "percentage of days abstinent" (Babor et al. 1994) or "percentage of heavy drinking days" (Allen 2003). However, a fundamental problem with such data is the probability of a high peak at one end of the distribution, in other words a point mass at "zero." For example, zero percent of days abstinent (common among participants in epidemiological studies) or zero percent days of heavy drinking (common among participants in epidemiological studies and alcoholism trials). Accordingly, researchers have regularly used various transformations to improve data distributions. For example, an arcsine transformation has been recommended and routinely adopted to improve the heteroscedasticity of the distribution of the percent days abstinent variable (Babor et al. 1994). However, the point mass remains because regardless of the transformation, the zeroes will be mapped to a different value (0 under the arcsine transformation), which will then cluster at end of the distribution of the transformed variable (0 under the arcsine transformation). Since the outcomes are in fact a mixture of degenerate zeros consisting of non-risk subjects and count responses from an at-risk group, it is natural to use mixture models. For example, under a zero-inflated Poisson regression model, one may apply a log-linear Poisson regression model for the at-risk group and logistic regression model for the non-risk group. Since zeros are not identified as structural or random, the two components of a zero-inflated model must be estimated jointly. There are many activities focused on zero-inflated models research and the zero-inflated models become more popular in practice. A search of "zero-inflated" in Google Scholar returned about 14,300 articles.

However, little attention has been paid on the issue of structural zeros when the count variables are treated as a predictor. Since the subjective nature of structural and random zeros can be quite different, their effects on the outcome may also be very different. Under conventional models, no matter the count variable is treated as continuous or transformed, the differences between structural and random zeros can't be assessed and thus biased inferences can be resulted.

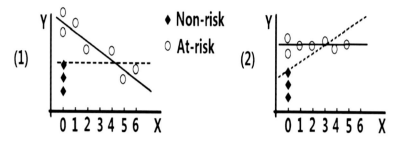

Fig. 1 Two hypothetic examples on the impact of structural zeros

For example, ignoring the structural zero issue, a linear regression of Y on X may fail to detect any association between X and Y for data (1) (dash line) in Fig. 1, although they are in fact associated in the at-risk subgroup (solid line) and there are differential effects between at-risk and non-risk groups on Y. For data (2), if the different effects of structural and random zeros are ignored, a conventional linear regression model may detect a false association between X and Y (dash line), but indeed there is no such association between the counts in X for the at-risk group and Y (solid line); the association between X and Y comes from the group difference between the at-risk and non-risk groups, instead of the counts for the at-risk group. Hence, it's very critical to distinguish the structural and random zeros in the predictor in order to achieve valid inferences. Moreover, a model with the structural zero issue addressed would allow us to understand the data more comprehensively. In the next section, we will introduce models to take care of the difference and assess more systematically the impact in terms of estimation bias and power analysis when such differences are ignored.

3   Modeling the Effects of Structural Zeros

For notational brevity, we consider only the cross-sectional data setting. The considerations as well as the conclusions obtained also apply for longitudinal study data. Given a sample of n subjects, let y_i denote the outcome of interest from the ith subject ($1 \leq i \leq n$). We are interested in assessing the effects of some personal trait such as alcohol dependency on the outcome, along with other covariates, collectively denoted by $\mathbf{z}_i = (z_{i1}, \ldots, z_{ip})^\top$. Suppose that the trait is measured by a count variable x_i with structural zeros.

Let r_i be the indicator of whether x_i is a structural zero, i.e., $r_i = 1$ if x_i is a structural zero and $r_i = 0$ otherwise. For simplicity, we assume that the structural zeros are observed, which we assume throughout the chapter unless stated otherwise. The indicator r_i partitions the study sample (population) into two distinctive groups, with one consisting of subjects corresponding to $r_i = 1$ and the other comprising of the remaining subjects with $r_i = 0$. Since the trait in many studies is often a risk factor such as alcohol use, the first group is often referred to as the non-risk group, while the second as the at-risk group.

3.1 Linear and Generalized Linear Models

Without distinguishing structural zeros from random zeros, one may apply generalized linear models (GLM) to model the association between the explanatory variables, the predictor of interest x_i plus the covariates z_i, and the outcome. For example, if y_i is continuous, we may use the following linear model:

$$E\left(y_i \mid x_i, \mathbf{z}_i\right) = \alpha x_i + \mathbf{z}_i^\top \boldsymbol{\beta}, \quad 1 \le i \le n. \tag{1}$$

Here one may include a covariate with a constant value 1 in $\mathbf{z}_i$ so that the intercept is included in $\boldsymbol{\beta}$ as well. In general, we may use generalized linear models

$$g\left(E\left(y_i \mid x_i, \mathbf{z}_i\right)\right) = \alpha x_i + \mathbf{z}_i^\top \boldsymbol{\beta}, \quad 1 \le i \le n, \tag{2}$$

where $g(\cdot)$ is a link function, such as a logarithm function for count responses and a probit or a logistic function for binary outcomes.

If the predictor x_i has structural zeros, the structural zeros have a quite different conceptual interpretation than their random zero counterparts and the conceptual difference carries a significant implication for the interpretation of the coefficient α in (1). For example, within the context of drinking outcomes, the difference in y_i between subjects with $x_i = 1$ and $x_i = 0$ has a different interpretation, depending on whether $x_i = 0$ is a structural or random zero. If $x_i = 0$ is a random zero, this difference represents the differential effects of drinking on y_i within the drinker subgroup when the drinking outcome changes from 0 to 1. For a structural zero, such a difference in y_i speaks to the effects of the trait of drinking on the response y_i. Thus, the model in (1) is flawed since it does not delineate the two types of effects and must be revised to incorporate the information of structural zeros.

One way to model the effects of a count variable with structural zeros as a predictor in regression analysis is to distinguish between random and structural zeros by including an indicator of structural zeros in the model, in addition to the count variable itself. By expanding $(x_i, \mathbf{z}_i)$ to include r_i, it follows from (1) that

$$E\left(y_i \mid x_i, \mathbf{z}_i, r_i\right) = \alpha x_i + \mathbf{z}_i^\top \boldsymbol{\beta} + \gamma r_i, \quad 1 \le i \le n. \tag{3}$$

Under the refined model above, the association between the trait and the response can be tested by checking whether both $\alpha = 0$ and $\gamma = 0$. This involves a composite linear contrast, $H_0 : \alpha = 0, \gamma = 0$. If the null H_0 is rejected, then either $\alpha \ne 0$ or $\gamma \ne 0$ or $\alpha \ne 0, \gamma \ne 0$. The coefficient γ is interpreted as the trait effects on the response y_i, all other things being equal. The coefficient α measures the change in y_i per unit increase in x_i within the at-risk group.

Similarly, we may introduce a link function to the linear model in (3) to extend it to generalized linear models to accommodate categorical and count responses.

3.2   Zero-Inflated Models

When the outcome y_i itself is a count response with structural zeros, it is not appropriate to apply Poisson or negative binomial (NB) log-linear models, the popular models for count responses. Instead, one needs to apply the zero-inflated Poisson (ZIP) or zero-inflated negative binomial (ZINB) model (Tang et al. 2012; Lambert 1992; Welsh et al. 1996). The ZIP model extends the Poisson model by including an additional logistic regression component so that it can model both the at- and non-risk groups. Estimates from the Poisson loglinear regression component assess the increased/reduced effects of an explanatory variable on the count response of interest within the at-risk subgroup, while those from the logistic regression component indicate increased/reduced likelihood of being in the non-risk group that an explanatory variable can affect on. By replacing Poison with NB, ZINB models also address the weakness of the Poisson component in ZIP to account for overdispersion, a common violation of Poisson models that restrict the variance to be the same as the mean.

By ignoring the structural zeros in x_i, one may model y_i using a ZIP model as following:

$$structural\ zero\ in\ y_i \mid x_i, \mathbf{z}_i \sim Bernoulli(v_i), \quad logit(v_i) = \alpha' x_i + \mathbf{z}_i^\top \boldsymbol{\beta}',$$

$$non-structural\ zero\ count\ in\ y_i \mid x_i, \mathbf{z}_i \sim Poisson(\mu_i), \quad \log(\mu_i) = \alpha x_i + \mathbf{z}_i^\top \boldsymbol{\beta},$$

$$(4)$$

where Bernoulli(v) (Poisson(μ)) denotes a Bernoulli (Poisson) distribution with mean v (μ), and $logit(v) = \frac{v}{1+v}$ is the logit function. Under the ZIP above, the effects of x_i on the outcome y_i is broken down into two parts, with one on the likelihood of being a structural zero, or being a member of the non-risk subgroup, determined by the logistic model in (4), and the other on the outcome y_i within the at-risk subgroup determined by the Poisson model in (4). Thus, one needs to test the null: $H_0 : \alpha = \alpha' = 0$, to check if the trait is associated with the outcome y_i.

Similarly, we can add the indicator r_i of structural zeros of x_i as an additional predictor for the ZIP in (4) to obtain:

$$structural\ zero\ in\ y_i \mid x_i, \mathbf{z}_i, r_i \sim Bernoulli(v_i),\ logit(v_i) = \alpha' x_i + \mathbf{z}_i^\top \boldsymbol{\beta}' + \gamma' r_i,$$

$$non-structural\ zero\ in\ y_i \mid x_i, \mathbf{z}_i, r_i \sim Poisson(\mu_i),\ \log(\mu_i) = \alpha x_i + \mathbf{z}_i^\top \boldsymbol{\beta} + \gamma r_i.$$

$$(5)$$

In this refined model, we need four coefficients to describe the relationship between the trait and the outcome. The coefficient γ measures the differential effects of the at- and non-risk group defined by x_i on the at-risk group defined by y_i, while the coefficient γ' captures the differential effects of the at- and non-risk group defined by x_i on the non-risk group defined by y_i. The coefficient α quantifies the increase in the outcome y_i within the at-risk group per unit increase in x_i within the at-risk subgroup defined by x_i, and the coefficient α' is the log odds ratio for the change of likelihood of being in the non-risk group defined by y per unit increase in x_i among the at-risk subjects defined by x_i. If the trait and the outcome are not related, then all the four coefficients are zero: $\alpha = \alpha' = \gamma = \gamma' = 0$.

Note that for notational brevity, we have assumed no interaction among the explanatory variables in the models discussed above. In practice, some of these variables may also create interaction effects on the response y_i. Such interactions are readily incorporated into all the models discussed.

4 Simulation Studies

We performed simulation studies to show the importance of addressing structural zeros issue in studying the effects of a count variable X on a response of interest Y. The count predictor X was generated from a ZIP consisting of a Poisson with mean μ and a point mass at zero, with a mixing probability of p (proportion of subjects with the trait). We considered two different types of response Y: continuous and zero-inflated Poisson count response. We simulated data using linear models for the first case. In the second case, we simulated data using ZIP models; a Poisson variate was first generated by a GLM and then mixed with a constant zero based on the mixing probability of a ZIP.

In both cases, the explanatory variables include X and the indicator R of the structural zeros of X. In addition to the true model, or Model I, which includes both X and R, we also considered Model II, which is identical to Model I, but with the indicator R removed. Since it is common to group the count variables into categories before they are analyzed in practice, we also dichotomized X according to whether X is positive. Thus, we also created Models III and IV by replacing X with such a dichotomized X in Models I and II, respectively.

A Monte Carlo (MC) size of 1,000 was used for all the models. We collected the point estimates of the coefficient of the count variable (X), and compared the bias and standard deviation of the estimates under the four different models. Further, we tested whether the trait was associated with the outcome Y and compared power across the models with type I error set at 0.05.

4.1 Continuous Response Y

For a continuous Y, the association of Y with X and R was specified as follows:

$$Y = c_0 + c_1 X + c_2 R + \varepsilon, \quad \varepsilon \sim N\left(0, \sigma^2\right), \tag{6}$$

where ε is the error term. If c_1 and c_2 have different signs, say $c_1 > 0 > c_2$, then the mean of the at-risk subgroup defined by positive X > the mean of the at-risk subgroup defined by the random zeros of X > the mean of the non-risk group defined by the structural zeros of X. In this case, this monotone relationship among the three subgroups will remain, even if the random and structural zeros are not distinguished between each other. However, if c_1 and c_2 have the same sign, say both are positive, $c_1, c_2 > 0$, then the mean of the at-risk subgroup defined by positive X > the mean of the at-risk group defined by the random zeros of X < the mean of the non-risk group defined by the structural zeros of X. In such cases, the mean of the non-risk group may be bigger than the at-risk subgroup defined by positive X, depending on the relationship between c_1 and c_2, and the monotone relationship among the three subgroups may fail, if random and structural zeros are combined. Thus, to assess power, we ran simulations to cover both situations, where c_1 and c_2 had the same and different signs.

The zero-inflated predictor X was simulated from a ZIP with the probability of being a structural zero $p = 0.2$ and the mean of the Poisson component $\mu = 0.3$. We simulated 1,000 samples with sample sizes of 100, 200, 500, and 1,000, for several sets of parameters:

$$c_0 = 0.5, \ c_1 = -0.5, \ -0.25, \ 0, \ 0.25, \ 0.5, \ c_2 = 0.5, \sigma^2 = 0.5. \tag{7}$$

For each simulated data, we fit the four aforementioned models, i.e.,

$$Model\ I : Y = c_0 + c_1 X + c_2 R + \varepsilon, \quad \varepsilon \sim N\left(0, \sigma^2\right), \tag{8}$$

$$Model\ II : Y = c_0 + c_1 X + \varepsilon, \quad \varepsilon \sim N\left(0, \sigma^2\right), \tag{9}$$

$$Model\ III : Y = c_0 + c_1 IX + c_2 R + \varepsilon, \quad \varepsilon \sim N\left(0, \sigma^2\right), \tag{10}$$

$$Model\ IV : Y = c_0 + c_1 IX + \varepsilon, \quad \varepsilon \sim N\left(0, \sigma^2\right), \tag{11}$$

where IX denotes the dichotomized X with $IX = 1$ (0) for $X > 0$ ($X \leq 0$).

To save space, we will only present some of the simulation results. Shown in Table 1 are the estimates (mean) of the parameters c_0, c_1, and c_2, and associated standard errors (Std err) averaged over the 1,000 MC replications when the sample size is 200. As expected the standard errors were similar between Models I and II as well as Models III and IV. However, the estimates from Model II (IV) were biased as compared to their counterparts from Model I (III). Although the estimates for parameters from Models I and III were not the same as their corresponding true

Table 1 Parameter estimates (Mean) and standard errors (Std err) averaged over 1,000 MC replications for the four models considered in the simulation study with a continuous response

Cases		c_0				c_1				c_2	
($c_1 =$)	Model	I	II	III	IV	I	II	III	IV	I	III
−0.5	Mean	0.50	0.62	0.50	0.63	−0.50	−0.60	−0.58	−0.70	0.49	0.49
	Std err	0.046	0.042	0.047	0.042	0.072	0.071	0.094	0.092	0.096	0.097
−0.25	Mean	0.50	0.62	0.50	0.63	−0.25	−0.35	−0.29	−0.42	0.49	0.49
	Std err	0.046	0.042	0.047	0.042	0.072	0.071	0.091	0.089	0.096	0.097
0	Mean	0.50	0.62	0.50	0.63	0.00	−0.10	0.00	−0.13	0.49	0.49
	Std err	0.046	0.042	0.047	0.042	0.072	0.071	0.090	0.088	0.096	0.097
0.25	Mean	0.50	0.62	0.50	0.63	0.25	0.15	0.29	0.16	0.49	0.49
	Std err	0.046	0.042	0.047	0.042	0.072	0.071	0.092	0.090	0.096	0.097
0.5	Mean	0.50	0.62	0.50	0.63	0.50	0.40	0.58	0.45	0.49	0.49
	Std err	0.046	0.042	0.047	0.042	0.072	0.071	0.096	0.094	0.096	0.097

values, the differences reflected the sampling variability. Note that the "true" value of the parameter c_1 under Model III should in fact be

$$E(Y \mid X > 0) - E(Y \mid X = 0 \, and R = 0) = \frac{\mu c_1}{\Pr(X > 0)} = \frac{0.3c_1}{1 - \exp(-0.3)}, \quad (12)$$

i.e., $-0.58, -0.29, 0.00, 0.29$, and 0.58, respectively, because of the grouping of subjects with $X > 0$.

Even if one does not care about the size of the effects of X on Y and just wants to detect association between the two variables, an application of incorrect models such as Models II and Model IV may still be quite problematic. For example, we also examined power in detecting association between the trait and the outcome for the different models, with a type I error of 0.05. For Models II and IV, we can simply test the null: $H_0 : c_1 = 0$ for this purpose. However, for Models I and III, there are two terms pertaining to the association of interest, one relating to the difference between the structural and random zero in X (c_2) and the other associated with difference between positive X and random zeros in X (c_1). So, we need to test a composite null: $H_0 : c_1 = c_2 = 0$ in Models I and III. We computed the proportions of p-values that were less than 0.05 for these hypothesis tests as the empirical power estimates. Shown in Table 2 are the estimated powers to test the effects of the trait based on 1,000 MC replications with sample sizes 100, 200, 500, and 1,000 in the range of values of c_1 (and c_2) considered. The models with the structural zero issue addressed (Models I and III) were much more powerful in detecting the association between Y and X than their counterparts (Models II and IV). Thus, models that do not account for structural zeros such as Models II and IV may not even be able to perform such a "crude" task.

Table 2 Estimated power in testing the association between the trait and the outcome based on 1,000 MC replications for the four models considered in the simulation study with a continuous response

Cases ($c_1 =$)	Sample size	Model I	Model II	Model III	Model IV
−0.5	100	1.000	0.999	1.000	0.998
	200	1.000	1.000	1.000	1.000
	500	1.000	1.000	1.000	1.000
	1,000	1.000	1.000	1.000	1.000
−0.25	100	0.997	0.879	0.997	0.872
	200	1.000	0.996	1.000	0.996
	500	1.000	1.000	1.000	1.000
	1,000	1.000	1.000	1.000	1.000
0	100	0.932	0.127	0.938	0.142
	200	0.999	0.227	0.999	0.249
	500	1.000	0.497	1.000	0.553
	1,000	1.000	0.818	1.000	0.870
0.25	100	0.964	0.312	0.949	0.231
	200	0.999	0.547	0.998	0.407
	500	1.000	0.888	1.000	0.778
	1,000	1.000	0.999	1.000	0.975
0.5	100	0.999	0.946	0.998	0.917
	200	1.000	0.999	1.000	0.999
	500	1.000	1.000	1.000	1.000
	1,000	1.000	1.000	1.000	1.000

4.2 Zero-Inflated Poisson Response Y

We considered a count response with structural zeros generated from the following ZIP:

$$non-structural zero count Y \mid X, R \sim Poisson(\mu), \ \log(\mu) = c_0 + c_1 X + c_2 R, \quad (13)$$

$$structural zero Y \mid X, R \sim Bernoulli(\nu), \ logit(\nu) = c_0' + c_1' X + c_2' R.$$

As in the previous cases, we fit four different ZIPs to the data simulated with the same set of parameter values (in addition to c_0, c_1, and c_2 are in previous cases, we set $c_0' = c_0$, $c_1' = c_1$ and $c_2' = c_2$). Again, we report the results for the case with sample size = 200 for the parameter estimates.

Shown in Table 3 are the averaged estimates of the parameters c_0, c_1, and c_2, and associated standard errors over the 1,000 MC replications. The same patterns of bias again emerged from the incorrect models (Models II and IV). The incorrect models also yielded much lower power than their correct counterparts. Shown in Table 4 are the estimated powers for testing the effects of the trait on the response. As seen, the

Table 3 Parameter estimates (Mean) and standard errors (Std err) averaged over 1,000 MC replications for the four models considered in the simulation study with a ZIP response

Cases		c_0				c_1				c_2	
($c_1 =$)	Model	I	II	III	IV	I	II	III	IV	I	III
−0.5	Mean	0.48	0.63	0.48	0.63	−0.55	−0.67	−0.60	−0.75	0.48	0.49
	Std err	0.155	0.126	0.155	0.126	0.370	0.360	0.425	0.416	0.298	0.299
−0.25	Mean	0.49	0.63	0.48	0.63	−0.30	−0.43	−0.33	−0.48	0.48	0.49
	Std err	0.152	0.125	0.155	0.126	0.330	0.325	0.392	0.383	0.297	0.299
0	Mean	0.49	0.63	0.48	0.63	−0.05	−0.17	−0.04	−0.19	0.48	0.49
	Std err	0.153	0.126	0.155	0.126	0.295	0.292	0.342	0.331	0.297	0.299
0.25	Mean	0.49	0.63	0.48	0.63	0.22	0.10	0.26	0.12	0.48	0.49
	Std err	0.150	0.125	0.155	0.126	0.266	0.263	0.315	0.302	0.295	0.299
0.5	Mean	0.49	0.63	0.48	0.63	0.49	0.37	0.57	0.42	0.48	0.48
	Std err	0.150	0.125	0.154	0.126	0.229	0.221	0.284	0.268	0.295	0.299

Table 4 Estimated power in testing the association between the trait and the outcome based on 1,000 MC replications for the four models considered in the simulation study with a ZIP response

Cases ($c_1 =$)	Sample size	Model I	Model II	Model III	Model IV
−0.5	100	0.377	0.245	0.378	0.231
	200	0.611	0.393	0.567	0.301
	500	0.970	0.848	0.957	0.799
	1,000	1.000	0.993	1.000	0.992
−0.25	100	0.276	0.115	0.274	0.112
	200	0.468	0.178	0.448	0.140
	500	0.903	0.468	0.900	0.439
	1,000	0.996	0.813	0.996	0.794
0	100	0.219	0.078	0.207	0.058
	200	0.354	0.052	0.347	0.052
	500	0.763	0.055	0.759	0.074
	1,000	0.969	0.136	0.969	0.154
0.25	100	0.213	0.090	0.201	0.081
	200	0.385	0.110	0.372	0.104
	500	0.783	0.190	0.748	0.117
	1,000	0.983	0.359	0.971	0.240
0.5	100	0.352	0.283	0.309	0.243
	200	0.641	0.501	0.570	0.416
	500	0.975	0.851	0.946	0.774
	1,000	1.000	0.993	0.999	0.966

ZIP seems to have similar power as the binary response Y, which is not surprising given that one of the components of ZIP is the binary response for modeling the structural zero of Y. Note that there are two components in ZIP models and thus the results are obtained from testing composite hypotheses. To see if the trait is associated with the outcome, we tested the null, $H_0 : c_1 = c_1' = 0$, for Models II and IV, but a different null, $H_0 : c_1 = c_1' = c_2 = c_2' = 0$, for Models I and III.

5 A Case Study Example

We now illustrate the effects of structural zeros with a real data example based on the 2009–2010 National Health and Nutrition Examination Survey (NHANES). In this database, we identified a measure of alcohol use to be examined as an explanatory variable for depressive symptoms (count response). Both the alcohol and depression outcomes show a preponderance of zeros because of a large percent of the surveyed population is not at risk for either of the health issues. The relationship between the two has been reported in a number of studies (Gibson and Becker 1973; Pettinati et al. 1982; Dackis et al. 1986; Willenbring 1986; Brown and Schuckit 1988; Penick et al. 1988; Davidson 1995; Merikangas et al. 1998; Swendsen et al. 1998; Hasin and Grant 2002).

The **NHANES** is an annual national survey of the health and nutritional status of adults and children in the United States. A nationally representative sample of about 5,000 persons participates each year. Interviews and assessments are conducted in respondents' homes. Health assessments are performed in equipped mobile centers, which travel to locations throughout the country. Starting in 2007, NHANES has been oversampling all Hispanics (previously Mexican Americans were oversampled). In the 2009–2010 data set, data were collected from 10,537 individuals of all ages during the 2-year period between January 2009 and December 2010. The race/ethnicity of the sample is 22.5 % Hispanic-Mexican American, 10.8 % Hispanic-other, 18.6 % non-Hispanic Black, 42.1 %, non-Hispanic White, and 6.1 % other.

Alcohol Use Measure In NHANES, for measurement of alcohol use, a different assessment was done for those aged 12–19 vs. those aged 20 and older; the assessment for the former age group asked only about the past 30 days, while the one administered to the latter age group asked about the past year. Therefore, for the current case study example we only used the data from the cohort aged 20 and older. Alcohol use (for those aged 20 or above) was assessed with a computer-assisted personal interview (CAPI). Specific questions of interest for the current work included number of days of any alcohol drinking (DAD) in the past year, which is commonly used in alcohol research. This variable was converted to average number of days drinking per month in our analysis. There were 6,218 subjects in the data set with age of 20 and older.

In NHANES, one question asks "In your entire life, have you had at least 12 drinks of any type of alcoholic beverage?". This variable has been used previously to differentiate lifetime abstainers, who answered "no" to this question and ex-drinkers, who answered "yes" (Tsai et al. 2012). Thus, an answer "no" to this question is a proxy of structural zeros. Hence the zeros were endorsed by two distinctive risk groups in this study population for the question about drinking.

Depression Symptoms Depression Symptoms were measured in those aged 12 and above in the 2009–2010 NHANES with the Patient Health Questionnaire (PHQ-9) administered by CAPI. The PHQ-9 is a multiple-choice self-report inventory of nine items specific to depression. Each item of the PHQ-9 evaluates the presence of one of the nine DSM-IV criteria for depressive disorder during the last 2 weeks. Each of the nine items can be scored 0 (not at all), 1 (few days), 2 (more than half the days) and 3 (nearly every day) and a total score is obtained. Among the 6,218 subjects with CAPI, 5,283 subjects reported PHQ-9, so there are about 935 subjects with missing values in the PHQ-9.

Covariates In epidemiological samples, several demographic characteristics, including female gender, older age, not being married, low education, low income level, poor physical health, social isolation, minority status, and urban residence, have been associated with higher levels of depressive symptoms or presence of a major depressive disorder, though overlap among some of these factors suggests that these may not all be independent influences (Oh et al. 2013; Roberts et al. 1997; Leiderman et al. 2012; Wilhelm et al. 2003; González et al. 2010; Rushton et al. 2002; Weissman et al. 1996). Based on these findings, in our analyses of the relationship of alcohol use to depressive symptoms, we incorporated relevant demographic variables available in NHANES (age, gender, education, race) as covariates.

Shown in Fig. 2 are the distributions of PHQ9 and DAD, both exhibiting a preponderance of zeros. Goodness of fit tests also rejected the fit of the data in

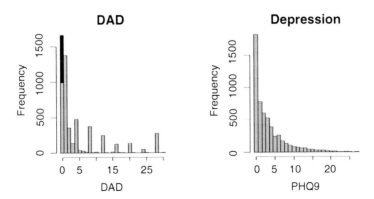

Fig. 2 Distributions of DAD and PHQ9 for the 2009–2010 NHANES data, with the *darker-shaded bar* in the distribution of DAD representing structural zeros

each case by the Poisson (p-value< 0.001). Further, the Vuong test showed that ZIP provided a much better fit than the Poisson (p-value<0.001). These findings are consistent with our prior knowledge that this study sample is from a mixed population consisting of an at-risk and non-risk subgroup for each of the behavioral and health outcomes.

Statistical Models We applied the ZIP to model the PHQ-9 score with DAD in the past month as the predictor, adjusting for age, gender, race, and education. Since we had the information to identify the non-risk group for the DAD variable, we conducted the analysis using two different models. In the first ZIP model, or Model I, we explicitly modeled the effects of structural zero of DAD on PHQ9 using a binary indicator (NeverDrink = 1 for structural and NeverDrink = 0 for sampling zero) and thus both the indicator of the non-risk group for drinking (NeverDrink) and DAD variable were included as predictors. As a comparison, we also fit the data with only the DAD predictor and thus the structural and sampling zeros were not distinguished in the second ZIP, or Model II. We used SAS 9.3 PROC GENMOD to fit the models, with parameter estimates based on the maximum likelihood approach.

Analysis Results Among the 5,283 subjects with both CAPI and PHQ-9, there were a small amount of missing values in the covariate and the actual sample size used for the analysis was 5,261. Shown in Tables 5 and 6 are the parameter estimates of the Poisson and Zero-Inflated components of the two ZIP models,

Table 5 Comparison of model estimates (Estimate), standard errors (Std err), and p-values (P-value) from the Poisson component for the count response (including random zeros) (Std err) for the real study data

Parameter estimates from Poisson component of ZIP							
Parameter		Model I			Model II		
		Estimate	Std err	P-value	Estimate	Std err	P-value
Intercept		2.2936	0.0495	<0.0001	2.2695	0.0490	<0.0001
NeverDrink	Yes	−0.0878	0.0253	0.0005			
NeverDrink	No	0.0000	0.0000	−			
DAD		−0.0023	0.0011	0.0423	−0.0017	0.0011	0.1409
Gender	Male	−0.1988	0.0164	<0.0001	−0.1890	0.0162	<0.0001
	Female	0.0000	0.0000	−	0.0000	0.0000	−
AGE		−0.0025	0.0005	<0.0001	−0.0026	0.0005	<0.0001
Race/ethnicity	Mexican American	−0.0954	0.0408	0.0192	−0.0928	0.0407	0.0228
	Other Hispanic	−0.0322	0.0425	0.4495	−0.0282	0.0425	0.5072
	Non-Hispanic white	−0.0952	0.0376	0.0114	−0.0864	0.0375	0.0213
	Non-Hispanic black	0.0030	0.0401	0.9402	0.0087	0.0401	0.8278
	Other race	0.0000	0.0000	−	0.0000	0.0000	−
Education		−0.1267	0.0067	<0.0001	−0.1246	0.0067	<0.0001
Scale		1.0000	0.0000		1.0000	0.0000	

Table 6 Comparison of model estimates (Estimate), standard errors (Std err), and p-values (P-value) from the Logistic component for the probability of occurrence of structural zeros for the real study data

Parameter estimates from logistic component of ZIP							
Parameter		Model I			Model II		
		Estimate	Std err	P-value	Estimate	Std err	P-value
Intercept		−1.9351	0.1998	<0.0001	−1.7999	0.1966	<0.0001
NeverDrink	Yes	0.4230	0.0945	<0.0001			
NeverDrink	No	0.0000	0.0000	–			
DAD		−0.0021	0.0043	0.6191	−0.0055	0.0042	0.1868
Gender	Male	0.5715	0.0641	<0.0001	0.5174	0.0626	<0.0001
	Female	0.0000	0.0000	–	0.0000	0.0000	–
AGE		0.0158	0.0018	<0.0001	0.0164	0.0018	<0.0001
Race/ethnicity	Mexican American	0.0883	0.1596	0.5799	0.0594	0.1590	0.7087
	Other Hispanic	−0.0904	0.1694	0.5934	−0.1209	0.1688	0.4739
	Non-Hispanic white	−0.2250	0.1471	0.1262	−0.2714	0.1463	0.0637
	Non-Hispanic black	0.0603	0.1563	0.6999	0.0309	0.1558	0.8428
	Other race	0.0000	0.0000	–	0.0000	0.0000	–
Education		0.0480	0.0261	0.0658	0.0394	0.0259	0.1284

respectively. The high statistical significance of the non-risk subgroup indicator in Model I indicates that Model I was more appropriate than Model II for the relationship of interest. In fact, Model I has a smaller AIC (28,998.1975 for Model II vs. 28,969.2253 for Model I) and BIC (29,116.4228 for Model II vs. 29,100.5868 for Model I).

Based on the tables, the model without the indicator of the non-risk subgroup (Model II) failed to detect any association between DAD and depression symptoms (p-value = 0.14 for the Poisson and 0.19 for the Zero-Inflated components), while the model with this indicator included (Model I) successfully identified a significant association between drinking and depression. The non-drinkers are less likely being at-risk of depression (p-value < 0.0001 for the Zero-Inflated component) and have less depressive symptoms (p-value = 0.0005 for the Poisson component). On the other hand, DAD is also a predictor of depressive symptoms for the at-risk drinking subgroup (p-value = 0.0423 for the Poisson component). However, the amount of drinking does not seem to increase the likelihood of depression (p-value = 0.6191 for the Zero-Inflated component).

6 Discussion

In this chapter, we discussed the importance of untangling the structural and random zeros for count variables with structural zeros in public health. Although older studies completely ignored structural zeros, many newer ones have attempted to address this issue. However, all efforts to date have focused on the statistical problems when the count outcomes are used as a response, or dependent variable, in regression analysis, with no attention paid to the equally important problem of biased estimates when such outcomes are used as an explanatory, or independent, variable. We failed to find any study in the extant literature that even acknowledged this problem. Our findings are significant in this respect since they show for the first time the critical importance of delineating the effects of the two different types of zeros in count outcomes like DAD.

Both our simulated and real study examples demonstrate that it is critical that we model and delineate the effects of structural and random zeros when using a zero-inflated count outcome as an explanatory variable in regression analysis. Otherwise, not only are we likely to miss opportunities to find associations between such a variable and an outcome of interest (due to significant loss of power), but also to obtain results that are difficult to interpret because of high bias in the estimate and dual interpretation of the value zero of such a count variable. For example, the estimated coefficient -0.0017 of DAD in the Poisson component of ZIP Model II for the relationship between PHQ9 and DAD had about 30 % upward bias as compared to -0.0023 for the same coefficient of the Poisson component of Model I ZIP of the analysis in the NHANES study. Even ignoring such bias, the estimate -0.0017 was difficult to interpret; without accounting for structural zeros as in ZIP Model I, the change in DAD from 0 to 1 has a dubious meaning, since it may mean the change in amount of drinking within alcohol users or it may mean the difference between alcohol users vs. lifetime abstainers.

In all the examples considered, we assumed linear functions of explanatory variables for notational brevity. In practice, more complex functions of explanatory variables may be considered utilizing piecewise linear, polynomial functions or even nonparametric methods such as local polynomial regression. Also, we limited our considerations to cross-sectional studies, but the same considerations are readily applied to longitudinal studies.

We assumed that structural zeros of a count explanatory variable are known in the simulation studies and the case study example. Although as in the case study example we sometimes may be able to provide concrete examples of structural zeroes (e.g., stable abstinence in a clinical trial), they are more appropriately conceptualized as latent (i.e., unobservable) variables and hence new statistical methods treating them as such are needed. Treating structural zeroes as latent or unobserved variables avoids the need to make a priori decisions associated with observed variables, for example in defining a cutoff to consider abstinence from drinking as "stable," a decision that involves subjective judgment and introduces error. Although lifetime abstainers in alcohol epidemiology studies represent a case where structural zeroes are conceptually more observable, this too is imperfect, for example a 23-year-old with no lifetime drinking history would be treated as a lifetime abstainer in such data. Further, in many studies, such proxies of structural zeros are not available. For example, no lifetime abstinence was collected in NHANES for heavy drinking. Thus, it is not possible to study the effects of structural zeros using the models considered in the study. Further research is needed to address this methodological issue to facilitate research in public health.

Acknowledgements The study was supported in part by National Institute on Drug Abuse grant R33DA027521, National Institute of General Medical Sciences R01GM108337, Eunice Kennedy Shriver National Institute of Child Health and Human Development grant R01HD075635, UR CTSI 8UL1TR000042-09, and a Faculty Research Support Grant from School of Nursing, University of Rochester.

References

Allen, J.P.: Measuring outcome in interventions for alcohol dependence and problem drinking: executive summary of a conference sponsored by the national institute on alcohol abuse and alcoholism. Alcohol. Clin. Exp. Res. **27**(10), 1657–1660 (2003)

Babor, T.F., Longabaugh, R., Zweben, A., Fuller, R.K., Stout, R.L., Anton, R.F., Randall, C.L.: Issues in the definition and measurement of drinking outcomes in alcoholism-treatment research. J. Stud. Alcohol Suppl. **12**, 101–111 (1994)

Brown, S.A., Schuckit, M.A.: Changes in depression among abstinent alcoholics. J. Stud. Alcohol Drugs **49**(05), 412–417 (1988)

Buu, A., Johnson, N.J., Li, R., Tan, X.: New variable selection methods for zero-inflated count data with applications to the substance abuse field. Stat. Med. **30**(18), 2326–2340 (2011)

Clifford Cohen, A. Jr.: Estimation in mixtures of discrete distributions. In: Classical and Contagious Discrete Distributions (Proc. Internat. Sympos., McGill Univ., Montreal, Que., 1963), pp. 373–378. Statistical Publishing Society, Calcutta (1965)

Connor, J.L., Kypri, K., Bell, M.L., Cousins, K.: Alcohol outlet density, levels of drinking and alcohol-related harm in new zealand: a national study. J. Epidemiol. Commun. Health **65**(10), 841–846 (2011)

Cranford, J.A., Zucker, R.A., Jester, J.M., Puttler, L.I., Fitzgerald, H.E.: Parental alcohol involvement and adolescent alcohol expectancies predict alcohol involvement in male adolescents. Psychol. Addict. Behav. **24**(3), 386–396 (2010)

Dackis, C.A., Gold, M.S., Pottash, A.L.C., Sweeney, D.R.: Evaluating depression in alcoholics. Psychiatry Res. **17**(2), 105–109 (1986)

Davidson, K.M.: Diagnosis of depression in alcohol dependence: changes in prevalence with drinking status. Br. J. Psychiatry **166**(2), 199–204 (1995)

Fernandez, A.C., Wood, M.D., Laforge, R., Black, J.T.: Randomized trials of alcohol-use interventions with college students and their parents: lessons from the transitions project. Clin. Trials **8**(2), 205–213 (2011)

Gibson, S., Becker, J.: Changes in alcoholics' self-reported depression. Q. J. Stud. Alcohol **34**, 829–836 (1973)

González, H.M., Tarraf, W., Whitfield, K.E., Vega, W.A.: The epidemiology of major depression and ethnicity in the united states. J. Psychiatr. Res. **44**(15), 1043–1051 (2010)

Hagger-Johnson, G., Bewick, B.M., Conner, M., O'Connor, D.B., Shickle, D.: Alcohol, conscientiousness and event-level condom use. Br. J. Health Psychol. **16**(4), 828–845 (2011)

Hall, D.B.: Zero-inflated Poisson and binomial regression with random effects: a case study. Biometrics **56**(4), 1030–1039 (2000)

Hall, D.B., Zhang, Z.: Marginal models for zero inflated clustered data. Stat. Model. **4**(3), 161–180 (2004)

Hasin, D.S., Grant, D.F.: Major depression in 6050 former drinkers - association with past alcohol dependence. Arch. Gen. Psychiatry **59**(9), 794–800 (2002)

He, H., Wang, W., Crits-Christoph, P., Gallop, R., Tang, W., Chen, D., Tu, X.: On the implication of structural zeros as independent variables in regression analysis: applications to alcohol research. J. Data Sci. (2013, in press)

Hernandez-Avila, C.A., Song, C., Kuo, L., Tennen, H., Armeli, S., Kranzler, H.R.: Targeted versus daily naltrexone: secondary analysis of effects on average daily drinking. Alcohol. Clin. Exp. Res. 30(5), 860–865 (2006)

Hildebrandt, T., McCrady, B., Epstein, E., Cook, S., Jensen, N.: When should clinicians switch treatments? an application of signal detection theory to two treatments for women with alcohol use disorders. Behav. Res. Therapy 48(6), 524–530 (2010)

Horton, N.J., Bebchuk, J.D., Jones, C.L., Lipsitz, S.R., Catalano, P.J., Zahner, G.E.P., Fitzmaurice, G.M.: Goodness-of-fit for GEE: an example with mental health service utilization. Stat. Med. 18(2), 213–222 (1999)

Johnson, N.L., Kotz, S.: Distributions in Statistics: Discrete Distributions. Houghton Mifflin, Boston (1969)

Lachenbruch, P.A.: Comparisons of two-part models with competitors. Stat. Med. 20(8), 1215–1234 (2001)

Lambert, D.: Zero-inflated poisson regression, with an application to defects in manufacturing. Technometrics 34(1), 1–14 (1992)

Leiderman, E.A., Lolich, M., Vázquez, G.H., Baldessarini, R.J.: Depression: point-prevalence and sociodemographic correlates in a buenos aires community sample. J. Affect. Disord. 136(3), 1154–1158 (2012)

Merikangas, K.R., Mehta, R.L., Molnar, B.E., Walters, E.E., Swendsen, J.D., Aguilar-Gaziola, S., Bijl, R., Borges, G., Caraveo-Anduaga, J.J., Dewit, D.J., et al.: Comorbidity of substance use disorders with mood and anxiety disorders: results of the international consortium in psychiatric epidemiology. Addict. Behav. 23(6), 893–907 (1998)

Neal, D.J., Sugarman, D.E., Hustad, J.T.P., Caska, C.M., Carey, K.B.: It's all fun and games. . . or is it? Collegiate sporting events and celebratory drinking. J. Stud. Alcohol. Drugs 66(2), 291–294 (2005)

Oh, D.H., Kim, S.A., Lee, H.Y., Seo, J.Y., Choi, B.-Y., Nam, J.H.: Prevalence and correlates of depressive symptoms in korean adults: results of a 2009 korean community health survey. J. Korean Med. Sci. 28(1), 128–135 (2013)

Pardini, D., White, H.R., Stouthamer-Loeber, M.: Early adolescent psychopathology as a predictor of alcohol use disorders by young adulthood. Drug Alcohol Depend. 88, S38–S49 (2007)

Penick, E.C., Powell, B.J., Liskow, B.I., Jackson, J.O., Nickel, E.J.: The stability of coexisting psychiatric syndromes in alcoholic men after one year. J. Stud. Alcohol Drugs 49(05), 395–405 (1988)

Pettinati, H.M., Sugerman, A.A., Maurer, H.S.: Four year mmpi changes in abstinent and drinking alcoholics. Alcohol. Clin. Exp. Res. 6(4), 487–494 (1982)

Roberts, R.E., Kaplan, G.A., Shema, S.J., Strawbridge, W.J.: Does growing old increase the risk for depression? Am. J. Psychiatry 154(10), 1384–1390 (1997)

Rushton, J.L., Forcier, M., Schectman, R.M.: Epidemiology of depressive symptoms in the national longitudinal study of adolescent health. J. Am. Acad. Child Adolesc. Psychiatry 41(2), 199–205 (2002)

Swendsen, J.D., Merikangas, K.R., Canino, G.J., Kessler, R.C., Rubio-Stipec, M., Angst, J.: The comorbidity of alcoholism with anxiety and depressive disorders in four geographic communities. Compr. Psychiatry 39(4), 176–184 (1998)

Tang, W., He, H., Tu, X.: Applied Categorical and Count Data Analysis. Chapman & Hall/CRC, Boca Raton (2012)

Tsai, J., Ford, E.S., Li, C., Zhao, G.: Past and current alcohol consumption patterns and elevations in serum hepatic enzymes among us adults. Addict. Behav. 37, 78–84 (2012)

Weissman, MM., et al.: Cross-national epidemiology of major depression and bipolar disorder. JAMA 276, 293–299 (1996)

Welsh, A.H., Cunningham, R.B., Donnelly, C.F., Lindenmayer, D.B.: Modelling the abundance of rare species: statistical models for counts with extra zeros. Ecol. Model. 88(1), 297–308 (1996)

Wilhelm, K., Mitchell, P., Slade, T., Brownhill, S., Andrews, G.: Prevalence and correlates of dsm-iv major depression in an australian national survey. J. Affect. Disord. **75**(2), 155–162 (2003)

Willenbring, M.L.: Measurement of depression in alcoholics. J. Stud. Alcohol **47**(5), 367–372 (1986)

Yu, Q., Chen, R., Tang, W., He, H., Gallop, R., Crits-Christoph, P., Hu, J., Tu, X.M.: Distribution-free models for longitudinal count responses with overdispersion and structural zeros. Stat. Med. **32**(14), 2390–2405 (2012)

Modeling Based on Progressively Type-I Interval Censored Sample

Yu-Jau Lin, Nan Jiang, Y.L. Lio, and Ding-Geng (Din) Chen

Abstract Progressively type-I interval censored data occurs very often in public health study. For example, 112 patients with plasma cell myeloma were admitted to be treated at the National Cancer Institute and all patients were under examination at time schedules (in terms of months), 5.5, 10.5, 15.5, 20.5, 25.5, 30.5, 40.5, 50.5, 60.5, respectively. The data reported by Carbone et al. (Am J Med 42:937–948, 1967) shows the number of patients at risk in each time interval and the number of withdrawn at each examination time schedule which is the most right end point of each time interval. After 60.5 months, the study was terminated. The patients withdrawn at the right end point of time interval have no follow-up study. This table did not provide any patient's exact lifetime. The data structure presented in the table is called progressively type-I interval censored data. In this chapter, many parametric modeling procedures will be discussed via maximum likelihood estimate, moment method estimate, probability plot estimate, and Bayesian estimation. Finally, model selection based on Bayesian concept will be addressed. The entire chapter will also include the model presentation of general data structure and simulation procedure for getting progressively type-I interval censored sample. Basically, this chapter will provide the techniques published by Ng and Wang (J Stat Comput Simul 79: 145–159, 2009), Chen and Lio (Comput Stat Data Anal 54:1581–1591, 2010), and Lin and Lio (2012). R and WinBUGS implementation for the techniques will be included.

Y.-J. Lin
Department of Applied Mathematics, Chung-Yuan Christian University,
Chung-Li, Taoyuan City, Taiwan
e-mail: yujaulin@cycu.edu.tw

N. Jiang (✉) • Y.L. Lio
Department of Mathematical Sciences, University of South Dakota, Vermillion, SD 57069, USA
e-mail: Yuhlong.Lio@gmail.com; Yuhlong.lio@usd.edu; Nan.Jiang@usd.edu

D.-G. Chen
School of Social Work, University of North Carolina, Chapel Hill, NC 27599, USA
e-mail: dinchen@email.unc.edu

© Springer International Publishing Switzerland 2015   117
D.-G. Chen, J. Wilson (eds.), *Innovative Statistical Methods for Public Health Data*,
ICSA Book Series in Statistics, DOI 10.1007/978-3-319-18536-1_7

1   Introduction

In industrial life testing and medical survival analysis, very often we encounter the situations that the object is lost or withdrawn before failure, or the object lifetime is only known within an interval. Hence, the obtained sample is called a censored sample (or an incomplete sample). The most common censoring schemes are type-I censoring, type-II censoring, and progressive censoring. The life testing is ended at a pre-scheduled time for the type-I censoring and for the type-II, the life testing is ended whenever the number of lifetimes is reached. In the type-I and type-II censoring schemes, the tested items are allowed to be withdrawn only at the end of life testing. However, in many real-life cases, subjects could be missing or withdrawn at some other times before the end of life testing, which motivated the progressive censoring scheme to be investigated. Balakrishnan and Aggarwala (2000) provided more information about progressive censoring in combined with type-I or type-II. Aggarwala (2001) introduced type-I interval and progressive censoring and developed the statistical inference for the exponential distribution based on progressive type-I interval censored data. Under progressive type-I interval censoring, lifetimes are only known within two consecutively pre-scheduled times and subjects would be allowed to withdraw at any time before the end of treatment.

Table 1 displays a typical progressively type-I interval censored data that consists of 112 patients with plasma cell myeloma treated at the National Cancer Institute. This data set was reported by Carbone et al. (1967) and discussed in Lawless (2003).

The most right side column in Table 1 shows the number of patients who were found to be dropped out from the study at the right end of each time interval. These dropped patients are known to be survived at the right end of each time interval but no further follow-up. Hence, the most right side column in Table 1 provides the numbers of withdraws, $R_i, i = 1, \cdots, m = 9$. The number of failures, $X_i, i = 1, \cdots, m$, can be easily calculated to be $X = (18, 16, 18, 10, 11, 8, 13, 4, 1)$ from the number at risk and the number of withdrawals.

Table 1 Plasma cell myeloma survival times

Interval in months	Number at risk	Number of withdrawals
[0, 5.5)	112	1
[5.5, 10.5)	93	1
[10.5, 15.5)	76	3
[15.5, 20.5)	55	0
[20.5, 25.5)	45	0
[25.5, 30.5)	34	1
[30.5, 40.5)	25	2
[40.5, 50.5)	10	3
[50.5, 60.5)	3	2
[60.5, ∞)	0	0

2 Data and Likelihood

Let n subjects be placed on a treatment or life testing simultaneously at time $t_0 = 0$ and under inspection at m pre-specified times $t_1 < t_2 < \ldots < t_m$, where t_m is the scheduled time to terminate the experiment. At the ith inspection time, t_i, the number, X_i, of failures occurred within $(t_{i-1}, t_i]$ is recorded and R_i surviving items are randomly removed from the treatment or life test, for $i = 1, 2, \ldots, m - 1$. At the time t_m, all surviving items are removed and the treatment or life test is terminated. Since the number, Y_i, of surviving subjects in $(t_{i-1}, t_i]$ is a random variable and the exact number of subjects withdrawn should not be greater than Y_i at schedule time t_i, R_i could be determined by the pre-specified percentage of the remaining surviving subjects at the time t_i for given $i = 1, 2, \ldots, m$. For example, given pre-specified percentage values, $p_1, \ldots, p_{m-1}$ and $p_m = 1$, for withdrawing at $t_1 < t_2 < \ldots < t_m$, respectively, $R_i = \lfloor p_i y_i \rfloor$ at each inspection time t_i where $i = 1, 2, \ldots, m$. Therefore, a progressively type-I interval censored sample can be denoted as $D = \{(X_i, R_i, t_i), i = 1, 2, \cdots, m\}$, where sample size $n = \sum_{i=1}^{m}(X_i + R_i)$. If $R_i = 0, i = 1, 2, \ldots, m - 1$, then the progressively type-I interval censored sample is a conventional type-I interval censored sample, $X_1, X_2, \ldots, X_m$, $X_{m+1} = R_m$.

2.1 Likelihood Function

Given a progressively type-I interval censored sample, $\{X_i, R_i, t_i\}, i = 1, 2, \ldots, m$, of size n, from a continuous lifetime distribution, which has probability density function and distribution function, $f(t, \Theta)$ and $F(t, \Theta), t \geq 0$, respectively, and population parameter vector θ, the likelihood function can be constructed as follows (see Aggarwala 2001):

$$L(\Theta) \propto \prod_{i=1}^{m} [F(t_i, \Theta) - F(t_{i-1}, \Theta)]^{X_i} [1 - F(t_i, \Theta)]^{R_i}, \tag{1}$$

where $t_0 = 0$. It can be seen easily that if $R_1 = R_2 = \cdots = R_{m-1} = 0$, the likelihood function (1) reduces to the corresponding likelihood function for the conventional type-I interval censoring. The maximum likelihood estimate (MLE) for the parameter can be carried out by maximizing the likelihood function of (1). Generally, it is often the case that we do not have a closed form formula for the MLE and therefore an iterative numerical search could be used to obtain the MLE from the above likelihood function. In the following, the mid-point approximation and Expectation-Maximization (EM) algorithm are discussed for getting the MLE. The estimations based on method of moments and based on probability plot will also be investigated for comparison.

2.2   Midpoint Approximation

Suppose that the X_i failure units in each subinterval $(t_{i-1}, t_i]$ occurred at the center of the interval $m_i = \frac{t_{i-1}+t_i}{2}$ and R_i censored items withdrawn at the censoring time t_i. Then the likelihood function (1) could be approximately represented as:

$$L_M(\Theta) \propto \prod_{i=1}^{m} (f(m_i, \Theta))^{X_i} [1 - F(t_i, \Theta)]^{R_i} .$$

The approximated likelihood function is usually simpler than the likelihood function of original progressive type-I interval censored sample. However, in many situations, the MLE of parameter vector, Θ, still cannot be solved by a closed form formula.

2.3   EM-Algorithm

The EM algorithm is a broadly applicable approach to the iterative computation of MLEs and useful in a variety of incomplete-data problems where algorithms such as the Newton-Raphson method may turn out to be more complicated to implement. On each iteration of EM algorithm, there are two steps that called the expectation step (E-step) and the maximization step (M-step). Therefore, the algorithm is called the EM algorithm. The detailed development of EM algorithm can be found in Dempster et al. (1977). The EM algorithm for finding the MLEs of population parameter vector, Θ, based on $\{X_i, R_i, t_i\}, i = 1, 2, \ldots, m$, of size n, starts with setting the likelihood function, $L^c(\Theta)$, for the corresponding lifetime random sample of size n.

Let $\tau_{i,j}, j = 1, 2, \ldots, X_i$, be the survival times within sub-interval $(t_{i-1}, t_i]$ and $\tau_{i,j}^*, j = 1, 2, \ldots, R_i$ be the survival times for those withdrawn items at t_i for $i = 1, 2, 3, \ldots, m$. The likelihood function, $L^c(\Theta)$, of the parameter θ based on the complete lifetimes, $\tau_{i,j}, j = 1, 2, \ldots, X_i$ and $\tau_{i,j}^*, j = 1, 2, \ldots, R_i$, of these n items is given as follows:

$$L^c(\Theta) = \prod_{i=1}^{m} \left[\prod_{j=1}^{X_i} f(\tau_{i,j}, \Theta) \prod_{j=1}^{R_i} f(\tau_{i,j}^*, \Theta) \right]. \tag{2}$$

To implement EM algorithm, the E-step is simply to update the likelihood function based on complete data set by replacing the missing data with the corresponding expected value using the previously updated population parameters; and the M-step is to find MLEs of population parameters from the updated likelihood function and to update the population parameters. The EM algorithm is the iterative procedure through these two steps until convergence occurs. Usually, the iterative procedure will be implemented by using the E-step first and then followed by the M-step. This iterative procedure can also be implemented by using the M-step first and then followed by the E-step. Then the algorithm is also called ME algorithm. In this chapter, ME algorithm will be used. More detailed procedure will be addressed in case by case situations.

2.4 Moment Method

Based on progressively type-I interval censored sample, $\{X_i, R_i, t_i\}, i = 1, 2, \ldots, m,$ of size n, the kth sample moment is defined as

$$\frac{1}{n}\left[\sum_i^m X_i E_\Theta(T^k | T \in [t_{i-1}, t_i)) + R_i E_\Theta(T^k | T \in [t_i, \infty))\right],$$

where $E_\Theta\left(T^k | T \in [a, b)\right) = \frac{\int_a^b t^k f(t,\Theta)dt}{F(b,\Theta) - F(a,\Theta)}$ for a given positive integer k and $0 \leq a < b \leq \infty$. Let L be the dimension of Θ. The moment method starts with setting the kth sample moment equal to the corresponding kth population moment, for $k = 1, 2, \ldots, L$. Then the moment method estimate of Θ will be obtained through solving the system of L equations. Since a closed form solution is usually not available, an iterative numerical process will be used to obtain the solution. More information will be provided in the case studies.

2.5 Method of Probability Plot

Given a progressive type-I interval censored data, $(X_i, R_i, t_i), i = 1, 2, \ldots, m$ of size n, the distribution function at time t_i can be estimated by the product-limit distribution and described as

$$\hat{F}(t_i) = 1 - \prod_{j=1}^{i}(1 - \hat{p}_j), i = 1, 2, \ldots, m, \tag{3}$$

where

$$\hat{p}_j = \frac{X_j}{n - \sum_{k=0}^{j-1} X_k - \sum_{k=0}^{j-1} R_k}, j = 1, 2, \ldots, m.$$

Let $\hat{F}(t_j)$ be the estimate of $F(t_j, \Theta)$, then the estimate of Θ based on probability plot can be obtained by minimizing $\sum_{i=1}^{m}\left[t_i - F^{-1}((\hat{F}(t_j)), \Theta)\right]^2$ with respect to Θ where $t = F^{-1}(p, \Theta)$ is the generalized inverse of $F(t_j, \Theta)$. A nonlinear optimization procedure will be applied to find the minimizer as the estimates of Θ.

3 Weibull Distribution Modeling

Ng and Wang (2009) introduced Weibull distribution into the progressive type-I interval data modeling. Weibull distribution has the probability density function, distribution function, and hazard function as follows:

$$f_W(t; \gamma, \beta) = \gamma \beta t^{\beta-1} e^{-\gamma t^\beta}, \tag{4}$$

$$F_W(t; \gamma, \beta) = 1 - e^{-\gamma t^\beta}, \tag{5}$$

$$h_W(t; \gamma, \beta) = \gamma \beta t^{\beta-1}, \tag{6}$$

where $\beta > 0$ is the shape parameter and $\gamma > 0$ is the scale parameter. When the shape parameter $\beta = 1$, the Weibull distribution reduces to the conventional exponential distribution. The Weibull hazard function can be increasing, decreasing, or constant depending upon the shape parameter. Therefore, the Weibull distribution has provided us with the flexibility in modeling lifetime data.

3.1 Maximum Likelihood Estimation

Given a progressive type-I interval censored sample $\{X_i, R_i, t_i\}, i = 1, 2, \ldots, m$ of size $n = \sum_{i=1}^{m}(X_i + R_i)$ from the two-parameter Weibull distribution defined by (4), the likelihood function (1) can be specified as follows:

$$L_W(\gamma, \beta) \propto \prod_{i=1}^{m} \left[e^{-\gamma t_{i-1}^\beta} - e^{-\gamma t_i^\beta} \right]^{X_i} e^{-\gamma t_i^\beta R_i}, \tag{7}$$

and the log-likelihood function is

$$l_W(\gamma, \beta) = ln L_W(\gamma, \beta) = \text{constant} + \sum_{i=1}^{m} X_i ln(e^{-\gamma t_{i-1}^\beta} - e^{-\gamma t_i^\beta}) - \sum_{i=1}^{m} \gamma t_i^\beta R_i. \tag{8}$$

Setting the derivatives with respect to parameters, γ and β, respectively, equal to zero, the likelihood equations for the Weibull modeling are

$$\sum_{i=1}^{m} \frac{X_i}{e^{-\gamma t_{i-1}^\beta} - e^{-\gamma t_i^\beta}} \left[-e^{-\gamma t_{i-1}^\beta} t_{i-1}^\beta + e^{-\gamma t_i^\beta} t_i^\beta \right] = \sum_{i=1}^{m} t_i^\beta R_i \tag{9}$$

and

$$\sum_{i=1}^{m} \frac{X_i}{e^{-\gamma t_{i-1}^{\beta}} - e^{-\gamma t_i^{\beta}}} \left[-e^{-\gamma t_{i-1}^{\beta}} ln(t_{i-1}) t_{i-1}^{\beta} + e^{-\gamma t_i^{\beta}} ln(t_i) t_i^{\beta} \right] = \gamma \sum_{i=1}^{m} ln(t_i) t_i^{\beta} R_i. \quad (10)$$

The MLEs of γ and β can be obtained by solving Eqs. (9) and (10) simultaneously. Since no closed form is available for the solution, a numerical iteration method could be used to evaluate the MLEs.

Next, let us apply EM-algorithm to obtain MLEs. When the lifetime is Weibull distributed, the likelihood function (2) based on the random sample of lifetimes, $\tau_{i,j}, j = 1, 2, \ldots, X_i$ and $\tau_{i,j}^*, j = 1, 2, \ldots, R_i$, of these n items can be represented as

$$L_W^c(\gamma, \beta) = \gamma^n \beta^n \prod_{i=1}^{m} \left[\prod_{j=1}^{X_i} \tau_{i,j}^{\beta-1} e^{-\gamma \tau_{i,j}^{\beta}} \prod_{j=1}^{R_i} (\tau_{i,j}^*)^{\beta-1} e^{-\gamma (\tau_{i,j}^*)^{\beta}} \right] \quad (11)$$

and the corresponding log likelihood is

$$l_W^c(\gamma, \beta) = nln(\gamma\beta) + \sum_{i=1}^{m} \left\{ \sum_{j=1}^{X_i} (\beta-1) ln(\tau_{i,j}) - \gamma \tau_{i,j}^{\beta} + \sum_{j=1}^{R_i} (\beta-1) ln(\tau_{i,j}^*) - \gamma (\tau_{i,j}^*)^{\beta} \right\}. \quad (12)$$

Let the derivatives of $l_W^c(\gamma, \beta)$ with respect to γ and β be equal to 0, respectively, the likelihood equations are given as,

$$\gamma = \frac{n}{\sum_{i=1}^{m} \left[\sum_{j=1}^{X_i} \tau_{i,j}^{\beta} + \sum_{j=1}^{R_i} (\tau_{i,j}^*)^{\beta} \right]}, \quad (13)$$

$$\beta = \frac{n}{\sum_{i=1}^{m} \left[\sum_{j=1}^{X_i} \gamma \tau_{i,j}^{\beta} ln(\tau_{i,j}) - ln(\tau_{i,j}) + \sum_{j=1}^{R_i} \gamma (\tau_{i,j}^*)^{\beta} ln(\tau_{i,j}^*) - ln(\tau_{i,j}^*) \right]}. \quad (14)$$

Given $t_0 < t_1 < \cdots < t_m$, the lifetime of the X_i failures in the ith interval $(t_{i-1}, t_i]$ are independent and follow a doubly truncated Weibull distribution from the left at t_{i-1} and from the right at t_i, and the lifetime of the R_i censored items in the ith interval $(t_{i-1}, t_i]$ are independent and follow a truncated Weibull distribution from the left at t_i, $i = 1, 2, \ldots, m$. The required expected values of a doubly truncated Weibull distribution from the left at a and from the right at b with $0 < a < b \le \infty$ for EM-algorithm are given by

$$E_{\gamma, \beta}(ln(Y)|Y \in [a, b)) = \frac{\int_a^b ln(y) f_W(y; \gamma, \beta) dy}{F_W(b; \gamma, \beta) - F_W(a; \gamma, \beta)} = \frac{\int_a^b \gamma \beta y^{\beta-1} ln(y) e^{-\gamma y^{\beta}} dy}{e^{-\gamma a^{\beta}} - e^{-\gamma b^{\beta}}},$$

$$E_{\gamma, \beta}(Y^{\beta}|Y \in [a, b)) = \frac{\int_a^b \gamma \beta y^{2\beta-1} e^{-\gamma y^{\beta}} dy}{e^{-\gamma a^{\beta}} - e^{-\gamma b^{\beta}}}$$

$$E_{\gamma, \beta}((ln(Y))Y^{\beta}|Y \in [a, b)) = \frac{\int_a^b \gamma \beta y^{2\beta-1} ln(y) e^{-\gamma y^{\beta}} dy}{e^{-\gamma a^{\beta}} - e^{-\gamma b^{\beta}}}.$$

Therefore, in this case the EM algorithm is given by the following iterative process:

1. Given starting values of γ and β say $\hat{\gamma}^{(0)}$ and $\hat{\beta}(0)$. Set $k = 0$.
2. In the $k + 1$th iteration,

   - E-step computes the following conditional expectations using numerical integration methods,

$$E_{1i} = E_{\hat{\gamma}^{(k)}, \hat{\beta}^{(k)}} \left[Y^{\hat{\beta}^{(k)}} | Y \in [t_{i-1}, t_i) \right],$$

$$E_{2i} = E_{\hat{\gamma}^{(k)}, \hat{\beta}^{(k)}} \left[Y^{\hat{\beta}^{(k)}} | Y \in [t_i, \infty) \right],$$

$$E_{3i} = E_{\hat{\gamma}^{(k)}, \hat{\beta}^{(k)}} \left[ln(Y) | Y \in [t_{i-1}, t_i) \right],$$

$$E_{4i} = E_{\hat{\gamma}^{(k)}, \hat{\beta}^{(k)}} \left[ln(Y) | Y \in [t_i, \infty) \right],$$

$$E_{5i} = E_{\hat{\gamma}^{(k)}, \hat{\beta}^{(k)}} \left[Y^{\hat{\beta}^{(k)}} ln(Y) | Y \in [t_{i-1}, t_i) \right],$$

$$E_{6i} = E_{\hat{\gamma}^{(k)}, \hat{\beta}^{(k)}} \left[Y^{\hat{\beta}^{(k)}} ln(Y) | Y \in [t_i, \infty) \right],$$

   and replace the likelihood Eqs. (13) and (14) by

$$\gamma = \frac{n}{\sum_{i=1}^{m} X_i E_{1i} + R_i E_{2i}}, \tag{15}$$

   and

$$\beta = \frac{n}{\sum_{i=1}^{m} [X_i \gamma E_{5i} + R_i \gamma E_{6,i} - X_i E_{3i} - R_i E_{4i}]}. \tag{16}$$

   - M-step solves the Eqs. (15) and (16) to obtain the next values, $\hat{\gamma}^{(k+1)}$ and $\hat{\beta}^{(k+1)}$ of γ and β

$$\hat{\gamma}^{(k+1)} = \frac{n}{\sum_{i=1}^{m} X_i E_{1i} + R_i E_{2i}}, \tag{17}$$

$$\hat{\beta}^{(k+1)} = \frac{n}{\sum_{i=1}^{m} \left[\hat{\gamma}^{(k+1)} (X_i E_{5i} + R_i E_{6i}) - (X_i E_{3,i} + R_i E_{4i}) \right]}. \tag{18}$$

3. Checking the convergence, if the convergence occurs then the current $\hat{\gamma}^{(k+1)}$ and $\hat{\beta}^{(k+1)}$ are the approximated MLEs of γ and β via EM algorithm; otherwise, set $k = k + 1$ and go to Step 2.

3.2 Midpoint Approximation

In the process of Weibull distribution modeling, the midpoint approximation, (2), of the likelihood function of (1), can be written as,

$$L_W^M(\gamma, \beta) = \prod_{i=1}^{m} \gamma^{X_i} \beta^{X_i} m_i^{X_i(\beta-1)} e^{-\gamma X_i m_i^{\beta}} e^{-\gamma R_i t_i^{\beta}} \tag{19}$$

and the corresponding log likelihood is

$$l_W^M(\gamma, \beta) = \sum_{i=1}^{m} X_i(ln(\gamma) + ln(\beta)) + X_i(\beta - 1)ln(m_i) - \gamma X_i m_i^{\beta} - \gamma R_i t_i^{\beta}. \tag{20}$$

Let the derivatives of $l_W^M(\gamma, \beta)$ with respect to γ and β be equal to 0, respectively, the likelihood equations are given as,

$$\gamma = \frac{\sum_{i=1}^{m} X_i}{\sum_{i=1}^{m} X_i m_i^{\beta} + R_i t_i^{\beta}} \tag{21}$$

and

$$\beta = \frac{\sum_{i=1}^{m} X_i}{\sum_{i=1}^{m} \gamma X_i m_i^{\beta} ln(m_i) + \gamma R_i t_i^{\beta} ln(t_i) - \sum_{i=1}^{m} X_i ln(m_i)} \tag{22}$$

3.3 Method of Moments

Let T be random variable which has Weibull distribution of (4). Then the kth moment of Weibull distribution is

$$E(T^k) = \gamma^{-k/\beta} \Gamma(1 + k/\beta),$$

where $\Gamma(\cdot)$ is the complete gamma function and k is a positive integer. Let the first and second sample moments, which were defined in Sect. 2.4, be equal to the corresponding population moments. The following two equations are obtained for solving the moment method estimates of γ and β

$$\gamma^{-1/\beta} \Gamma(1 + 1/\beta) = \frac{1}{n} \left[\sum_{i}^{m} X_i E_{\gamma,\beta}(T | T \in [t_{i-1}, t_i)) + R_i E_{\gamma,\beta}(T | T \in [t_i, \infty)) \right], \tag{23}$$

and

$$\gamma^{-2/\beta}\Gamma(1+2/\beta) = \frac{1}{n}\left[\sum_{i}^{m} X_i E_{\gamma,\beta}(T^2|T \in [t_{i-1}, t_i)) + R_i E_{\gamma,\beta}(T^2|T \in [t_i, \infty))\right].$$

(24)

Since the solutions to Eqs. (23) and (24) cannot be obtained in a closed form, an iterative numerical process to obtain the parameter estimates is described as follows:

1. Let the initial estimates of γ and β be $\gamma^{(0)}$ and $\beta^{(0)}$ and $k = 0$.
2. In the $(k+1)$th iteration,

   - computing $E_{\gamma^{(k)},\beta^{(k)}}\left[T^j|T \in [t_{i-1}, t_i)\right]$ and $E_{\gamma^{(k)},\beta^{(k)}}\left[T^j|T \in [t_i, \infty)\right]$ for $j = 1, 2$, and solving the following equation, which is derived from Eqs. (23) and (24), for β, say $\beta^{(k+1)}$:

$$\frac{[\Gamma(1+1/\beta)]^2}{[\Gamma(1+2/\beta)]}$$

$$= \frac{\left\{\sum_{i}^{m} X_i E_{\gamma^{(k)},\beta^{(k)}}\left[T|T \in [t_{i-1}, t_i)\right] + R_i E_{\gamma^{(k)},\beta^{(k)}}\left[T|T \in [t_i, \infty)\right]\right\}^2}{n\left\{\sum_{i}^{m} X_i E_{\gamma^{(k)},\beta^{(k)}}\left[T^2|T \in [t_{i-1}, t_i)\right] + R_i E_{\gamma^{(k)},\beta^{(k)}}\left[T^2|T \in [t_i, \infty)\right]\right\}}.$$

   - The solution for γ, say $\gamma^{(k+1)}$, is obtained based on Eq. (23)

$$\gamma = \left\{\frac{n\Gamma(1+1/\beta^{(k+1)})}{\sum_{i}^{m} X_i E_{\gamma^{(k)},\beta^{(k)}}\left[T|T \in [t_{i-1}, t_i)\right] + R_i E_{\gamma^{(k)},\beta^{(k)}}\left[T|T \in [t_i, \infty)\right]}\right\}^{\beta^{(k)}}.$$

3. Checking the convergence, if the convergence occurs then the current $\gamma^{(k+1)}$ and $\beta^{(k+1)}$ are the estimates of γ and β by the method of moments; otherwise, set $k = k + 1$ and go to Step 2.

3.4 Estimation Based on Probability Plot

Let the product-limit distribution, $\hat{F}(t)$, described in Sect. 2.5 be the estimate of the Weibull distribution function of (5), then the estimates of γ and β in the Weibull distribution based on probability plot can be obtained by minimizing $\sum_{i=1}^{m}\left[t_i - (\frac{-\ln(1-\hat{F}(t_i))}{\gamma})^{1/\beta}\right]^2$ with respect to γ and β. A nonlinear optimization procedure will be applied to find the minimizers as the estimates of γ and β.

In addition, Ng and Wang (2009) mentioned that the estimates of γ and β based on probability plot can also be obtained by least square fit of linear regression model

$$y = ln(\gamma) + \gamma x + \epsilon, \tag{25}$$

with data set $(x_i, y_i) = (ln(t_i), ln(-ln(1 - \hat{F}(t_i))))$ for $i = 1, 2, \cdots, m$, and ϵ is an error term.

4 Generalized Exponential Distribution Modeling

Mudholkar and Srivastava (1993) introduced a two-parameter generalized exponential (GE) distribution as an alternative to the commonly used gamma and Weibull distribution. The GE distribution has a probability density function, a distribution function, and a hazard function as follows:

$$f_{GE}(t; \alpha, \lambda) = \alpha\lambda(1 - e^{-\lambda t})^{\alpha-1}e^{-\lambda t}, \tag{26}$$

$$F_{GE}(t; \alpha, \lambda) = (1 - e^{-\lambda t})^{\alpha}, \tag{27}$$

$$h_{GE}(t; \alpha, \lambda) = \frac{\alpha\lambda(1 - e^{-\lambda t})^{\alpha-1}e^{-\lambda t}}{1 - (1 - e^{-\lambda t})^{\alpha}}, \quad t > 0, \ \alpha > 0, \tag{28}$$

where $\theta = (\alpha, \lambda)$, $\alpha > 0$ is the shape parameter and $\lambda > 0$ is the scale parameter. If $\alpha = 1$, then the GE defined above reduces to the conventional exponential distribution. If $\alpha < 1$, then the density function (26) is decreasing and if $\alpha > 1$, then the density function (26) is a unimodal function. Similar to Weibull distribution, GE hazard function can be increasing, decreasing, or constant depending upon the shape parameter α. The GE distribution has been studied by numeral authors, for example, Chen and Lio (2010); Gupta and Kundu (1999, 2001a,b, 2002, 2003). Gupta and Kundu (2001a, 2003) mentioned that the two-parameter GE distribution could be used quite effectively in analyzing many lifetime data sets and provide a better fit than the two-parameter Weibull distribution in many situations. An extensive survey of recent developments for the two-parameter GE distribution based on a complete random sample can be found from Gupta and Kundu (2007).

4.1 Maximum Likelihood Estimation

Given a progressively type-I interval censored sample, $\{X_i, R_i, t_i\}$ for $i = 1, 2, \cdots, m$, of size $n = \sum_{i=1}^{m} X_i + R_i$ from the GE defined by Eqs. (26) and (27), the likelihood function, (1), can be specified as follows:

$$L_{GE}(\alpha, \lambda) \propto \prod_{i=1}^{m} \left[(1 - e^{-t_i \lambda})^\alpha - (1 - e^{-t_{i-1} \lambda})^\alpha \right]^{X_i} \left[1 - (1 - e^{-t_i \lambda})^\alpha \right]^{R_i}, \quad (29)$$

and the log likelihood is

$$l_{GE}(\alpha, \lambda) = constant + \sum_{i=1}^{m} X_i ln((1 - e^{-t_i \lambda})^\alpha - (1 - e^{-t_{i-1} \lambda})^\alpha) + R_i ln(1 - (1 - e^{-t_i \lambda})^\alpha).$$
$$(30)$$

By setting the derivatives of the log likelihood function with respect to α or λ to zero, the MLEs of α and λ are the solutions of the following likelihood equations

$$\sum_{i=1}^{m} \frac{R_i t_i (1 - e^{-\lambda t_i})^{\alpha-1}}{1 - (1 - e^{-\lambda t_i})^\alpha} = \sum_{i=1}^{m} \frac{X_i [(1 - e^{-\lambda t_i})^{\alpha-1} t_i - (1 - e^{-\lambda t_{i-1}})^{\alpha-1} t_{i-1}]}{(1 - e^{-\lambda t_i})^\alpha - (1 - e^{-\lambda t_{i-1}})^\alpha}, \quad (31)$$

and

$$\sum_{i=1}^{m} \frac{R_i [ln(1 - e^{-\lambda t_i})](1 - e^{-\lambda t_i})^\alpha}{1 - (1 - e^{-\lambda t_i})^\alpha}$$
$$= \sum_{i=1}^{m} \frac{X_i [(1 - e^{-\lambda t_i})^\alpha ln(1 - e^{-\lambda t_i}) - (1 - e^{-\lambda t_{i-1}})^\alpha ln(1 - e^{-\lambda t_{i-1}})]}{(1 - e^{-\lambda t_i})^\alpha - (1 - e^{-\lambda t_{i-1}})^\alpha} \quad (32)$$

No closed form solution can be found to the above equations, and an iterative numerical search can be used to obtain the MLEs. Let $\hat{\alpha}$ and $\hat{\lambda}$ be the solution to the above equations. Since there is no closed form of the MLE, the EM-algorithm and a mid-point approximation are introduced as follows for finding the MLEs of α and λ.

Similarly to Sect. 3.1, let $\tau_{i,j}, j = 1, 2, \cdots, X_i$, be the survival times within subinterval $(t_{i-1}, t_i]$ and $\tau_{i,j}^*, j = 1, 2, \cdots, R_i$ be the survival times for withdrawn items at t_i for $i = 1, 2, 3, \cdots, m$, then the likelihood $L_G^c(\alpha, \lambda)$ and log likelihood $l_G^c(\alpha, \lambda) = ln(L_G^c(\alpha, \lambda))$, for the complete lifetimes of n items from the two-parameter GE, are given by:

$$L_{GE}^c(\alpha, \lambda) = (\alpha \lambda)^n \prod_{i=1}^{m} \left\{ \prod_{j=1}^{X_i} \left[(1 - e^{-\tau_{i,j} \lambda})^{\alpha-1} e^{-\lambda \tau_{i,j}} \right] \prod_{j=1}^{R_i} \left[(1 - e^{-\tau_{i,j}^* \lambda})^{\alpha-1} e^{-\lambda \tau_{i,j}^*} \right] \right\},$$

and

$$l_{GE}^c(\alpha, \lambda) = [ln(\alpha) + ln(\lambda)]n - \lambda \sum_{i=1}^{m} (\sum_{j=1}^{X_i} \tau_{i,j} + \sum_{j=1}^{R_i} \tau_{i,j}^*)$$

$$+(\alpha - 1) \sum_{i=1}^{m} \left[\sum_{j=1}^{X_i} ln(1 - e^{-\lambda\tau_{i,j}}) + \sum_{j=1}^{R_i} ln(1 - e^{-\lambda\tau_{i,j}^*}) \right]. \quad (33)$$

Setting the derivative of Eq. (33) with respective to α and λ equal to 0, respectively, the following likelihood equations are obtained:

$$\frac{n}{\alpha} = -\sum_{i=1}^{m} \left[\sum_{j=1}^{X_i} ln(1 - e^{-\lambda\tau_{i,j}}) + \sum_{j=1}^{R_i} ln(1 - e^{-\lambda\tau_{i,j}^{*2}}) \right], \quad (34)$$

and

$$\frac{n}{\lambda} = \sum_{i=1}^{m} \left[\sum_{j=1}^{X_i} \tau_{i,j} + \sum_{j=1}^{R_i} \tau_{i,j}^* \right] - (\alpha - 1) \sum_{i=1}^{m} \left[\sum_{j=1}^{X_i} \frac{\tau_{i,j} e^{-\lambda\tau_{i,j}}}{(1 - e^{-\lambda\tau_{i,j}})} + \sum_{j=1}^{R_i} \frac{\tau_{i,j}^* e^{-\lambda\tau_{i,j}}}{(1 - e^{-\lambda\tau_{i,j}})} \right]$$

$$= \sum_{i=1}^{m} \left[\sum_{j=1}^{X_i} \tau_{i,j} + \sum_{j=1}^{R_i} \tau_{i,j}^* \right] - (\alpha - 1) \sum_{i=1}^{m} \left[\sum_{j=1}^{X_i} \frac{\tau_{i,j}}{(e^{\lambda\tau_{i,j}} - 1)} + \sum_{j=1}^{R_i} \frac{\tau_{i,j}^*}{(e^{\lambda\tau_{i,j}^*} - 1)} \right]. \quad (35)$$

The lifetimes of the X_i failures in the ith interval $(t_{i-1}, t_i]$ are independent and follow a doubly truncated GE from the left at t_{i-1} and from the right at t_i. The lifetimes of the R_i censored items in the ith interval $(t_{i-1}, t_i]$ are independent and follow a truncated GE from the left at t_i, $i = 1, 2, \ldots, m$. The required expected values of a doubly truncated GE from the left at a and from the right at b with $0 < a < b \le \infty$ for EM algorithm are given by

$$E_{\alpha,\lambda}[Y|Y \in [a, b]] = \frac{\int_a^b y f_{GE}(y; \alpha, \lambda) dy}{F_{GE}(b; \alpha, \lambda) - F_{GE}(a; \alpha, \lambda)},$$

$$E_{\alpha,\lambda}\left[ln\left(1 - e^{-\lambda Y}\right)|Y \in [a, b]\right] = \frac{\int_a^b ln(1 - e^{-\lambda y}) f_{GE}(y; \alpha, \lambda) dy}{F_{GE}(b; \alpha, \lambda) - F_{GE}(a; \alpha, \lambda)},$$

$$E_{\alpha,\lambda}\left[\frac{Y}{e^{\lambda Y} - 1}|Y \in [a, b]\right] = \frac{\int_a^b \frac{y}{e^{\lambda y} - 1} f_{GE}(y; \alpha, \lambda) dy}{F_{GE}(b; \alpha, \lambda) - F_{GE}(a; \alpha, \lambda)}.$$

Therefore the EM algorithm is given by the following iterative process:

1. Given starting values of α and λ, say $\hat{\alpha}^{(0)}$ and $\lambda^{(0)}$. Set $k = 0$.
2. In the $k + 1$th iteration,

   - the E-step computes the following conditional expectations using numerical integration methods,

$$E_{1i} = E_{\hat{\alpha}^{(k)}, \hat{\lambda}^{(k)}} \left[Y | Y \in [t_{i-1}, t_i) \right],$$

$$E_{2i} = E_{\hat{\alpha}^{(k)}, \hat{\lambda}^{(k)}} \left[\ln \left(1 - e^{-Y\hat{\lambda}^{(k)}} \right) | Y \in [t_{i-1}, t_i) \right],$$

$$E_{3i} = E_{\hat{\alpha}^{(k)}, \hat{\lambda}^{(k)}} \left[Y | Y \in [t_i, \infty) \right],$$

$$E_{4i} = E_{\hat{\alpha}^{(k)}, \hat{\lambda}^{(k)}} \left[\ln \left(1 - e^{-Y\hat{\lambda}^{(k)}} \right) | Y \in [t_i, \infty) \right],$$

$$E_{5i} = E_{\hat{\alpha}^{(k)}, \hat{\lambda}^{(k)}} \left[\frac{Y}{e^{Y\hat{\lambda}^{(k)}} - 1} | Y \in [t_{i-1}, t_i) \right],$$

$$E_{6i} = E_{\hat{\alpha}^{(k)}, \hat{\lambda}^{(k)}} \left[\frac{Y}{e^{Y\hat{\lambda}^{(k)}} - 1} | Y \in [t_i, \infty) \right],$$

and the likelihood Eqs. (34) and (35) are replaced by

$$\frac{n}{\alpha} = - \sum_{i=1}^{m} [X_i E_{2i} + R_i E_{4i}] \tag{36}$$

and

$$\frac{n}{\lambda} = \sum_{i=1}^{m} [X_i E_{1i} + R_i E_{3i}] - (\alpha - 1) \sum_{i=1}^{m} [X_i E_{5i} + R_i E_{6i}]; \tag{37}$$

   - the M-step solves the Eqs. (36) and (37) and obtains the next values, $\hat{\alpha}^{(k+1)}$ and $\hat{\lambda}^{(k+1)}$, of α and λ, respectively, as follows:

$$\hat{\alpha}^{(k+1)} = \frac{-n}{\sum_{i=1}^{m} (X_i E_{2i} + R_i E_{4i})} \tag{38}$$

$$\hat{\lambda}^{(k+1)} = \frac{n}{\sum_{i=1}^{m} (X_i E_{1i} + R_i E_{3i}) - \left[\hat{\alpha}^{(k+1)} - 1 \right] \sum_{i=1}^{m} (X_i E_{5i} + R_i E_{6i})}. \tag{39}$$

3. Checking the convergence, if the convergence occurs then the current $\hat{\alpha}^{(k+1)}$ and $\hat{\lambda}^{(k+1)}$ are the approximated MLEs of α and λ via EM algorithm; otherwise, set $k = k + 1$ and go to Step 2.

It can be easily seen that EM algorithm has no complicated likelihood equations involved for solving MLEs of α and λ as does Equations (31) and (32). Therefore, it can be efficiently implemented through a computing program.

4.2 Mid-Point Approximation Method

Suppose that X_i failure units in each subinterval $(t_{i-1}, t_i]$ occurred at the center of the interval $m_i = \frac{t_{i-1}+t_i}{2}$ and R_i censored items withdrawn at the censoring time t_i. Then the log likelihood function (30) could be approximately represented as:

$$ln(L_{GE}^M) \propto \sum_{i=1}^{m} [X_i ln\,(f(m_i, \theta)) + R_i ln\,(1 - F(t_i, \theta))]$$

$$= [ln(\alpha) + ln(\mu)] \sum_{i=1}^{m} X_i - \lambda \sum_{i=1}^{m} X_i m_i$$

$$+ (\alpha - 1) \sum_{i=1}^{m} \left[X_i ln(1 - e^{-m_i \lambda})\right] + \sum_{i=1}^{m} \left[R_i ln(1 - (1 - e^{-t_i \lambda})^\alpha)\right]. \quad (40)$$

The MLEs, $\hat{\alpha}$ and $\hat{\lambda}$, of α and λ are the solutions of the following system of equations,

$$\hat{\alpha} \sum_{i=1}^{m} X_i ln(1 - e^{-m_i \hat{\lambda}}) + \sum_{i=1}^{m} X_i = \hat{\alpha} \sum_{i=1}^{m} \left[R_i \frac{(1 - e^{-t_i \hat{\lambda}})^{\hat{\alpha}} ln(1 - e^{-t_i \hat{\lambda}})}{1 - (1 - e^{-t_i \hat{\lambda}})^{\hat{\alpha}}}\right], \quad (41)$$

and

$$\sum_{i=1}^{m} X_i / \hat{\lambda} + (\hat{\alpha} - 1) \sum_{i=1}^{m} \frac{X_i m_i e^{-m_i \hat{\lambda}}}{1 - e^{-m_i \hat{\lambda}}} = \sum_{i=1}^{m} X_i m_i + \hat{\alpha} \sum_{i=1}^{m} \frac{t_i R_i e^{-t_i \hat{\lambda}} (1 - e^{-t_i \hat{\lambda}})^{\hat{\alpha}-1}}{1 - (1 - e^{-t_i \hat{\lambda}})^{\hat{\alpha}}}. \quad (42)$$

There is no closed form for the solutions and an iterative numerical search is needed to obtain the parameter estimates, $\hat{\alpha}_{Mid}$ and $\hat{\lambda}_{Mid}$, from the above equation(s). Although there is no closed form of solution, the mid-point likelihood equations are simpler than the original likelihood equations.

4.3 Method of Moments

Let T be random variable which has the pdf (26). Gupta and Kundu (1999) had shown that the mean and the variance are:

$$\mu = E(T) = \frac{\varphi(\alpha + 1) - \varphi(1)}{\lambda},$$

$$\sigma^2 = E[(T - \mu)^2] = \frac{-\varphi'(\alpha + 1) + \varphi'(1)}{\lambda^2},$$

where $\varphi(t)$ is the digamma function and $\varphi'(t)$ is the derivative of $\varphi(t)$. The kth moment of a doubly truncated GE in the interval (a, b) with $0 < a < b \le \infty$ is given by

$$E_{\alpha,\lambda}\left(T^k | T \in [a, b)\right) = \frac{\int_a^b t^k f_{GE}(t) dt}{F_{GE}(b) - F_{GE}(a)}.$$

Equating the sample moments to the corresponding population moments, the following equations can be used to find the estimates of moment method.

$$\frac{\varphi(\alpha + 1) - \varphi(1)}{\lambda} = \frac{1}{n}\left[\sum_i^m X_i E_{\alpha,\lambda}(T | T \in [t_{i-1}, t_i)) + R_i E_{\alpha,\lambda}(T | T \in [t_i, \infty))\right], \tag{43}$$

$$\sigma^2 + \mu^2 = \frac{1}{n}\left[\sum_i^m X_i E_{\alpha,\lambda}(T^2 | T \in [t_{i-1}, t_i)) + R_i E_{\alpha,\lambda}(T^2 | T \in [t_i, \infty))\right]. \tag{44}$$

Since no closed form of the solutions of Eqs. (43) and (44) can be derived, an iterative numerical process to obtain the parameter estimates is described as follows:

1. Let the initial estimates of α and λ be $\alpha^{(0)}$ and $\lambda^{(0)}$. Set $k = 0$.
2. In the $(k + 1)$th iteration,

   - computing $E_{1i} = E_{\alpha^{(k)},\lambda^{(k)}}(T | T \in [t_{i-1}, t_i))$, $E_{3i} = E_{\alpha^{(k)},\lambda^{(k)}}(T | T \in [t_i, \infty))$, $E_{7i} = E_{\alpha^{(k)},\lambda^{(k)}}(T^2 | T \in [t_{i-1}, t_i))$ and $E_{8i} = E_{\alpha^{(k)},\lambda^{(k)}}(T^2 | T \in [t_i, \infty))$ and solving the following equation for α, say $\alpha^{(k+1)}$:

   $$\frac{[\varphi(\alpha + 1) - \varphi(1)]^2}{[\varphi(\alpha + 1) - \varphi(1)]^2 + \varphi'(1) - \varphi'(\alpha + 1)} = \frac{[\sum_i^m X_i E_{1i} + R_i E_{3i}]^2}{n\left[\sum_i^m X_i E_{7i} + R_i E_{8i}\right]}; \tag{45}$$

   - the solution for λ is obtained through the following equation and labeled by $\lambda^{(k+1)}$,

   $$\frac{\varphi(\alpha^{(k+1)} + 1) - \varphi(1)}{\lambda} = \frac{1}{n}\left[\sum_i^m X_i E_{1i} + R_i E_{3i}\right]. \tag{46}$$

3. Checking the convergence, if the convergence occurs then the current $\alpha^{(k+1)}$ and $\lambda^{(k+1)}$ are the estimates of α and λ by the method of moments; otherwise, set $k = k + 1$ and go to Step 2.

4.4   Estimation Based on Probability Plot

From (27), we have $t = \frac{-ln(1-p^{1/\alpha})}{\lambda}$. Let $\hat{F}(t_j)$ defined by (3) be the estimate of $F_{GE}(t;\alpha,\lambda)$, then the estimates of α and λ of GE distribution based on probability plot can be obtained by minimizing $\sum_{i=1}^{m}\left[t_i + ln\left(1 - (\hat{F}(t_j))^{1/\alpha}\right)/\lambda\right]^2$ with respect to α and λ. A nonlinear optimization procedure will be applied here to find the minimizers as the estimates of α and λ.

5   Real Data Analysis: Non-Bayesian Approach

5.1   The Data

The data set which consists of 112 patients with plasma cell myeloma treated at the National Cancer Institute (See [21]) is used for modeling two-parameter Weibull and two-parameter GED.

5.2   Model Selection

The three-parameter exponential Weibull distribution (EWD) proposed by Mudholkar et al. (1995, 1996) extended the classical Weibull distribution (WD) and the generalized exponential distribution (GE). The EWD has probability density function which is defined as,

$$f(t,\alpha,\lambda,\beta) = \alpha\lambda\beta t^{\beta-1} e^{-\lambda t^\beta}\left[1 - e^{-\lambda t^\beta}\right]^{\alpha-1}, \tag{47}$$

where $\alpha > 0$, $\lambda > 0$, and $\beta > 0$. It is clear that the EWD of (47) reduces to the GE distribution defined by (26) when $\beta = 1$, the Weibull distribution (WD) when $\alpha = 1$ and the classical exponential distribution (ED) when both $\beta = 1$ and $\alpha = 1$. Here, the three-parameter EWD will be used to fit the given data set and statistically tested whether it can be reduced to the WD model or the GE model for the given data set.

Fitting the EWD of (47) to the given data, the estimated parameters are $\hat{\theta} = (\hat{\alpha},\hat{\lambda},\hat{\beta}) = (1.064, 0.026, 1.185)$ and log likelihood, logL(EWD), has -2logL(WED) = 460.693. Fitting the classical Weibull distribution yields the estimated parameters $(\hat{\lambda},\hat{\beta}) = (0.021, 1.227)$ and log likelihood, logL(WD), with $-2\log L(WD) = 460.681$. Fitting the GE distribution results the estimated parameters $(\hat{\alpha},\hat{\lambda}) = (1.433, 0.057)$ and log likelihood, logL(GE), with $-2\log L(GE) = 460.941$. Therefore, the log likelihood ratio statistic between EWD and WD is

$[-2logL(WD)] - [-2logL(EWD)] = 0.013$, and the log likelihood ratio statistic between EWD and GED is $[-2logL(GED)] - [-2logL(EWD)] = 0.248$. By using χ^2 test with 1-degree of freedom, both comparisons are not statistically significant with p value of 0.909 and p value of 0.618, respectively. Fitting the classical exponential distribution with the given data set reveals that the estimated parameter $\hat{\alpha} = 0.045$ and log likelihood, $logL(ED)$, has $-2\log L(ED) = 465.562$. Hence, the log likelihood ratio statistic between the ED and the WD is $[-2logL(ED)] - [-2logL(WD)] = 4.881$, and the log likelihood ratio statistic between the ED and the GED is $[-2logL(ED)] - [-2logL(GE)] = 4.621$. By using χ^2 test with 1-degree of freedom, both comparisons show that the WD is better model than the classic exponential distribution with p value of 0.027, and the GE distribution is better model than the classic exponential distribution with p value of 0.032.

5.3   Model Comparison

Since the GE distribution and classical Weibull distribution have no sub-model relation, the chi-square test cannot be directly applied to select GE or Weibull distribution. In view of $-2\log L(WD) = 460.681$ and $-2\log L(GE) = 460.941$, there is no virtual difference between GE model fitting and the WD model fitting. Gupta and Kundu (2001a, 2003) mentioned that in many situations two-parameter GE distribution provides a better fit than the two-parameter Weibull distribution for the data from a right tailed distribution. It should be noticed that process to discriminate the two-parameter Weibull distribution from the two-parameter GE distribution has not been developed for the progressively type-I interval censored data.

In order to apply the Kolmogorov-Smironov goodness-of-fit test for fitting a given complete data set with a distribution, $F(x|\theta)$, the maximum distance, $D_n(F) = \sup_{0 \leq x < \infty} |\hat{F}_n(x) - F(x|\hat{\theta})|$, of the empirical distribution, $\hat{F}_n(x)$, of the given data set and the population distribution, $F(x|\hat{\theta})$ with $\hat{\theta}$ as the MLE of θ, must be obtained. When a progressively censored data is given, the empirical distribution is replaced by the product-limit distribution defined through Eq. (3) in the formula $D_n(F)$. Fitting the given data set with the Weibull distribution F_W, $D_n(F_W) = 0.4595$, with the GE distribution F_{GE}, $D_n(F_{GE}) = 0.1524$. The sampling distribution of $D_n(F)$ should have been applied to find the critical values for the goodness-of-fit tests mentioned. Although the sampling distribution for $D_n(F)$ under any progressive censoring has not been developed, we can see that the GE distribution provides a better fit than the Weibull distribution for the given data set in the sense of smaller $D_n(F)$.

5.4 Model Fitting

Applying the estimation processes developed in Sect. 3, the parameter estimates are $\gamma = (0.021, 0.019, 0.021, 0.020, 0.021)$ and $\beta = (1.231, 1.263, 1.227, 1.248, 1.224)$ for maximum likelihood estimate, midpoint approximation estimates, EM-algorithm estimates, moment method estimate and probability plot estimates, respectively, for Weibull distribution modeling procedure with the given data set. Meanwhile, applying the estimation processes developed in Sect. 4, the parameter estimates are $\alpha = (1.433, 1.514, 1.433, 1.513, 1.499)$ and $\lambda = (0.057, 0.059, 0.057, 0.059, 0.059)$ for maximum likelihood estimate, midpoint approximation estimates, EM-algorithm estimates, moment method estimate and probability plot estimates, respectively, for GE distribution modeling procedure with the given data set. It can be seen that these are virtually identical, so do the estimated GE density function, distribution function, and hazard function. Since all the estimates for α are greater than 1, the estimated GE densities are unimodal functions and the estimated GE hazard functions are increasing functions.

6 Markov Chain Monte Carlo for Bayesian Estimation

6.1 Likelihood Function and Bayes Estimation

Let the likelihood function of (1), based on progressively type-I interval censored data $D = \{(X_i, R_i, t_i), i = 1, 2, \cdots, m\}$, be represented as follows:

$$L(\Theta|D) \propto \prod_{i=1}^{m} [F(t_i, \Theta) - F(t_{i-1}, \Theta)]^{X_i} [1 - F(t_i, \Theta)]^{R_i}, \tag{48}$$

and the joint prior distribution for Θ in the likelihood function, $L(\Theta|D)$, be denoted by $h(\Theta)$. Then, the posterior joint likelihood for a given progressively type-I censored data D of size n can be obtained as follows:

$$\Pi(\Theta|D) \propto L(\Theta|D) \times h(\Theta)$$

$$\propto \left\{ \prod_{i=1}^{m} [F(t_i, \Theta) - F(t_{i-1}, \Theta)]^{X_i} [1 - F(t_i, \Theta)]^{R_i} \right\} \times h(\Theta). \tag{49}$$

Hence, the marginal posterior density function of $\theta_j, j = 1, 2, \ldots, k$, is given as

$$\Pi_j(\theta_j|D) = \int \Pi(\Theta|D) d\theta_1 d\theta_2 \ldots d\theta_{j-1} d\theta_{j+1} \ldots d\theta_k. \tag{50}$$

Given $\theta_1, \theta_2, \ldots, \theta_{j-1}, \theta_{j+1}, \ldots, \theta_k$, the full conditional posterior for θ_j could be written as

$$\Pi_j(\theta|D, \theta_1, \theta_2, \ldots, \theta_{j-1}, \theta_{j+1}, \ldots, \theta_k) \propto L(\theta_1, \theta_2, \ldots, \theta_{j-1}, \theta, \theta_{j+1}, \theta_k)|D)$$

$$\times h(\theta_1, \theta_2, \ldots, \theta_{j-1}, \theta, \theta_{j+1}, \theta_k), \quad (51)$$

where $L(\theta_1, \theta_2, \ldots, \theta_{j-1}, \theta, \theta_{j+1}, \theta_k)|D)$ is Eq. (48) and $h(\theta_1, \theta_2, \ldots, \theta_{j-1}, \theta, \theta_{j+1}, \theta_k)$ is the joint priors. Under the square error loss function, Bayesian estimation for unknown parameter is marginal posterior mean and under the absolute value of error loss, Bayesian estimation for unknown parameter is unconditional posterior median. However, the posterior likelihood usually does not have a closed representation for a given progressively type-I interval censored data. Moreover, a numerical integration cannot be easily applied in this situation. Hence, to derive Bayesian estimation for population parameter, Markov Chain Monte Carlo process through the application of Metropolis-Hastings (M-H) algorithm (Metropolis et al. 1953; Hastings 1970) to draw a sample of θ_j, given $j = 1, 2, \ldots, k$, via Gibbs scheme (Geman and Geman 1984) is introduced in the following subsection.

6.2 A Markov Chain Monte Carlo Process

Given $j = 1, 2, \ldots, k$, the Markov Chain $\theta_j^{(i)}, i = 1, 2, \ldots,$ of the jth parameter, θ_j, is constructed by applying the M-H algorithm described as following:

0. Propose $q_j(\theta_j^{(*)}|\theta_j^{(i)})$ as a transition probability from $\theta_j^{(i)}$ to $\theta_j^{(*)}$ for $j = 1, 2, \ldots, k$. Set $i = 0$ and initial states of $\theta_j^{(0)}, j = 1, 2, \ldots, k$, respectively.
1. Let $i = i$ and $j = 1$.
2. Let $j = j$ and generate $\theta_j^{(*)}$ from the proposed density $q_j(\theta_j^{(*)}|\theta_j^{(i)})$ and u_1 from uniform distribution over $(0, 1)$ interval independently, then

$$\theta_j^{(i+1)} = \begin{cases} \theta_j^{(*)} & \text{if } u_1 \leq \min\{1, \frac{\Pi_j(\theta_j^*|D, \theta_1^{(i)}, \theta_2^{(i)}, \ldots, \theta_{j-1}^{(i)}, \theta_{j+1}^{(i)}, \ldots, \theta_k^{(i)})q_j(\theta_j^{(*)}|\theta_j^{(i)})}{\Pi_j(\theta_j^{(i)}|D, \theta_1^{(i)}, \theta_2^{(i)}, \ldots, \theta_{j-1}^{(i)}, \theta_{j+1}^{(i)}, \ldots, \theta_k^{(i)})q_j(\theta_j^{(i)}|\theta_j^{(*)})}\} \\ \theta_j^{(i)} & \text{otherwise.} \end{cases}$$

3. Set $j = j + 1$.
4. Repeat Step (2) to Step (3) until $j = k + 1$.
5. Set $i = i + 1$
6. Repeat Step (1) to Step (5) for a huge number, say $i = N + 1$, of periods.

Given $j = 1, 2, \ldots, k$, the empirical distribution of θ_j can be then described by the realizations of θ_j from the constructed Markov chain after "some" burn-in period, N_b. The Bayesian estimation of θ_j can be approximated by using the empirical distribution of $\left\{\theta_j^{(l)} | l = N_b, \ldots, N\right\}$ for given $j = 1, 2, \ldots, k$. For example: if the loss function is the square error, then the Bayesian estimate of θ_j is the mean of $\left\{\theta_j^{(l)} | l = N_b, \ldots, N\right\}$; and if the loss function is the absolute value of difference, then the Bayesian estimate of θ_j is the median of the empirical distribution of $\left\{\theta_j^{(l)} | l = N_b, \ldots, N\right\}$.

It should be mentioned that the iterative processes described in this section could be implemented without priors imposed. When no priors are used, $\Pi_j(\theta | D, \theta_1, \theta_2, \ldots, \theta_{j-1}, \theta_{j+1}, \ldots, \theta_k)$ can be replaced by $L(\theta_1, \theta_2, \ldots, \theta_{j-1}, \theta, \theta_{j+1}, \theta_k) | D)$ in the Step (2) of M-H algorithm described above.

To implement the GE distribution modeling and Weibull distribution modeling through Bayesian procedure, the joint prior distribution for the parameters need to be selected. Following the suggestion by Kundu and Gupta (2008) for random sample as well as Kundu and Pradhan (2009) for progressively type-II censored data, to study the Bayesian estimations for GE parameters, the priors used could be independent gamma distributions,

$$g_1(\alpha)g_2(\lambda) \propto \alpha^{b-1} e^{-a\alpha} \lambda^{d-1} e^{-c\lambda}. \tag{52}$$

Since no any prior information provided along with the real data set, the improper priors of α and λ with hyper parameters $a = b = c = d = 0$ maybe used for the investigation of the MCMC process in the study. Sun (1997) had a detailed discussion about the Jeffreys priors for the parameters, γ and β of Weibull distribution in the Bayesian estimation procedure based on random sample. However, the Jeffreys priors, which is proportional to the square root of the determinant of the Fisher information matrix, is difficulty derived based on a progressively type-I interval censored data. For simplicity, the Jeffreys priors under random sample could be adopted to demonstrate the MCMC process. The Jeffreys priors for the Weibull distribution of (4) have the following form,

$$h_1(\beta)h_2(\gamma) \propto \frac{1}{\gamma\beta}. \tag{53}$$

Lin and Lio (2012) studied the GE distribution modeling and Weibull distribution modeling by using Bayesian approach based on progressive type-I interval censored data under the same pre-specified inspection times (in terms of month) as the given read data set and had a detailed discussion about the Bayesian estimation based on progressive type-I interval censored data.

7   Real Data Analysis: Bayesian Approach

7.1   The Data

The data set which contains 112 patients with plasma cell myeloma treated at the National Cancer Institute (Carbone et al. 1967) has been used for the two-parameter GE distribution modeling and the two-parameter Weibull distribution modeling through non-Bayesian approach in Sect. 5. It had been mentioned that the two-parameter GE distribution and two-parameter Weibull distribution modelings were virtually indistinguishable for modeling the data set in Table 1 through likelihood process. In this section, model selection between GE and Weibull distributions will be investigated through Bayesian framework.

7.2   Model Selection

Bayesian model comparison and selection is commonly accomplished through the utilization of Bayes factor, that is a ratio of two posterior probabilities of models, say M_1 and M_2, given data D. Here, we briefly describe how the posterior probability is evaluated. Let M indicate either GE distribution or Weibull distribution and $f(D|\Theta, M)$ is the likelihood (48) with $F(t|\Theta)$ replaced by either $F_{GE}(t, \Theta)$ or $F_W(t, \Theta)$. Then for a given progressively type-I censored data $D = \{(X_i, R_i, t_i),$ $i = 1, 2, \ldots, m\}$ of size n, the posterior marginal likelihood of the model M is defined as

$$L(D|M) = \int f(D|\Theta, M) \Pi(\Theta|M) d\Theta. \tag{54}$$

The Eq. (54) can be viewed as the expectation $E(f(D|\Theta, M))$ taken with respect to the prior distribution $\Pi(\Theta|M)$ and can be approximated by the Monte Carlo method as follows:

$$L(D|M) \approx \frac{1}{N - N_b} \sum_{i=N_b}^{N} f(D|\Theta^{(i)}, M), \tag{55}$$

where $\Theta^{(i)} = (\alpha^{(i)}, \lambda^{(i)})$ or $\Theta^{(i)} = (\beta^{(i)}, \gamma^{(i)})$ with the index i from the burn-in period N_b to Gibbs sampler size N.

However, there are some difficulties with the approximation of the likelihood of parameters, see, for example, Robert and Marin (2008). In this study, the approximation by (55) is infeasible, because the size of Monte Carlo simulation should be very large, say 10^{10} or more, to guarantee the convergence of the desired quantity. Regarding the model selection, we also try to find the limiting model probabilities of reversible jump MCMC between two models' posterior likelihoods [for more information about reversible jump MCMC, reader may refer to Green (1995)]. Yet, we never know when two competing models' transition probabilities reach balance. Instead, we come up with a novel idea dealing with such "mixed" type of data. The novel approach is that a "supervised" mixture model M_m containing both GE and Weibull distributions is proposed. And then the MCMC method is employed to calculate the mix proportions, π_w and π_G, for both components that can be served as the weight of two models' posterior probabilities and the criterion for model selection. Through the process, we find the calculation is fast and simple. More detail is given as follows:

Assume the interval censoring data $\{X_i : i = 1, 2, \cdots, m\}$ came from the mixture model of GE and Weibull distributions as follows:

$$X_i \sim \pi_w \cdot f_W(t, \gamma, \beta) + \pi_G \cdot f_{GE}(t, \alpha, \lambda)$$

with $\pi_w + \pi_G = 1$. Then $D = \{(X_i, R_i, t_i), i = 1, 2, \ldots, m\}$ has the posterior likelihood

$$L(D|M_m) = \pi_w \cdot L(D|M_w) + \pi_G \cdot L(D|M_G) \tag{56}$$

where $L(D|M_G)$ and $L(D|M_w)$ are the posterior likelihoods of GE and Weibull models defined in (54). When π_w is 0, then we see $X_i \sim$ GE model and when π_w is 1, then $X_i \sim$ Weibull model. Also notice that if $\pi_w > 1/2$, Weibull model is preferred since Weibull distribution has more mix weight in the mixture model M_m; otherwise, GE model is preferred. Next, the estimation of π_w can be done by usual MCMC process.

Assume the prior distribution of π_w is uniformly distributed over (0,1), then the Gibbs scheme to estimate π_w in the mixture model is given as follows.

- Set the initial values of all parameters.
- For $i = 1$ to N_w, do

    1. Update the parameters $\Theta^{(i)} = (\alpha^{(i)}, \lambda^{(i)})$ of GE distribution using the posterior likelihood $L(D|M_m)$ in (56).
    2. Update the parameters $\Theta'^{(i)} = (\beta^{(i)}, \gamma^{(i)})$ of Weibull distribution using the posterior likelihood $L(D|M_m)$ in (56).
    3. Update the parameter π_w using the M-H algorithm through the posterior likelihood in (56) and set the proposal density $q_w(\pi_w^*|\pi_w) \sim U(0, 1)$ to avoid the local extrema. Specifically, draw the candidate π_w^* from $q^* \sim U(0, 1)$, then accept π_w^* as the ith state value, $\pi_w^{(i)}$, with probability

$$\min \left\{ 1, \frac{\pi_w^* \cdot L(D|M_w, \Theta'^{(i)}) + (1 - \pi_w^*) \cdot L(D|M_G, \Theta^{(i)})}{\pi_w^{(i-1)} \cdot L(D|M_w, \Theta'^{(i)}) + (1 - \pi_w^{(i-1)}) \cdot L(D|M_G, \Theta^{(i)})} \right\},$$

otherwise, the ith state value, $\pi_w^{(i)}$, is $\pi_w^{(i-1)}$.

- The Bayes estimate of π_w is the sample mean of $\{\pi_w^{(i)}\}$ after some burn-in period N_b'',

Time series of MCMC outputs
after 50,000 buru-in period

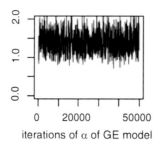

iterations of α of GE model

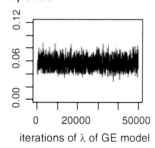

iterations of λ of GE model

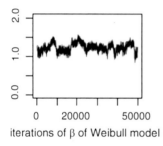

iterations of β of Weibull model

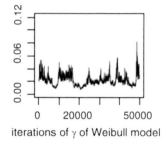

iterations of γ of Weibull model

Fig. 1 Time series plots of the MCMC samplers

The simulation study shows that when the progressively type-I censored data $\{X_i : i = 1, 2, \cdots, 8\}$ is generated from GE distribution or from Weibull distribution, the MCMC estimate of π_w correctly identifies the correct model about 989 out 1000 times for each situation.

Given the real data set in Table 1, we apply the proposed Bayesian procedure with the improper priors for GE model and the Jeffreys priors for Weibull model, and make the time series plots of the MCMC samplers of parameters (α, λ) in GE distribution and (β, γ) in Weibull distribution shown in Fig. 1. Even with different initial values of parameters, the times series plots are stable and have a similar pattern. The Bayes estimate of $\alpha = 1.547$ (variance= 0.00482) and $\lambda = 0.0592$ (variance= 0.01362) if data are assumed from GE distribution. On the other hand, the Bayes estimate of $\beta = 1.2789$ (variance = 0.00032) and $\gamma = 0.0189$ (variance= 0.0000013) if data are assumed from Weibull distribution.

With the aid of the above mixture model, the MCMC estimate of π_w ($N = 200,000, N_b = 100,000$) is 0.128294 (with standard deviation 0.103). Also, a

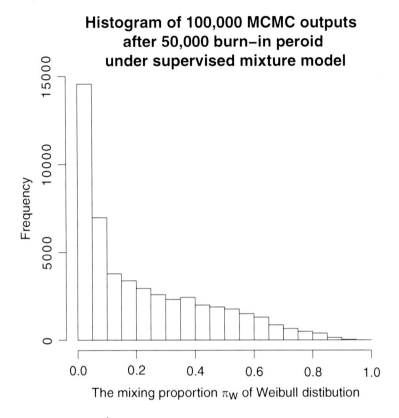

Fig. 2 Histogram plot for $\hat{\pi}_w$

histogram of π_w's MCMC outputs after 50,000 burn-in period is plotted in Fig. 2. We can see the empirical distribution of π_w is skewed to the right. Therefore, we would conclude that the GE model is more likely to be chosen for the data set of Table 1.

Appendix

```
############################################
#Random sample from Generalized exponential distribution(GED)
#    n: sample size; alpha, lambda: parameters
############################################
# random number for GED
rGexp=function(n,alpha,lambda){
U=runif(n, min=0, max=1)
return(-1/lambda*log(1.0-U^(1/alpha)))
}
# density for GED
dGexp=function(x,alpha,lambda){
alpha *lambda*(1.0-exp(-lambda *x))^(alpha -1)*exp(-lambda *x)
```

```
}
#   Distribution function of GED
#   x is input; alpha, lambda: parameters
pGexp=function(x,alpha,lambda) (1.0 - exp(-x*lambda))^alpha

# 3 function calls for the EM and moment under GED
ydg   = function(x,alpha,lambda) x*dGexp(x,alpha,lambda)
y2dg  = function(x,alpha,lambda) x^2*dGexp(x,alpha,lambda)
lndg  = function(x,alpha,lambda)
              log(1-exp(-lambda*x))*dGexp(x,alpha,lambda)
y2Edg = function(x,alpha,lambda){
   x*exp(-lambda*x)/(1-exp(-lambda*x))*dGexp(x,alpha,lambda)
}


######################################
# Procedure for Maximum Likelihood Estimate
######################################
estMLE = function(x,R,T,inita,initb)
{
m=length(x)
# make the mle objective function
obj.mle = function(parm)
{
    alpha=parm[1];lambda= parm[2]
    tmpFi  = pGexp(T[-1],alpha,lambda)
    tmpFi1 = pGexp(T[-(m+1)],alpha,lambda)
      tmp  = (tmpFi-tmpFi1)^x*(1-tmpFi)^R
      logL = log(tmp)
      -sum(logL[is.finite(logL)])
 #logL could be infinite since of the log
}
pa  = c(inita,initb)
tmp = optim(pa,obj.mle,method="L-BFGS-B",lower=c(0.001,0.001) )

}


#################################################
#      Procedure for Mid-point Module from DC
#################################################
MidPT=function(x,R,T,inita,initb)
{
  m=length(R)
  mi= (T[-1]+T[-(m+1)])/2

  obj.MLE=function(parm){
  alpha = parm[1];lambda= parm[2]
  logL = x*log(dGexp(mi,alpha,lambda))
           +R*log(1-pGexp(T[-1],alpha,lambda))
  -sum(logL)
} # end of the obj.MLE

pa=c(inita,initb)
tmp=optim(pa,obj.MLE,method="L-BFGS-B",lower=c(0.001,0.001))

}


###################################################
# Proceudre for  EM algorithm
###################################################

EM=function(x,R,T,inal,inlam)
{
 m=length(R)
 n=sum(x) + sum(R)
 all=inal
 lam1=inlam
 E1=E2=E3=E4=E5=E6= numeric(m)
```

```
 mm=m+1
 Cont=TRUE
 while( Cont ){
  alp=all
  lam=lam1
#  E-step
  for(i in 2:mm){
   d1=pGexp(T[i],alp,lam)-pGexp(T[i-1],alp,lam)
   d2=1.0 - pGexp(T[i],alp,lam)
   EMval=integrate(ydg,lower=T[i-1],upper=T[i],alpha=alp,
                                         lambda=lam)
 E1[i-1]=EMval$value/d1
   EMval=integrate(lndg,lower=T[i-1],upper=T[i],alpha=alp,
                                          lambda=lam)
   E2[i-1]=EMval$value/d1
   EMval=integrate(ydg,lower=T[i],upper=Inf,alpha=alp,
                                         lambda=lam)
 E3[i-1]=EMval$value/d2
   EMval=integrate(lndg,lower=T[i],upper=Inf,alpha=alp,
                                          lambda=lam)
 E4[i-1]=EMval$value/d2
   EMval=integrate(y2Edg,lower=T[i-1],upper=T[i],alpha=alp,
                                          lambda=lam)
 E5[i-1]=EMval$value/d1
   EMval=integrate(y2Edg,lower=T[i],upper=Inf,alpha=alp,
                                          lambda=lam)
 E6[i-1]=EMval$value/d2
   }
  #M step
  all=-n/sum(x*E2 + R*E4)
  lam1=n/( sum(x*E1+R*E3)-(all-1)*sum(x*E5+R*E6) )

#Convergence checking

   if( abs(all - alp)<exp(-10)&&abs(lam1-lam)<exp(-10)){
         Cont= FALSE; }
     }
cbind(all,lam1)
}

##########################################
# Procedure for Moment method
#########################################3
MMM=function(x,R,T,inal,inlam)
{
   m=length(R)
   n=sum(x) + sum(R)
   all=inal
   lam1=inlam
   E1= numeric(m)
   E2=numeric(m)
   E3=numeric(m)
   E4=numeric(m)
   mm=m+1
   Cont=TRUE
   while( Cont ){
     alp=all
     lam=lam1
    # next step
    for(i in 2:mm){
      d1=pGexp(T[i],alp,lam)-pGexp(T[i-1],alp,lam)
      d2=1.0 - pGexp(T[i],alp,lam)
      MMEva=integrate(ydg,lower=T[i-1],upper=T[i],alpha=alp,
                                          lambda=lam)
E1[i-1]=MMEva$value/d1
      E2[i-1]=integrate(y2dg,lower=T[i-1],upper=T[i],alpha=alp,
                                          lambda=lam)
```

```
E2[i-1]=MMEva$value/d1
      E3[i-1]=integrate(ydg,lower=T[i],upper=Inf,alpha=alp,
                                               lambda=lam)
E3[i-1]=MMEva$value/d2
      E4[i-1]=integrate(y2dg,lower=T[i],upper=Inf,alpha=alp,
                                               lambda=lam)
E4[i-1]=MMEva$value/d2
      }
#   continue next step
#------------------------------------------------
#   psigamma(x, deriv=1) is the derivative of digamma function
#------------------------------------------------
 MMEq=function(b){
   n*(sum(x*E2+R*E4))/(sum(x * E1 +R*E3))^2 - 1.0-
      (psigamma(1,deriv=1)-psigamma(b+1,deriv=1))
  /( digamma(b+1)-digamma(1) )^2
  }

#   Use the uniroot to find the solution of alpha
      al1= uniroot(MMEq,interval=c(1E-10,1E50))root
      lam1=n*(digamma( al1 +1 )-digamma(1))/(sum(x*E1+R*E3))

#   Convergence checking

    if( abs(al1 - alp)<exp(-10)&&abs(lam1-lam)<exp(-10)){
          Cont= FALSE; }
    }
cbind(al1,lam1)

}

###################################################
#    Procedure of Probability-plot Estimation Method
###################################################
Pplot=function(x,R,Ti,inita,initb)
{
 n = sum(x)+sum(R)
 m=length(R)
 p= numeric(m)
 T =numeric(m)
 hatF=numeric(m)
 cux=0.0
 cur=0.0
 mm = m+1
 for(i in 2:mm){T[i-1]=Ti[i]}

 for (j in 1:m){
  sur = n- cux -cur
  if ( sur <= 0 ) { p[j]=1}
  else{
   p[j]=x[j]/sur

   cux=cux+x[j]; cur=cur + R[j]
  }
 }
 pd=1.0
 for (j in 1:m){
   pd= pd * (1.0 -p[j])
   hatF[j] = 1.0 - pd
 }
 obj.f=function(parm){
   alpha =parm[1]
   lambda= parm[2]
   return( sum( (T + log(1.0 - (hatF)^(1.0/alpha))/lambda )^2) )
 }

 pa=c(inita,initb)
```

```
 tmp=nlminb(pa, obj.f, gradient = NULL, hessian = NULL,
        lower =c(0.001,0.001), upper =c(Inf,Inf))
}

#########################################################
#Ox program code to implement Model Selection
# Between WB and GED from Mixture Model
#########################################################

#include<oxstd.h>
#include<oxprob.h>
WBCDF(xt, beta, gamma) {return (1-exp(-gamma*(xt^beta)));}
GEDF(xt, alpha, lambda) {return (1-exp(-lambda*xt))^alpha;}
Mixed(xt, beta, gamma, alpha, lambda, probWB)
 {return probWB*(1-exp(-gamma*(xt^beta)))+(1- probWB)*
     (1-exp(-lambda*xt))^alpha;}

rWBtypeI(T,pp, beta, gamma, N_size)
// Generate WB type I interval censored data
{decl i, N_left=N_size, iInt=rows(T), icXR=zeros(iInt,2);
 for (i=0; i<iInt;i++){
  if (i==0){
   icXR[i][0]=ranbinomial(1,1,N_left,  WBCDF(T[0], beta, gamma));
   N_left=N_left-icXR[i][0];
   icXR[i][1]=floor(pp[i]*N_left);
   N_left=N_left-icXR[i][1];} // end of if i==0
   else{
    icXR[i][0]=ranbinomial(1,1,N_left, (WBCDF(T[i], beta, gamma)
                -WBCDF(T[i-1], beta, gamma))
  /(1-WBCDF(T[i-1], beta, gamma)));
    N_left=N_left-icXR[i][0];
    icXR[i][1]=floor(pp[i]*N_left);
    N_left=N_left-icXR[i][1];
       }// end of if i>0
}// end of for i loop
 return icXR;
}//

rGEDtypeI(T,pp, alpha, lambda, N_size)
{ decl i, N_left=N_size, iInt=rows(T), icXR=zeros(iInt,2);
// Generate GE type I interval censored data
  for (i=0; i<iInt;i++){
   if (i==0){
    icXR[i][0]=ranbinomial(1,1,N_left,  GEDF(T[i], alpha, lambda));
    N_left=N_left-icXR[i][0];
    icXR[i][1]=floor(pp[i]*N_left);
    N_left=N_left-icXR[i][1];}
   else{
    icXR[i][0]=ranbinomial(1,1,N_left,(GEDF(T[i], alpha, lambda)
 -GEDF(T[i-1], alpha, lambda))/(1-GEDF(T[i-1],
                                    alpha, lambda)));
    N_left=N_left-icXR[i][0];
    icXR[i][1]=floor(pp[i]*N_left);
    N_left=N_left-icXR[i][1];
   }// end of if i>0
  }// end of for i loop
    return icXR;
}//

logLtypeIWB(icX,icR,T,beta,gamma){
  decl i,j, iInterval=rows(T), logLL=0 ;
  decl logProb=zeros(iInterval,1),logProbR=zeros(iInterval,1);
  logProb[0] =log(1-exp(-gamma*(T[0])^beta));
  logProbR[0]=log(1-WBCDF(T[0],beta,gamma));
  for(i=1;i<iInterval;i++){ //begin of for i loop
    logProb[i] =log(WBCDF(T[i],beta,gamma)-WBCDF(T[i-1],
                                          beta,gamma));
```

```
    logProbR[i]=log(1-WBCDF(T[i],beta,gamma));
  } // end of for i loop
  logLL=sumc(logProb.*icX)+sumc(logProbR.*icR);
  return logLL;
} // end of  logLtypeI

logLMixed(icX,icR,T,alpha,lambda,beta,gamma,probWB){
// This function compute the loglikelihood of given counts
//   to be used in M-H algorithm
 decl i,j, iInterval=rows(T), logLL=0 ;
 decl logProb=zeros(iInterval,1),logProbR=zeros(iInterval,1);
 logProb[0] =log(Mixed(T[0],beta,gamma,alpha,lambda,probWB));
 logProbR[0]=log(1-Mixed(T[0],beta,gamma,alpha,lambda,probWB));
 for(i=1;i<iInterval;i++){ //begin of for i loop
   logProb[i]=log(Mixed(T[i],beta,gamma,alpha,lambda,probWB)
               -Mixed(T[i-1], beta,gamma,alpha, lambda, probWB));
   logProbR[i]=log(1-Mixed(T[i],beta,gamma,alpha,lambda,probWB));
 } // end of for i loop
 logLL=sumc(logProb.*icX)+sumc(logProbR.*icR);
 return logLL;
} // end of  logLtypeIGE

logLtypeIGE(icX,icR,T,alpha,lambda){
 decl i,j, iInterval=rows(T), logLL=0 ;
 decl logProb=zeros(iInterval,1),logProbR=zeros(iInterval,1);
 logProb[0] =alpha*log(1-exp(-lambda*T[0]));
 logProbR[0]=log(1-GEDF(T[0],alpha,lambda));
 for(i=1;i<iInterval;i++){ //begin of for i loop
   logProb[i] =log(GEDF(T[i],alpha,lambda)
                   -GEDF(T[i-1],alpha,lambda));
   logProbR[i]=log(1-GEDF(T[i],alpha,lambda));
 } // end of for i loop
 logLL=sumc(logProb.*icX)+sumc(logProbR.*icR);
   return logLL;
} // end of  logLtypeIGE

main()
{ decl seed=182632;
  decl simmodel=2;
  //simmodel=0,if WB;simmodel=1,if GE;simmodel=2 if real data
  decl alpha_sim=1.56,lambda_sim=.06;
  // targeted values if simmodel=1
  decl beta_sim=1.12,gamma_sim=.03;
  // targeted values if simmodel==0
  decl N_mcmc=1000*100; // length of MCMC
  decl burninperiod=1000*50; //the burn-in period in MCMC
  decl censorT=<5.5,10.5,15.5,20.5,25.5,30.5,40.5,50.5,60.5>';
  //decl prob=<0.25,0.25,0.25,0.25,0.25,0.25,0.25,0.25,1>;
                 //the prob of withdrawals
  decl prob=<0,0,0,0,0,0,0,0,1>; // the prob of withdrawals
  decl N_obsn=112;//sample size if simmodel=0 or 1, disabled
                                 if THE real data is applied
  decl beta_start=beta_sim+0.1*rann(1,1)[0]; //starting points
decl gamma_start=gamma_sim+.0013*+rann(1,1)[0];
        // starting points
  decl alpha_start=alpha_sim+0.1*rann(1,1)[0];
        // starting points
decl lambda_start=lambda_sim+.000125*+rann(1,1)[0];
        // starting points
  decl cXF,vec,cXR,i,hh,hh1=.001, sum_Like=0,iInt=rows(censorT);
  decl logL, logLcand;
  decl gamma_mc,beta_mc,alpha_mc,lambda_mc;
  decl invgamma_cand,invlambda_cand;
  decl gamma_cand,beta_cand,alpha_cand,lambda_cand;
  decl nowstate,newstate;
  decl alpha_rjmc, lambda_rjmc,beta_rjmc, gamma_rjmc;
  decl cGE=0, cWB=0,cRJMCMC=0,probGE=1/5, probWB=1/2;
```

```
  decl probWB_mc, probWB_cand;
  decl file, file1;
  file = fopen("WB_mixing_mc.txt", "w");
 file1 = fopen("beta_gamma_alpha_lambda.txt", "w");
  ranseed(seed); // change the random seed to get different simulations
  print("\n the seed=", seed, "\n");
  // generate data (simmodel <=1) or use real data (simmodel>1)
  if(simmodel==1){vec=rGEDtypeI(censorT,prob, alpha_sim,
                                       lambda_sim, N_obsn);
     cXF=vec[][0]; cXR=vec[][1];        }
  if(simmodel==0){ vec=rWBtypeI(censorT,prob, beta_sim,
                                     gamma_sim, N_obsn);
     cXF=vec[][0]; cXR=vec[][1];}
  if(simmodel >1){cXF=<18;16;18;10;11;8;13;4;1>;
            cXR=<1 ;1 ;3 ; 0; 0;1; 2;3;2>;}
  if(simmodel==1){ print("\n a data set of progessive type-I interval
                    censored count is simulated from GED,\n");}
  if(simmodel==0){print("\n a data set of progessive type-I interval
                    censored count is simulated from WEIBULL,\n");}
  if(simmodel>1) print("\n We're using the REAL DATA. \n");
  //print("The staring points of beta MCMC= ",beta_start,
        "\t and lamba=", gamma_start);
  print(" \n The total MCMC iteration is ", N_mcmc, "\n ");
  print(" \n Sum of failures and withdrawls=",
                          sumc(cXF+cXR)[0],"\n");
  print("\n The censoring time is \n\t\t\t\t", "d", "\t")  ;
  for ( i=0;i<iInt;i++) print("2.2f", censorT[i],"\t");
  if (simmodel<2){
    print("\n The withdral prob is \n\t\t\t\t")  ;
    for( i=0;i<iInt;i++) print("1.2f", prob[i],"\t");}
//end of NO printing prob
     print("\n the count of X =");
    for ( i=0;i<iInt;i++) print("4d", cXF[i][0],"\t");
    print("\n the count of R =");
    for ( i=0;i<iInt;i++) print("4d", cXR[i][0],"\t");
    print("\n");
// Construct Markov Chains of beta and gamma
// by applying the M-H step (Gibbs sampling)
   beta_mc=ones(N_mcmc,1)*beta_sim;
   gamma_mc=ones(N_mcmc,1)*gamma_sim;
   gamma_mc[0]=gamma_start; beta_mc[0]=beta_start;
  // starting points of parameters
   sum_Like=0; //compute the averaged (posterior)
             //likelihood based on the MCMC outputs
   for (i=1;i<N_mcmc;i++) { // estimate the parameters of WB
     // update gamma_mc by M-H algorithm
     if (i<2000) hh=hh1*2; else hh=hh1;
     gamma_cand= 1/(1/gamma_mc[i-1] +1*rann(1,1) );
     if (i<2000) beta_cand=beta_mc[i-1]+.05*(rann(1,1));
     else  beta_cand=beta_mc[i-1]+.05*(rann(1,1));
     while( beta_cand<0) beta_cand=beta_mc[i-1]+.02*rann(1,1);
     logL = logLtypeIWB(cXF,cXR,censorT,beta_mc[i-1],
                                       gamma_mc[i-1]);
     logLcand = logLtypeIWB(cXF,cXR,censorT,beta_cand,
                                       gamma_cand);

     if(log(ranu(1,1)) < logLcand-logL) {beta_mc[i]= beta_cand;
                   gamma_mc[i]= gamma_cand;}
     else { beta_mc[i]= beta_mc[i-1]; gamma_mc[i]= gamma_mc[i-1];
      if(i>burninperiod) {if(i==burninperiod)
      sum_Like=1/exp(logLtypeIWB(cXF,cXR,censorT,beta_mc[i],
                                       gamma_mc[i]))[0];
        else sum_Like=sum_Like +
1/exp(logLtypeIWB(cXF,cXR,censorT,beta_mc[i],
                                       gamma_mc[i]))[0]  ;
      }// end of if> burninperiod-1
    } // end of else,
```

```
    if (imod(i,5000*2)==0)print(".") ;
}// end of for loop
print("\n The likelihood of Weibull model =",
        1/((sum_Like)/(N_mcmc-burninperiod)[0]),"\n");
alpha_mc=ones(N_mcmc,1);
lambda_mc=ones(N_mcmc,1);
lambda_mc[0]=lambda_start; alpha_mc[0]=alpha_start;
            // starting points of parameters
sum_Like=0;
 //compute the averaged (posterior) likelihood
 // based on the MCMC outputs
for (i=1;i<N_mcmc;i++){
    // estimate the parameters of GE model
    if (i<2000) hh=hh1*5;else hh=hh1;
    lambda_cand=     1/(1/lambda_mc[i-1] + rann(1,1) );
    alpha_cand=alpha_mc[i-1]+.05*rann(1,1);
    // in case lambda_cand is negative
    while( alpha_cand>2.8)alpha_cand=alpha_mc[i-1]+hh*rann(1,1);
    logL = logLtypeIGE(cXF,cXR,censorT,alpha_mc[i-1],
                                            lambda_mc[i-1]);
    logLcand = logLtypeIGE(cXF,cXR,censorT,alpha_cand,
                                            lambda_cand);
    if(log(ranu(1,1)) < logLcand-logL)
      {alpha_mc[i]= alpha_cand; lambda_mc[i]= lambda_cand; }
    else{alpha_mc[i]= alpha_mc[i-1];
                            lambda_mc[i]= lambda_mc[i-1];}
    if (imod(i,5000*2)==0) print(".");
    if(i>burninperiod){
     if(i==burninperiod)
      sum_Like=1/exp(logLtypeIGE(cXF,cXR,censorT,alpha_mc[i],
         lambda_mc[i]))[0];
      else sum_Like=sum_Like+1/exp(logLtypeIGE(cXF,cXR,censorT,
         alpha_mc[i], lambda_mc[i]))[0];       }
                        }
    print("\n The likelihood of GE model=",
        1/((sum_Like)/(N_mcmc-burninperiod)),"\n");
    for (i=0; i<N_mcmc;i++)
        fprint(file1," ", "\t",beta_mc[i],"\t",
gamma_mc[i],"\t", alpha_mc[i],"\t", lambda_mc[i],"\n");
    alpha_mc=ones(N_mcmc,1)*alpha_sim;
    lambda_mc=ones(N_mcmc,1)*lambda_sim;
    lambda_mc[0]=0.06;  alpha_mc[0]=1.6;
    beta_mc=ones(N_mcmc,1)*beta_sim;
    gamma_mc=ones(N_mcmc,1)*gamma_sim;
    gamma_mc[0]=0.03;//meanc(gamma_mc[burninperiod:N_mcmc-1])[0];
    beta_mc[0]=1.2;//meanc(beta_mc[burninperiod:N_mcmc-1])[0];
    probWB_mc= ones(N_mcmc,1)*.5;
  for (i=1;i<N_mcmc;i++){ // estimate the parameters of WB
   gamma_cand= 1/(1/gamma_mc[i-1] + rann(1,1) );
   beta_cand=beta_mc[i-1]+.01*(rann(1,1));
   logL=logLMixed(cXF,cXR,censorT,alpha_mc[i-1],lambda_mc[i-1],
    beta_mc[i], gamma_mc[i], probWB_mc[i-1]);
   logLcand = logLMixed(cXF,cXR,censorT,alpha_mc[i-1],
   lambda_mc[i-1],beta_cand, gamma_cand, probWB_mc[i-1]);

   if(log(ranu(1,1)) < logLcand-logL) {gamma_mc[i]= gamma_cand;
                                      beta_mc[i]= beta_cand;}
    else { gamma_mc[i]= gamma_mc[i-1];
                                       beta_mc[i]= beta_mc[i-1]; }
   alpha_cand=alpha_mc[i-1]+.005*(rann(1,1));
   while( alpha_cand>2.0)alpha_cand=alpha_mc[i-1]+.01*rann(1,1);
    lambda_cand=1/(1/lambda_mc[i-1] + rann(1,1) );
    while( lambda_cand<0)
                   lambda_cand=lambda_mc[i-1]+hh1*100*rann(1,1);
    logL= logLMixed(cXF,cXR,censorT,alpha_mc[i-1],
lambda_mc[i-1],beta_mc[i], gamma_mc[i], probWB_mc[i-1]);
    logLcand = logLMixed(cXF,cXR,censorT,alpha_cand,
```

```
lambda_cand,beta_mc[i], gamma_mc[i], probWB_mc[i-1]);

  if(log(ranu(1,1)) < logLcand-logL) {alpha_mc[i]= alpha_cand;
                lambda_mc[i]= lambda_cand;}
  else{lambda_mc[i]=lambda_mc[i-1];alpha_mc[i]=alpha_mc[i-1];}

  probWB_cand=ranu(1,1);
  while( probWB_cand<0 ||probWB_cand>1)  probWB_cand=
                        probWB_mc[i-1]+.05*(rann(1,1));
   logL = logLMixed(cXF,cXR,censorT,alpha_mc[i], lambda_mc[i],
        beta_mc[i], gamma_mc[i], probWB_mc[i-1]);
   logLcand=logLMixed(cXF,cXR,censorT,alpha_mc[i],lambda_mc[i],
         beta_mc[i], gamma_mc[i], probWB_cand);
   if(log(ranu(1,1))<logLcand-logL){probWB_mc[i]=probWB_cand;}
   else { probWB_mc[i]= probWB_mc[i-1];  }
   if (imod(i,5000*2)==0) print(".");
  }// end of for loop
alpha_rjmc=meanc(alpha_mc[burninperiod:N_mcmc-1])[0];
lambda_rjmc=meanc(lambda_mc[burninperiod:N_mcmc-1])[0];
gamma_rjmc=meanc(gamma_mc[burninperiod:N_mcmc-1])[0];
beta_rjmc=meanc(beta_mc[burninperiod:N_mcmc-1])[0];
print("\n The MCMC estimates for WeiBull is ");
print("\n beta hat=",beta_rjmc);
print("\t gamma hat=",gamma_rjmc);
print("\n The MCMC estimates for GE is ");
print("\n alpha hat=", alpha_rjmc);
print("\t lambda hat=",lambda_rjmc);
if(simmodel==0) print("\n\n The true model is Weibull");
if(simmodel==1) print("\n\n The true model is GED");
if(simmodel>1) print("\n\n THE real data is applied.");
print("\t The  last  20 obsn of probWB is=",
      probWB_mc[N_mcmc-20:N_mcmc-1]');
print("\t min probWB hat=",
           min(probWB_mc[burninperiod:N_mcmc-1])[0],"\n" );
print("\t max probWB hat=",
           max(probWB_mc[burninperiod:N_mcmc-1])[0],"\n" );
print("\t probWB hat=",
           meanc(probWB_mc[burninperiod:N_mcmc-1])[0],"\n" );
print("\t sd probWB hat=",
           varc(probWB_mc[burninperiod:N_mcmc-1])[0]^.5,"\n" );
for (i=0; i<N_mcmc;i++) fprint(file," ", probWB_mc[i], "\n");
  fclose(file);      fclose(file1);
}

################################################################
# Using WinBUGS to implement Built-in probability transition jump
# Selecting Probability Model between WB and GED
################################################################
model {  # Define the mixture model using the Poison zerostrick
const<- 5; zero<-0; zero ~ dpois(zero.mean)
zero.mean <- const + (-1)*logL
logL<- log( rho*exp(sum(logLGEx[])+sum(logLGEr[]))
          +(1-rho)*exp(sum(logLWBx[])+sum(logLWBr[])) )
# compute the likelihood of GE model
pr[1] <- pow(1-exp(-lambda*tt[1]), alpha)
for (i in 2:9) {
 pr[i] <-pow(1-exp(-lambda*tt[i]),alpha)
                     -pow(1-exp(-lambda*tt[i-1]), alpha)
}
pr[10] <- 1-pow(1-exp(-lambda*tt[9]), alpha)
xxsum <- sum(xx[1:10]) ;xx[1:10] ~ dmulti (pr[], xxsum)
for (i in 1:8) {
prob[i]<-equals(rr[i],0)*1/2+
               (1-equals(rr[i],0))*sum(pr[(i+1):10])
nn [i] <-rr[i]+equals(rr[i],0);rr[i]~dbin(prob[i],nn[i])}
for (i in 1:10) {logLGEx[i]<-xx[i]*log(pr[i])}
for (i in 1:8) {logLGEr[i]<-rr[i]*log(prob[i])}
```

```
# compute the likelihood of WB model
prw[1] <- 1-exp(-gamma*pow(tt[1],beta) )
for (i in 2:9) {
prw[i]<-exp(-gamma*pow(tt[i-1],beta))-exp(-gamma*pow(tt[i],beta))}
prw[10] <- exp(-gamma*pow(tt[9],beta) )
xx[1:10] ~ dmulti (prw[], xxsum)
for (i in 1:8) {
prow[i]<-equals(rr[i],0)*1/2+(1-equals(rr[i],0))*sum(pr[(i+1):10])
nw [i] <- rr[i]+equals(rr[i],0)
rr[i] ~ dbin( prow[i], nw[i]) }
for (i in 1:10) {logLWBx[i]<-xx[i]*log(prw[i])}
for (i in 1:8) {logLWBr[i]<-rr[i]*log(prow[i])}
  # prior distributions of parameters
alpha~dunif(1, 2); lambda~dunif(0,1); beta~dunif(1,2)
gamma~dunif(0,1); rho~dbeta(1,1)
}
DATA list(xx=c(18,16,18,10,11,8,13,4,1,0),
       rr= c(1,1,3,0,0,1,2,3,2),
       tt=c(5.5,10.5,15.5,20.5,25.5,30.5,40.5,50.5,60.5))
# Initial values
INITIAL list(alpha=1.5,lambda=0.06,beta=1.2,gamma=0.02,rho=0.25)
INITIAL list(alpha=1.5,lambda=0.06,beta=1.2,gamma=0.02,rho=0.75)
INITIAL list(alpha=1.5,lambda=0.06,beta=1.2,gamma=0.02,rho=0.50)
```

References

Aggarwala, R.: Progressively interval censoring: some mathematical results with application to inference. Commun. Stat. Theory Methods **30**, 1921–1935 (2001)

Balakrishnan, N., Aggarwala, R.: Progressive Censoring: Theory, Methods and Applications. Birkhauser, Boston (2000)

Carbone, P.P., Kellerhouse, L.E., Gehan, E.A.: Plasmacytic myeloma: A study of the relationship of survival to various clinical manifestations and anomalous protein type in 112 patients. Am. J. Med. **42**, 937–948 (1967)

Chen, D.G., Lio, Y.L.: Parameter estimations for generalized exponential distribution under progressive type-I interval censoring. Comput. Stat. Data Anal. **54**, 1581–1591 (2010)

Dempster, A.P., Laird N.M., Rubin, D.B.: Maximum likelihood from incomplete data via the EM algorithm. J. R. Stat. Soc. Ser. B **39**, 1–38 (1977)

Geman, S., Geman, D.: Stochastic relaxation, Gibbs distributions and the Bayesian restoration of images. IEEE Trans. Pattern. Anal. Mach. Intell. **6**, 721–741 (1984)

Green, P.: Reversible jump Markov chain Monte Carlo computation and Bayesian model determination. Biometrika **82**, 711–732 (1995)

Gupta, R.D., Kundu, D.: Generalized exponential distributions. Aust. N. Z. J. Stat. **41**, 173–188 (1999)

Gupta, R.D., Kundu, D.: Exponentiated exponential distribution: an alternative to gamma and Weibull distributions. Biom. J. **43**, 117–130 (2001a)

Gupta, R.D., Kundu, D.: Generalized exponential distributions: different method of estimations. J. Stat. Comput. Simul. **69**, 315–338 (2001b)

Gupta, R.D., Kundu, D.: Generalized exponential distributions: statistical inferences. J. Stat. Theory Appl. **1**, 101–118 (2002)

Gupta, R.D., Kundu, D.: Discriminating between Weibull and generalized exponential distributions. Comput. Stat. Data Anal. **43**, 179–196 (2003)

Gupta, R.D., Kundu, D.: Generalized exponential distributions: existing results and some recent developments. J. Stat. Plann. Inference **137**, 3537–3547 (2007)

Hastings, W.K.: Monte Carlo sampling methods using Markov chains and their applications. Biometrika **57**, 97–109 (1970)

Kundu, D., Gupta, R.D.: Generalized exponential distribution: Bayesian inference. Comput. Stat. Data Anal. 52, 1873–1883 (2008)

Kundu, D., Pradhan, B.: Bayesian inference and life testing plans for generalized exponential distribution. Sci. China Ser. A Math. **52**, 1373–1388 (2009)

Lawless, J.F.: Statistical models and methods for lifetime data, 2nd edn. Wiley, New Jersey (2003)

Lin, Y.-J., Lio, Y.L.: Bayesian inference under progressive type-I interval censoring. J. Appl. Stat. **39**, 1811–1824 (2012)

Metropolis, N., Rosenbluth, A., Rosenblith, M., Teller, A., Teller, E.: Equations of state calculations by fast computing machines. J. Chem. Phys. **21**, 1087–1092 (1953)

Mudholkar, G.S., Srivastava, D.K.: Exponentiated Weibull family for analyzing bathtub failure data. IEEE Trans. Reliab. **42**, 299–302 (1993)

Mudholkar, G.S., Srivastava, D.K., Friemer, M.: The exponentiated Weibull family: a reanalysis of the bus-motor-failure data. Technometrics **37**, 436–445 (1995)

Mudholkar, G.S., Srivastava, D.K., Kollia, G.D.: A generalization of the Weibull distribution with application to the analysis of survival data. J. Am. Stat. Assoc. **91**, 1575–1583 (1996)

Ng, H., Wang, Z.: Statistical estimation for the parameters of Weibull distribution based on progressively type-I interval censored sample. J. Stat. Comput. Simul. **79**, 145–159 (2009)

Robert, C.P., Marin, J.M.: On some difficulties with a posterior probability approximation technique. Bayesian Anal. **3**, 427–442 (2008)

Sun, D.: A note on noninformative priors for Weibull distributions. J. Stat. Plann. Inference **61**, 319–338 (1997)

Techniques for Analyzing Incomplete Data in Public Health Research

Valerie Pare and Ofer Harel

Abstract Statistical inference of incomplete data has been an obstacle in numerous areas of research, and public health studies are no exception. Since studies in this field are often survey-based and can center around sensitive personal information, it can make them susceptible to missing records. This chapter discusses the causes and problems created by incomplete data and recommends techniques for how to handle it through multiple imputation.

1 Introduction

There are several resources available which offer suggestions on how to prevent or reduce non-response and attrition that should be considered in advance of data collection (Little et al. 2012; Chang et al. 2009). There should be a sincere attempt to avoid unplanned non-response when possible, but it is not realistic to assume it can be avoided all together. Even the most well-designed studies are susceptible to missing values! In a research setting in public health, the challenge is even greater. Participants could miss appointments, refuse to respond, become unwell, or simply lose interest in the study.

Since missing values are difficult to control, it is important to know how to move forward and to understand what assumptions you are willing (or unwilling) to make. It should be mentioned that many statistical analysis and estimation procedures were not designed to handle missing values. Conventional statistical methods assume that all variables of a particular model are measured for all cases. Therefore, the software being used, simply by default, may discard all incomplete cases and proceed. A lot of research has been devoted to demonstrating that this approach is only reasonable under some very strict assumptions regarding the nature of the missing data, but is very unreasonable and misleading otherwise. For this reason, a lot of emphasis should be placed on what assumptions are reasonable to make with your data.

V. Pare • O. Harel (✉)
Department of Statistics, University of Connecticut, 215 Glenbrook Road,
Storrs, CT 06269, USA
e-mail: vlpare@gmail.com; ofer.harel@uconn.edu

© Springer International Publishing Switzerland 2015
D.-G. Chen, J. Wilson (eds.), *Innovative Statistical Methods for Public Health Data*,
ICSA Book Series in Statistics, DOI 10.1007/978-3-319-18536-1_8

The first part of this chapter is devoted to the missing data theory, as described by Rubin (1976). It continues with an overview of some ad hoc approaches to handling missing values and describes the inherent faults with these techniques. Likelihood-based methods and multiple imputation are then discussed with particular attention given towards multiple imputation. Next, an overview of useful R packages for visualization of missing data and analysis through multiple imputation are presented. An example in public health is also used to demonstrate the impact of missing data and the utility of multiple imputation for obtaining unbiased and efficient estimates.

2   Overview of Missing Data

A key component in understanding how to treat missing data is to first understand the nature of how and why it is missing. This is important since all the missing data techniques that we discuss require some assumptions regarding the missing values. Unfortunately, it may not always be straightforward what assumptions are viable. Data can be missing for a variety of reasons; including equipment failure, extreme weather conditions, or a participant's refusal to provide a response. While it is unlikely to know the exact reason why each piece of data is missing, it is often necessary to examine the *pattern of missingness* and to make assumptions regarding the *mechanism of missingness*.

2.1   Pattern of Missingness

Let the complete data be denoted by $Y_{n \times p}$ where n denotes the number of observational units and p represents the number of variables. The pattern of missingness describes which variables are missing and where the missing data are located. Schafer and Graham (2002) describe some of the patterns of missingness which include univariate, monotone, and arbitrary patterns. A univariate pattern describes the situation in which missingness occurs in only one of the variables while all other variables are completely observed. A monotone pattern is often used to describe a dropout pattern. That is, an observational unit has observed values up until the ith position, but has all subsequent values missing. Finally, an arbitrary pattern describes when missing values occur in no particular pattern.

Figure 1 shows some examples of each type of missingness pattern. These plots are available with the R package VIM and are a useful initial assessment of your data. Evaluating these plots can illustrate the frequency at which particular variables are missing and can show particular patterns in the data. In Fig. 1a, 59 % of experimental units have observed data for variables $x_1 - x_4$, whereas 41 % of experimental units have observed data for variables $x_1 - x_3$, but have missing values for x_4. This is a univariate missingness pattern since the only missing values in that particular data set occurred in one of the variables, in our case, x_4.

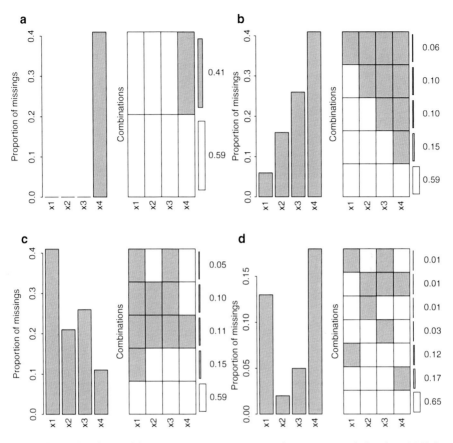

Fig. 1 Examples of potential non-response patterns: *gray* regions represent missing data. (**a**) Univariate missingness. (**b**) Monotone missingness (i). (**c**) Monotone missingness (ii). (**d**) Arbitrary missingness

In Fig. 1b, 59 % of experimental units have observed data for variables $x_1 - x_4$, whereas 41 % of experimental units have some occurrence of missing data. It is considered a monotone pattern since if we arrange the variables from least amount of missing values to most amount of missing values, the following pattern holds: if x_1 is missing, it automatically implies that x_2, x_3, and x_4 are missing, and if x_2 is missing, it automatically implies that x_3 and x_4 are missing, and if x_3 is missing, it automatically implies that x_4 is missing. If the variables, x_1, x_2, x_3, x_4, represented time point measurements, this would describe the different patterns of dropout. Figure 1c shows monotone missingness in a less obvious way, when there is no meaningful ordering of the variables. Re-arranging the variables from the least amount of missing to the most amount of missing would allow you to see the same pattern. Figure 1d shows an example of arbitrary missing values where no particular pattern can be deciphered.

An indicator matrix $R_{n \times p}$ can also be used to indicate the pattern of non-response. The entries in R are defined as $r_{ij} = 1$, $i = 1, \ldots, n$ and $j = 1, \ldots, p$, if the observation for the jth variable of subject i is missing (y_{ij}), and $r_{ij} = 0$ for observations that are observed.

2.2 Missingness Mechanisms

In order to implement any missing data method, assumptions need to be made on how the data came to be missing. The mechanism of missingness gives a probabilistic definition for the missing values. Let Y be partitioned into its observed and missing components as (Y_{obs}, Y_{mis}). The statistical model for missing data is $P(R|Y, \varphi)$ where φ is the parameter for the missing data process. The mechanism of missingness is determined by the dependency of R on the variables in the data set.

Typically, there are three missingness mechanisms that are considered including missing completely at random (MCAR), missing at random (MAR), and missing not at random (MNAR) (Rubin 1976; Little and Rubin 2002).

2.2.1 Missing Completely at Random

The strongest of the missing data assumptions is MCAR. It implies that the probability of missing values is unrelated to observed and unobserved values. This mechanism of missingness is given by

$$P(R|Y_{obs}, Y_{mis}, \varphi) = P(R|\varphi),$$

for all values of φ and at the realized values of R and Y_{obs}. In other words, the missing values are a random sample of all data values.

Little (1988) lists a number of important instances where verification of MCAR is important. One reason is that many methods for handling incomplete data will work well when this assumption is valid.

Is MCAR a realistic assumption for your data? It depends. Imagine a situation where the collection of all data is costly. Therefore, researchers may design a study in which the data on particular variables is only collected on a complete random sample of participants. This refers to a study that is missing by design (Graham et al. 1996) and since the data is not missing for any reason related to the given variable or other observed values, then missing completely at random can be considered a reasonable assumption. If the data is not missing due to a known and completely random process, then MCAR may be difficult to justify. We will discuss some methods used for determining types of missingness in Sect. 2.2.4.

2.2.2 Missing at Random

Data are missing at random if the probability of missing values can be described through observed values only. This mechanism is given by

$$P(R|Y_{obs}, Y_{mis}, \varphi) = P(R|Y_{obs}, \varphi),$$

for all values of φ and at realized values of R and Y_{obs}. This mechanism requires that the missing values are a random sample of all values within a subclass defined by the observed data. Notice that MCAR is a special case of MAR.

Is MAR a realistic assumption for your data? Again, it depends. Consider a study where particular variables of interest can only be measured through biopsies. Since biopsies can be costly, invasive, and risky, it may only be ethical to perform a biopsy if the participant is considered high risk. If risk is an observed and measured characteristic of all participants and if the probability that a participant is biopsied can be fully explained by risk, then the missing biopsy data could be considered MAR. This is another case of data that is missing by design. However, if the data is missing for reasons not controlled (or fully understood) by the experimenter, then the assumption of missing at random may be difficult to justify.

In Bayesian or likelihood-based inference, if the parameters that govern the missingness mechanism (φ) are distinct from the parameters of the data model (θ) and if the data is MAR or MCAR, then the missing data mechanism is said to be ignorable (Little and Rubin 2002). These parameters are considered distinct if the joint prior distribution for θ and φ is equal to the product of two independent priors. From a frequentist perspective, the parameters are distinct if the joint parameter space is the Cartesian cross-product of the individual parameter spaces of θ and φ (Schafer 1997). There is a marked benefit to being able to classify the missingness mechanism as ignorable in that one does not have to model the mechanism by which the data became missing.

2.2.3 Missing Not at Random

If the relationship of MAR does not hold, then data are missing not at random. This implies that the probability that a value is missing cannot be described fully by observed values. MNAR data automatically implies that the missing data mechanism is non-ignorable. That means that valid estimation would require that the missing data mechanism be modeled. Unfortunately, this is not an easy task and inferences could be highly sensitive to any misspecification. Non-ignorable missing data techniques are not covered in this chapter. Some resources to consider in the event of non-ignorable missingness are Little and Rubin (2002), Fitzmaurice et al. (2011), and Diggle and Kenward (1994).

2.2.4 Supporting Assumptions of Non-Response

It may be difficult to decipher whether data are missing completely at random, missing at random, or missing not at random . Plots may aid in this process. One type of plot that can be potentially enlightening is a matrix plot that helps to detect dependencies and patterns in the missing values. This plot can be constructed using the R package VIM (Templ et al. 2013). Missing values are colored in red and observed values are sorted from lowest to highest and assigned a shade of gray. White and light shades of gray correspond to relatively smaller values, and dark shades of gray and black correspond to larger values. The data matrix can be sorted by the magnitude of a specified variable.

Figure 2 shows one example. The upper left plot is sorted by variable x_1. Here you can see that there is a clear relationship between the value of x_1 and whether x_4 is missing. That is, smaller values of x_1 are associated with missing values of x_4, and larger values of x_1 are associated with observed values of x_4. Hence, it is clear that the data is not missing completely at random. If it was fair to assume that the missingness was deterministic based on the value of x_1, then we can assume that the data is missing at random. Examining the upper right and lower left plots (which are sorted by x_2 and x_3 respectively), there is no obvious relationship between the values of x_2 and x_3 with regard to whether x_4 is observed. Again, the lower right plot shows that there is a clear relationship between the value of x_1 and the missingness of x_4. These plots help capture whether missingness depends on one of the variables,

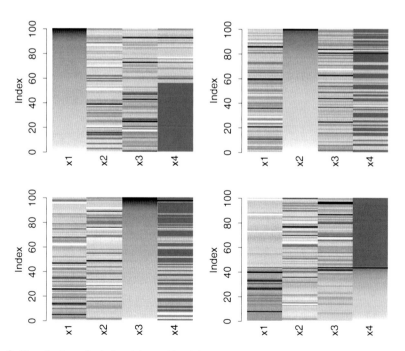

Fig. 2 Visualization of missing data: matrix plots

but it may be more challenging to detect whether missingness depends on a linear combination of observed variables. Therefore, use caution when interpreting these plots to make any definitive statement regarding the nature of the missing values.

Is there any other way to check the plausibility of MCAR? One possibility is to compare the observed variable means for participants with complete data against those with incomplete data. For example, suppose we have a data set with variables age, alcohol consumption, and sexual risk. Participants with and without missing values on sexual risk could be compared on age and alcohol consumption via t-tests. Significant differences between participants with complete data and participants with incomplete data would suggest that the data was not MCAR.

Little (1988) proposed an omnibus chi-square test for MCAR to control for inflated Type I error rates when multiple t-tests would be required. Jamshidian and Jalal (2010) proposed a normal-theory test and a nonparametric test of homoscedasticity to be used for testing for MCAR. This test is available in the R package MissMech (Jamshidian et al. 2014). If the p-value of this test is less than 0.05, then the data should not be assumed to be MCAR.

Another possibility is to run a logistic regression of R on the predictor variables. If any of the coefficients of the logistic regression model are significantly different from 0, then it would imply that data is not MCAR.

It should be noted that the above methods will only detect whether the values are missing due to the values that are observed and will not detect whether the values are missing due to values that are not observed. Therefore, these tests may help justify the plausibility of MCAR, but still require assumptions beyond what can be tested.

Is there a way to test the data for MAR? Unfortunately, unless there was a way to follow up with non-responders, then the answer is no. An expert may have reason to suspect that data is missing for a particular known and measured reason, but there is nothing in the data that will allow us to test whether or not this is actually the case. Despite this, it may be reasonable assumption if there are variables available that are highly correlated with the missing variable. Schafer and Graham (2002) discuss many cases where the MAR assumption is reasonable.

In the remainder of this chapter, we focus on situations of ignorable missingness and offer a brief overview of options available for non-ignorable missingness. Additional resources are available for the latter case.

3 Missing Data Methods

It is well documented that ad hoc treatments for missing data can lead to serious problems including loss of efficiency, biased results, and underestimation of error variation (Belin 2009; White and Carlin 2010; Harel et al. 2012). Many methods have been discounted for leading to one of those aforementioned problems.

One such method is complete case analysis (CCA) which deletes observational units with any missing values. Therefore, if the data is not MCAR, then implementing such a procedure may fail to account for the systematic difference between observed and not fully observed cases. This will potentially cause bias in inferences of parameters. Even if the data is MCAR, CCA will result in a marked loss of efficiency depending on the proportion of incomplete cases.

A second missing data method is single imputation in which researchers replace missing values with some plausible values. There are a wide range of procedures which seek to fill in these missing values including mean imputation, hot deck imputation, regression imputation, or, in longitudinal settings, last observation carried forward. All of these methods have been shown to underestimate the error variation which will lead to inflated Type I error. These imputation methods are discussed in detail by Schafer and Graham (2002).

There are several more sophisticated methods for treating incomplete data that perform much better than the above methods including maximum likelihood estimation via the EM algorithm (Dempster et al. 1977), Bayesian analysis (Gelman et al. 2003), and multiple imputations (Rubin 1987). This chapter focuses on multiple imputation and will therefore be discussed in detail in the following section.

4 Multiple Imputation

One principled method for handling incomplete data is with multiple imputation (Rubin 1987). This method can be applied to an array of different models, which can make it more appealing than other principled missing data techniques. The procedure entails creating several data sets by replacing missing values with a set of plausible values that represent the uncertainty about the true unobserved values. There are three stages of multiple imputation: (1) Imputation: Replace each missing value with $m > 1$ imputations under a suitable model, (2) Analysis: Analyze each of the completed data sets using complete data techniques, and (3) Combination: Combine the m sets of estimates and standard errors using Rubin's (1987) rules.

4.1 Imputation Stage

There are some considerations that should be made during the imputation stage. You will need to decide on appropriate variables to use for imputation, the type of imputation approach you will use, and how many imputations you should make.

4.1.1 Approaches

There are two general approaches to imputing multivariate data-joint modeling and chained equations (van Buuren and Oudshoorn 2000). Both approaches should begin by deciding on what variables should be used for imputation. Collins et al.

(2001) found that including all auxiliary variables in the imputation model prevents one from inadvertently omitting important causes of missingness. This will aid in the plausibility of the missing at random assumption. That is, there is evidence which suggests that the imputation model should utilize all available variables, including those that are not of specific interest for the analysis. At the very least you should include all variables that will be used in your analysis.

The first approach, joint modeling, involves specifying a multivariate distribution for the data, and drawing imputations from the conditional distributions of $Y_{mis}|Y_{obs}$ usually by MCMC techniques. The multivariate normal distribution is the most widely used probability model for continuous multivariate data (Schafer 1997). Schafer (1997) mentions that even when data sets deviate from this distribution, the multivariate normal model may still be useful in the imputation framework. One obvious reason for this is that a suitable transformation may help make the assumption of multivariate normality seem more realistic. Further, in many settings it is believed that inference by multiple imputation is relatively robust to departures from the imputation model, particularly when there are small amounts of missing information (Schafer 1997).

Suppose we have a set of variables $x_1, x_2, \ldots, x_k$ that are believed to follow a multivariate normal distribution. The parameters of this joint distribution are estimated from the observed data. Then, the missing values are imputed from the conditional distribution (also multivariate normal) of the missing values given the observed values for each missing data pattern. Under the assumption of multivariate normality, we can use the R package norm (Schafer 2012) to perform these imputations.

The chained equation approach specifies a multivariate imputation model by a series of univariate conditional regressions for each incomplete variable. For example, suppose we have a set of variables, $x_1, x_2, \ldots, x_k$, where x_1, x_2, x_3 have some missing values. Suppose further that x_1 is binary, x_2 is count, and x_3 is continuous. The chained equations approach would proceed in the following steps:

- Initially, all missing values are filled in at random
- Then, for all cases where x_1 is observed, a logistic regression is performed where x_1 is regressed on $x_2, \ldots, x_k$.
- Missing values for x_1 are then replaced by simulated draws from the posterior predictive distribution of x_1.
- Then, for all cases where x_2 is observed, a Poisson regression is performed where x_2 is regressed on $x_1, x_3, \ldots, x_k$
- Missing values for x_2 are then replaced by simulated draws from the posterior predictive distribution of x_2.
- Then, for all cases where x_3 is observed, a linear regression is performed where x_3 is regressed on $x_1, x_2, x_4, \ldots, x_k$
- Missing values for x_3 are then replaced by simulated draws from the posterior predictive distribution of x_3.
- The process is repeated several times

The R package mice (van Buuren and Groothuis-Oudshoorn 2011) can be used for the chained equations approach and the documentation covers additional scenarios.

4.2   Analysis and Combination Stage

Next, each of the M data sets can be analyzed using complete data methods. Suppose that Q is a quantity of interest—an example might be a mean or a regression coefficient. Assume that with complete data, inference about Q would be based on the statement that $Q - \hat{Q} \sim N(0, U)$ where $\hat{Q}$ is the complete-data statistic estimating parameter Q, and U is the complete-data statistic providing the variance of $Q - \hat{Q}$. Since each missing value is replaced by M simulated values, we have M complete data sets and M estimates of Q and U. The overall estimate of Q is

$$\bar{Q} = \frac{1}{M} \sum_{m=1}^{M} \hat{Q}^{(m)},$$

which is simply the average of $\hat{Q}$ across each imputed data set.

To get the variance estimate for $\bar{Q}$, there are two sources of variability which must be appropriately combined. These two sources of variability are the within-imputation variance $(\bar{U})$ and the between-imputation variance (B), where

$$\bar{U} = \frac{1}{M} \sum_{m=1}^{M} U^{(m)} \text{ and}$$

$$B = \frac{1}{M-1} \sum_{m=1}^{M} (\hat{Q}^{(m)} - \bar{Q})^2,$$

and where $U^{(m)}$ is the variance across each imputed data set. The total variance (T) of $(Q - \bar{Q})$ is then

$$T = \bar{U} + (1 + \frac{1}{M})B.$$

In the equation above, $\bar{U}$ estimates the variance if the data were complete and $(1 + \frac{1}{M})B$ estimates the increase in variance due to the missing data (Rubin 1987).

Interval estimates and significance levels for the scalar Q are based on a Student-t reference distribution

$$T^{-1/2}(Q - \bar{Q}) \sim t_v,$$

where the degrees of freedom follows from

$$v = (M - 1)\left(1 + \frac{\bar{U}}{(1 + M^{-1})B}\right)^2.$$

Various improved estimates for v have been proposed over the years (Barnard and Rubin 1999; Reiter 2007; Marchenko and Reiter 2009). Wagstaff and Harel (2011) compared the various estimates and found those of Barnard and Rubin (1999) and Reiter (2007) performed satisfactorily.

Thankfully, draws from the posterior predictive distribution, along with combination of parameter estimates (including the extension to multivariate parameter estimates) can be accomplished with R packages mice and norm and are discussed in the example to follow.

4.3 Rates of Missing Information

One way to describe the impact of missing data uncertainty is in a measure called rate of missing information (Rubin 1987). This measure can be used in diagnostics to indicate how missing data influences the quantity being estimated (Schafer 1997). If Y_{mis} carries no information about Q, then the estimates of $\hat{Q}$ across each imputed data set are identical. Thus, the total variance (T) reduces to $\bar{U}$. Therefore, $(1 + M^{-1})B/\bar{U}$ estimates the relative increase in variance due to missing data. An estimate of the rate of missing information due to Y_{mis} is

$$\hat{\gamma} = \frac{B}{\bar{U} + B},$$

which does not tend to decrease as the number of imputations increases (Rubin 1987).

Harel (2007) establishes the asymptotic behavior of $\hat{\gamma}$ to help determine the number of imputations necessary when accurate estimates of the missing-information rates are of interest. From this distribution, an approximate 95 % confidence interval for the population rate of missing information is

$$\hat{\gamma} \pm \frac{1.96\hat{\gamma}(1 - \hat{\gamma})}{\sqrt{M/2}},$$

which can aid in determining the approximate number of imputations necessary under a desired level of precision. Since the maximum number of required imputations is for $\hat{\gamma} = 0.5$, it is a safe estimate when we do not have an understanding of how influential the missing values are on the quantity being estimated.

When the main interest is point estimates (and their variances), it is sufficient to use only a modest number of imputations (5–10) (Rubin 1987). However, as we just illustrated, when the rates of missing information are of interest, more imputations are required. In addition, there is a general trend to increase the number of imputations particularly when p-values are of interest (Graham et al. 2007; Bodner 2008; White et al. 2011).

5   Example

Let's look at a study of sexual risk behavior in South Africa. Cain et al. (2012) studied the effects of patronizing alcohol serving establishments (shebeens) and alcohol use in predicting HIV risk behaviors. For the data of this particular analysis, men and women were recruited from inside shebeens and in the surrounding areas near shebeens in 8 different communities. Surveys were administered to measure demographic characteristics, alcohol use, shebeen attendance, and sexual risk behaviors. It was of interest to determine whether social influences and environmental factors in shebeens attribute to sexual risk behavior independently of alcohol consumption. The variables of interest are:

GENDER	1 if female, 0 if male
AGE	Age of survey participant
UNEMP	1 if unemployed, 0 if employed
ALC	alcohol index
SHEBEEN	1 if attends shebeen, 0 if does not attend
RBI	risk behavior index

The alcohol index was measured as the product of alcohol use frequency and alcohol consumption quantity. The risk behavior index was measured as the logarithm of one plus the product of number of sexual partners in the past 30 days and number of unprotected sex acts in the past 30 days. The ultimate goal is to predict this risky behavior index from all other independent variables.

The original analysis utilized 1,473 people, which will serve as our completely observed data. We deliberately introduce missing data on several of the variables under the missing at random assumption for illustrative purposes. For AGE, 24 % of observations were removed conditional on GENDER. For ALC, 29 % of observations were removed conditional on GENDER and RBI. For RBI, 49 % of observations were removed conditional on Shebeen attendance and auxiliary information regarding the community where recruited. Suppose community 4 had a much higher prevalence of missing RBI responses. Data was imposed as missing based on the probabilities derived from the following models:

$\text{Logit}(P(\text{AGE missing})) = 0.10 + 0.15 \times \text{GENDER}$
$\text{Logit}(P(\text{ALC missing})) = -0.35 + 0.65 \times \text{GENDER} - 0.05 \times \text{RBI}$
$\text{Logit}(P(\text{RBI missing})) = -0.5 + 1.03 \times \text{SHEBEEN} + 1.5 \times \text{COMM4}$

Listwise deletion on this set of variables leaves 399 records, which is less than one-third the original sample size.

Now, let's forget for a moment that we understand the nature of how the data came to be missing. Ordinarily, we would be uncertain of this process and would be required to make some assumptions. Initial visualizations on our data set 'risk' are performed using the following R code:

```
>   # load required package
>   require(VIM)
>   # create pattern of missingness plot
>   aggr(risk, delimiter = NULL, col=c('grey'), plot = TRUE, numbers=T, prop=t)
>   # adjust plot settings
>   par(mfrow=c(3,2))
>   # construct matrix plots sorting by each variable of interest to the analysis
>   matrixplot(risk, sortby='GENDER', interactive=F)
>   matrixplot(risk, sortby='AGE', interactive=F)
>   matrixplot(risk, sortby='UNEMP', interactive=F)
>   matrixplot(risk, sortby='RBI', interactive=F)
>   matrixplot(risk, sortby='SHEBEEN', interactive=F)
>   matrixplot(risk, sortby='ALC', interactive=F)
```

Figures 3 and 4 show the resulting output. We see that there is an arbitrary pattern of missingness and that there are no clearly visible relationships in the matrix plots that might explain why the data came to be missing. Next, we may want to examine the plausibility of the MCAR assumption:

```
>   # load required package
>   require(MissMech)
>   # test for MCAR
>   TestMCARNormality(risk)
```

The output for this test states that the hypothesis of MCAR is rejected at the 0.05 significance level. This indicates that missing values are unlikely due to complete random chance (no surprise to us!). Further, this tells us that if we ran an analysis of just the complete cases, that our estimates may be biased. The following code could be used in the event that CCA is appropriate and if there is little concern for the reduction in sample size:

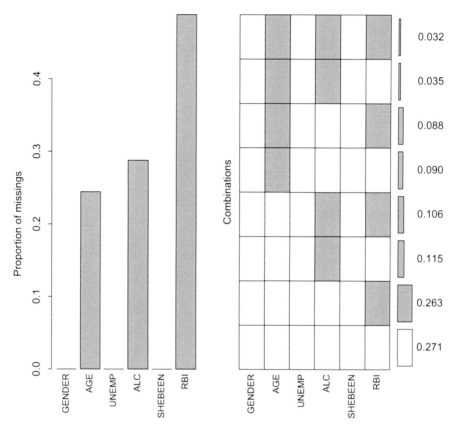

Fig. 3 Data example: missingness pattern

```
>  CCAModel=lm(RBI ~ GENDER + AGE + UNEMP + ALC +SHEBEEN, data=risk)
>  summary(CCAModel)
```

Suppose that subject experts feel that MAR is a reasonable assumption. Since we have auxiliary information available, we will proceed with constructing imputations with all available variables in the data set. In addition to the variables of primary interest in our model, we also include:

COMM   Identifies location of recruitment (1–8)
STRESS   Index measure of self-perceived feelings of stress (rated low to high)
GBV   Index measure of attitude towards gender based violence

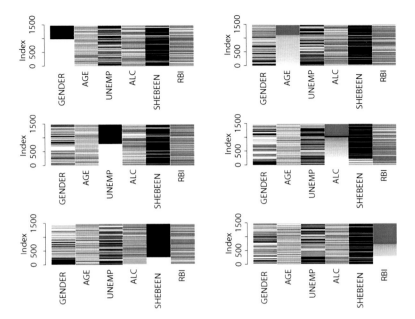

Fig. 4 Data example: matrix plots

Using the recommendation from Sect. 4.3, if we are also interested in obtaining the rates of missing information for our estimates of interest with 95 % confidence and margin of error 0.04, then approximately 300 imputations are required.

Under the joint modeling approach, we would now have to decide on a joint model for our data. Suppose we assume that the variables form a multivariate normal model. We could then obtain imputations with the following code:

```
> # install required package for generating imputations
> require(norm)
> # install required package for pooling results
> require(mice)
> # required preliminary manipulations of data
> risk←as.matrix(risk)
> s=prelim.norm(risk)
> # find the MLE for a starting value
> thetahat=em.norm(s)
> # set a random seed
> rngseed(1217)
> # set number of imputations
> M=300
> # where we store the M fit objects of our analysis
```

(continued)

```
>  results=list()
>  # generate imputations using data augmentation
>  for(i in 1:M){
       imps=da.norm(s, start=thetahat, steps=100,
           showits=FALSE, return.ymis=TRUE)$ymis
       imputeddata← risk
           for(j in 1:length(imps)){
               imputeddata[which(is.na(risk))[j]]=imps[j]
               }
       imputeddata←data.frame(imputeddata)
       results[[i]]=lm(RBI ~ AGE + GENDER+ UNEMP+ ALC +
           SHEBEEN, data=imputeddata)
               }
>  # take the results of complete-data analysis from the imputed data sets,
>  # and turn it into a mira object that can be pooled
>  results←as.mira(results)
>  # combine results from M imputed data sets with df estimate from Barnard and Rubin
   (1999)
>  analysis←summary(pool(results, method="small sample"))
>  # view results
>  analysis
```

While multivariate normality may not seem the most realistic model (we have several dichotomous variables), more complex models are not as readily available. This is where the chained equations approach makes sense to use. For our data, GENDER and SHEBEEN are fully observed. We impute our data assumed to be normally distributed using Bayesian linear regression, our dichotomous variables using logistic regression, and our categorical variables using predictive mean matching. Specifically, we impute AGE, ALC, RBI, STRESS, and GBV using Bayesian linear regression, UNEMP using logistic regression, and COMM using predictive mean matching. These methods are specified in the mice function on the 5th line of the code below. There are many other methods available and details can be found in van Buuren and Groothuis-Oudshoorn (2011). The following displays our code for generating imputations under this approach:

```
>  # load required package
>  require(mice)
>  # generate multiple imputations using chained equations
>  mids←mice(risk, m=M, printFlag=F,
       method=c('', 'norm','logreg','norm','','norm','pmm','norm','norm'))
>  fit←with(data=mids, exp=lm(RBI ~ GENDER + AGE + UNEMP + ALC +SHE-
   BEEN, data=risk))
```

(continued)

Many longitudinal studies suffer from missing data due to subjects dropping into or out of a study or not being available at some measurement times, which can cause bias in the analysis if the missingness are informative. For likelihood procedures of estimating linear mixed models, we may generally ignore the distribution of missing indicators when the missing data are MAR (or ignorable likelihood estimation), that is missingness depends only on observed information. However, when the missing data mechanism is related to the unobservable missing values, the missing data are non-ignorable and the distribution of missingness has to be considered. To account for informative missingness, a number of model based approaches have been proposed to jointly model the longitudinal outcome and the non-ignorable missing mechanism. Little and Rubin (2002) described three major formulations of joint modeling approaches: selection model, pattern-mixture model, and shared-parameter model, while Verbeke and Molenberghs (2000) provided applications for these models in their book. Other researchers have extended this field in the last decade. Some authors have incorporated latent class structure into pattern-mixture models to jointly describe the pattern of missingness and the outcome of interest (Lin et al. 2004; Muthén et al. 2003; Roy 2003). Lin et al. (2004) proposed a latent pattern-mixture model where the mixture patterns are formed from latent classes that link a longitudinal response with a missingness process. Roy (2003) investigated latent classes to model dropouts in longitudinal studies to effectively reduce the number of missing-data patterns. Muthén et al. (2003) also discussed how latent classes could be applied to non-ignorable missingness. Jung et al. (2011) extended traditional latent class models, where the classes are defined by the missingness indicators alone.

All the above extensions are from the family of pattern-mixture models, and these models stratify the data according to time to dropout or missing indicators alone and formulate a model for each stratum. This usually results in under-identifiability since we need to estimate many pattern-specific parameters, even though the eventual interest is usually on the marginal parameters. Further, there is a controversial and also important practical modeling issue in using latent class models, which is determining a suitable number of latent classes. Some authors suggested a criterion approach as a way of comparing models with different number of classes. In our work using simulation studies, we found that the selection of latent classes is sensitive to many factors that relate to missing data, and a simulation study on selection latent classes is strongly recommended if one wants to apply latent class modeling for missing data. Moreover, the uncertainty of model selection makes latent class models inefficient in estimating population parameters. Instead of modeling missing indicators with latent categorical classes, one possible alternative approach is to model missingness as continuous latent variables.

As the alternative, Guo et al. (2004) extended pattern-mixture to a random pattern-mixture model for longitudinal data with dropouts. The extended model works effectively on the case where a good surrogate for the dropout can be representative for the dropout process. In most real studies, however, it maybe impossible to find good measures for the missing mechanism. For instance, in a longitudinal study with many intermittent missing values, time to dropout is not necessarily a good measure, and it probably would not capture most features of missingness. That is, this measurement cannot represent for subjects who have drop-in responses. Instead, modeling for missing indicators is necessary in this case. Further, models other than the normal distribution will be required to describe the missingness process. The violation of joint multivariate normality will lead to an increase of computation difficulties. In the proposed new model, missing indicators are directly modeled with a continuous latent variable, and this latent factor is treated as a predictor for latent subject-level random effects in the primary model of interests. Some informative variables related with missingness (e.g. time to first missing, number of switches between observed and missing responses) will serve as covariates in the modeling of missing indicators. A detailed description of the new model will be given in the next section.

2.1   Review of Continuous Latent Factor Model for Binary Outcomes

For analyzing multivariate categorical data, continuous latent factor modeling which is often referred to as categorical variable factor analysis (Muthén 1978) and item response modeling (Lord 1980; Embretson and Reise 2000) probably is the most widely used method. In the terminology of educational testing, the involved binary variables are called items and the observed values are referred to as binary or dichotomous responses. In this paper, we will extend this model to describe missing data procedure.

Let $r_{i1}, \ldots, r_{iJ}$ be the J binary responses (missing indicators) on J given time points for a given individual i out of a sample of n individuals, $i = 1, \ldots, n$ and $j = 1, \ldots, J$. In concrete cases 1 and 0 may correspond to an observed or unobserved outcome in a longitudinal study. In the continuous latent factor model there are two sets of parameters. The probability of r_{ij} being 1 or 0 can depend on an individual parameter u_i, specific and characteristic for the individual in study. This parameter is also referred to as a latent parameter. In addition, the probability may depend on a parameter for different time points (items) τ_j, characteristic for the particular time point.

We use the following notation to define the probability of a missing outcome as a function of the latent individual factor:

$$\pi_{ij}(\tau_j) = Pr(r_{ij} = 1 | u_i).$$

It is usually assumed that $\pi_{ij}(\tau_j)$ is monotonously increasing from 0 to 1 as u_i runs from $-\infty$ to ∞, and that ξ_j is the 50%-point, i.e. $\pi_{ij}(\xi_j) = 0.5$. A typical latent trait plot is shown in Fig. 1.

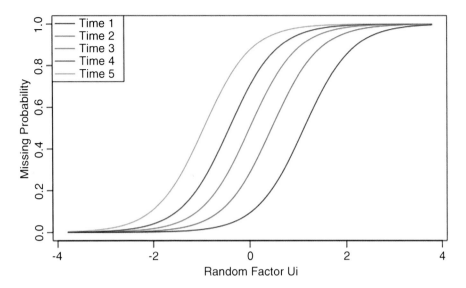

Fig. 1 A typical latent trait plot

In the literature two main models for a latent trait have been suggested. The normal ogive or probit model is given by

$$\pi_{ij}(u_i) = \Phi(u_i - \tau_j),$$

where $\Phi(x)$ is the cumulative normal distribution function. Alternatively we may use the logistic or logit model,

$$\pi_{ij}(u_i) = \Psi(u_i - \tau_j),$$

where $\Psi(x) = e^x/(1 + e^x)$ $(-\infty < x < \infty)$ is the cumulative distribution function of the standard logistic random variable.

There is a series of continuous latent variable models for different kinds of categorical data. Here, we present the two-parameter (2PL) item response model for binary data, which could be reduced to the model discussed above. The 2PL model is used to estimate the probability (π_{ij}) of a missing response for subject i and time point j while considering the item (time)-varying parameters, τ_{2j} for item (time) location parameters, and τ_{1j} for item (time) slope parameters, which allow for different weights for different times, and the person-varying latent trait variables u_i. The 2PL model is expressed as

$$logit(\pi_{ij}) = \tau_{1j}(u_i - \tau_{2j}).$$

As τ_{1j} increases, the item (time) has a stronger association with the underlying missingness. When τ_{1j} is fixed to be 1, the 2PL model is reduced to be a Rasch model (Rasch 1960) or a 1PL model. As τ_{2j} increases, the response is more likely to be observed. This 2PL model has been shown to be mathematically equivalent to be confirmatory factor analysis model for binary data (Takane and de-Leeuw 1987). The IRT models can be expressed as generalized mixed or multilevel models (Adams et al. 1997; Rijmen et al. 2003). Considering a mixed logistic regression model for binary data:

$$Pr(r_{ij} = 1|\mathbf{x}_{ij}, \mathbf{z}_{ij}, \boldsymbol{\beta}, \mathbf{u}_i) = \frac{exp(\mathbf{x}_{ij}^T\boldsymbol{\beta} + \mathbf{z}_{ij}^T\mathbf{u}_i)}{1 + exp(\mathbf{x}_{ij}^T\boldsymbol{\beta} + \mathbf{z}_{ij}^T\mathbf{u}_i)}$$

where r_{ij} is the binary response variable for subject i at time j, $i = 1,\ldots,n$; $j = 1,\ldots,J$; $\mathbf{x}_{ij}$ is a known P-dimensional covariate vector for the P fixed effects; $\mathbf{z}_{ij}$ is a known Q dimensional design vector for the Q random effects; $\boldsymbol{\beta}$ is the P-dimensional parameter vector of fixed effects; and $\mathbf{u}_i$ is the Q-dimensional parameter vector of random effects for subject i. In this model, the binary responses are assumed to be independent Bernoulli conditional on the covariates, the fixed effects, as well as the random effects. This conditional independence assumption is often referred to in the latent variable model literature as the assumption of local independence. The described model comes from the family of the generalized linear mixed models in which the observations are relations from a Bernoulli distribution (belonging to the exponential family), mean $\mu_{ij} = p(r_{ij} = 1|\mathbf{x}_{ij})$, and the canonical link function is the logit function. The IRT model is formally equivalent to a nonlinear mixed model, where the latent variable $\mathbf{u}_i$ is the random effect; time covariate τ_{2j} and slope parameter τ_{1j} are treated as fixed effects. Raudenbush et al. (2003) also reexpressed the Rasch model and the 2PL model as a two-level logistic model by including dummy variables indicating item numbers (time locations).

2.2 Proposed Model

In this section we present a continuous latent factor model (CLFM) for longitudinal data with non-ignorable missingness. For a J-time period study which may have as many as 2^J possible missing patterns, modeling the relationship among the missing indicators and their relationships to the observed data is a challenge. The underlying logic of our new model comes from the assumption that a continuous latent variable exists and allows flexibly for modeling missing indicators. Suppose we have a data set with n independent individuals. For individual i ($i = 1,\cdots,n$), let $\mathbf{Y}_i = (Y_{i1},\cdots,Y_{iJ})'$ be a J-dimensional observed vector with continuous elements used to measure a q-dimensional continuous latent variable $\mathbf{b}_i$. Let $\mathbf{R}_i = (r_{i1},\cdots,r_{iJ})'$ be a J-dimensional missing data indicator vector with binary elements and u_i be a continuous latent variable, which is used to measure $\mathbf{R}_i$. The primary

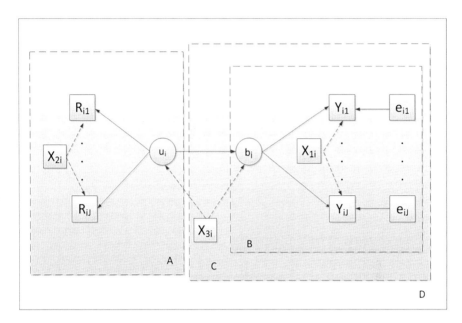

Fig. 2 Proposed model diagram: observed quantities are described in *squared boxes*, latent quantities are in *circled boxes*

model of interest will be the joint distribution of $\mathbf{Y}_i$ and $\mathbf{R}_i$, given u_i and possibly additional observed covariates $\mathbf{X}_i$, where $\mathbf{X}_i$ represents p-dimensional fully observed covariates. Figure 2 provides a diagram representing the proposed model for all the observed and latent variables. As indicated in Fig. 2, $\mathbf{X}_{1i}$, containing both time-variant and time-invariant attributes for subject i, is the p_1 dimensional covariates and used in model B; $\mathbf{X}_{2i}$ is the p_2 dimensional covariates used in model A; a p_3 dimensional time-invariant covariate vector $\mathbf{X}_{3i}$ is used in modeling link function between $\mathbf{b}_i$ and u_i. These three covariate-vectors form the covariates for the model, i.e. $p = p_1 + p_2 + p_3$.

One of the fundamental assumptions of this new model is that $\mathbf{Y}_i$ is conditionally independent of $\mathbf{R}_i$ given the latent variables u_i and $\mathbf{b}_i$. This is a natural assumption when modeling relationships between variables measured with error, i.e., we want to model the relationship between the underlying variables, not the ones with error. Finally, we assume that $\mathbf{Y}_i$ is conditionally independent of u_i given $\mathbf{b}_i$, and likewise, $\mathbf{R}_i$ is conditionally independent of $\mathbf{b}_i$ given u_i. Hence, we introduce the following model for the joint distribution of the responses $\mathbf{Y}_i$ and missing indicators $\mathbf{R}_i$,

$$f(\mathbf{Y}_i, \mathbf{R}_i|\mathbf{X}_i) = \iint f(\mathbf{Y}_i|\mathbf{b}_i, \mathbf{X}_{1i})f(\mathbf{R}_i|u_i, \mathbf{X}_{2i})f(\mathbf{b}_i|u_i, \mathbf{X}_{3i})f(u_i)du_id\mathbf{b}_i \quad (1)$$

with specific parametric models specified as follows: ($N_p(\mathbf{a}, B)$ denotes the p-variate normal distribution with mean $\mathbf{a}$ and covariance matrix B)

$$(\mathbf{Y}_i|\mathbf{b}_i, \mathbf{X}_{1i}) \sim_{ind} N_J(\mathbf{X}_{1i}\boldsymbol{\beta} + \mathbf{Z}_{1i}\mathbf{b}_i, \Sigma_\epsilon) \tag{2}$$

$$(\mathbf{b}_i|u_i, \mathbf{X}_{3i}) \sim_{ind} N_q(\mathbf{X}'_{3i}\boldsymbol{\gamma}, \zeta_i) \tag{3}$$

$$u_i \sim_{ind} N_1(0, \sigma_u^2) \tag{4}$$

$$f(\mathbf{R}_i|u_i, \mathbf{X}_{2i}) = \prod_{j=1}^{J} \pi_{ij}^{r_{ij}}(1 - \pi_{ij})^{1-r_{ij}} \tag{5}$$

A linear mixed model (growth curve) is used for the relationship between $\mathbf{Y}_i$ and $\mathbf{b}_i$, where $\mathbf{X}_{1i}$ is a known ($J \times p_1$) design matrix containing fixed within-subject and between-subject covariates (including both time-invariate and time-varying covariates), with associated unknown ($p_1 \times 1$) parameter vector $\boldsymbol{\beta}$, $\mathbf{Z}_{1i}$ is a known ($J \times q$) matrix for modeling random effects, and $\mathbf{b}_i$ is an unknown ($q \times 1$) random coefficient vector. We specify $\mathbf{Y}_i = \mathbf{X}_{1i}\boldsymbol{\beta} + \mathbf{Z}_i\mathbf{b}_i + \boldsymbol{\epsilon}_i$, where the random error term $\boldsymbol{\epsilon}_i$ is a J-dimensional vector with $E(\boldsymbol{\epsilon}_i) = \mathbf{0}$, $Var(\boldsymbol{\epsilon}_i) = \Sigma_\epsilon$, and $\boldsymbol{\epsilon}_i$ is assumed independent of $\mathbf{b}_i$. Furthermore, the $J \times J$ covariance matrix Σ_ϵ is assumed to be diagonal, that any correlations found in the observation vector $\mathbf{Y}_i$ are due to their relationship with common $\mathbf{b}_i$ and not due to some spurious correlation between $\boldsymbol{\epsilon}_i$. A continuous latent variable model is assumed for the relationship between $\mathbf{R}_i$ and u_i with $\pi_{ij} = Pr(r_{ij} = 1)$ representing the probability that the response for subject i at time point j is missing. We apply the logit link for the probability of the missingness, i.e., $log(\frac{\pi_{ij}(u_i, \mathbf{X}_{2i})}{1-\pi_{ij}(u_i, \mathbf{X}_{2i})}) = u_i - \tau_j \equiv X_{2i}\boldsymbol{\alpha} + Z_{2i}u_i$, where τ_j are unknown parameters for determining an observation at time point j is missing. As discussed earlier, this relationship is equivalent to a random logistic regression, with appropriate design matrices $\mathbf{X}_{2i}$ and Z_{2i}. A latent variable regression, $\mathbf{b}_i = \mathbf{X}'_{3i}\boldsymbol{\gamma} + \zeta_i$, is used to establish the relationship between latent variable $\mathbf{b}_i$ and u_i, where $\mathbf{X}'_{3i} = [\mathbf{X}_{3i} \ u_i]$ is a $p_3 + 1$ dimensional vector combining $\mathbf{X}_{3i}$ and u_i, $\boldsymbol{\gamma}$ is the ($p_3 + 1$) $\times q$ unknown regression coefficients for $\mathbf{X}'_{3i}$ and the $q \times q$ matrix Ψ determines variance–covariance structure for error term ζ_i. Finally the latent continuous variable u_i is assumed to be normally distributed with mean 0 and variance σ_u^2.

Note that the maximum likelihood (ML) estimation of the model (2)–(4) requires the maximization of the observed likelihood, after integrating out missing data $\mathbf{Y}^{mis}$ and latent variables $\mathbf{b}$ and $\mathbf{u}$ from complete-data likelihood function. Detail of the ML estimation technique will be given in next section.

3 Maximum Likelihood Estimation

The main objective of this section is to obtain the ML estimate of parameters in the model and standard errors on the basis of the observed data $\mathbf{Y}^{\mathbf{obs}}$ and $\mathbf{R}$. The ML approach is an important statistical procedure which has many optimal properties such as consistency, efficiency, etc. Furthermore, it is also the foundation of many important statistical methods, for instance, the likelihood ratio test, statistical diagnostics such as Cook's distance and local influence analysis, among others. To perform ML estimation, the computational difficulty arises because of the need to integrate over continuous latent factor $\mathbf{u}$, random subject-level effects $\mathbf{b}$, as well as missing responses $\mathbf{Y}^{mis}$. The classic Expectation-Maximization (EM) algorithm provides a tool for obtaining maximum likelihood estimates under models that yield intractable likelihood equations. The EM algorithm is an iterative routine requiring two steps in each iteration: computation of a particular conditional expectation of the log-likelihood (E-step) and maximization of this expectation over the parameters of interest (M-step). In our situations, in addition to the real missing data $\mathbf{Y}^{mis}$, we will treat the latent variables $\mathbf{b}$ and $\mathbf{u}$ as missing data. However, due to the complexities associated with the missing data structure and the nonlinearity part of the model, the E-step of the algorithm, which involves the computations of high-dimensional complicated integrals induced by the conditional expectations, is intractable. To solve this difficulty, we propose to approximate the conditional expectations by sample means of the observations simulated from the appropriate conditional distributions, which is known as Monte Carlo Expectation Maximization algorithm. We will develop a hybrid algorithm that combines two advanced computational tools in statistics, namely the Gibbs sampler (Geman and Geman 1984) and the Metropolis Hastings (MH) algorithm (Hastings 1970) for simulating the observations. The M-step does not require intensive computations due to the distinctness of parameters in the proposed model. Hence, the proposed algorithm is a Monte Carlo EM (MCEM) type algorithm (Wei and Tanner 1990). The description of the observed likelihood function is given in the following.

Given the parametric model (2)–(4) and the i.i.d. $J \times 1$ variables $\mathbf{Y}_i$ and $\mathbf{R}_i$, for $i = 1, \ldots, n$, estimation of the model parameters can proceed via the maximum likelihood method. Let $\mathbf{W}_i = (\mathbf{Y}_i^{obs}, \mathbf{R}_i)$ be the observed quantities, $\mathbf{d}_i = (\mathbf{Y}_i^{mis}, \mathbf{b}_i, u_i)$ be the missing quantities, and $\boldsymbol{\theta} = (\boldsymbol{\alpha}, \boldsymbol{\beta}, \tau_j, \boldsymbol{\gamma}, \Psi, \sigma_u^2, \Sigma_\epsilon)$ be the vector of parameters relating $\mathbf{W}_i$ with $\mathbf{d}_i$ and covariates $\mathbf{X}_i$. Under Birch's (1964) regularity conditions for parameter vector $\boldsymbol{\theta}$, the observed likelihood function for the model (2)–(4) can be written as

$$L_o(\boldsymbol{\theta} \,|\, \mathbf{Y}^{\mathbf{obs}}, \mathbf{R}) = \prod_{i=1}^{n} f(\mathbf{W}_i | \mathbf{X}; \boldsymbol{\theta}) = \prod_{i=1}^{n} \int f(\mathbf{W}_i, \mathbf{d}_i | \mathbf{X}_i; \boldsymbol{\theta}) d\mathbf{d}_i \qquad (6)$$

where the notation for the integral over $\mathbf{d}_i$ is taken generally to include the multiple continuous integral for u_i and $\mathbf{b}_i$, as well as missing observations $\mathbf{Y}_i^{mis}$. In detail, the above function can be rewritten as following:

$$L_o(\theta|\mathbf{Y}^{\mathbf{obs}},\mathbf{R}) = \prod_{i=1}^{n}$$

$$\iiint \frac{1}{\sqrt{2\pi}}|\Sigma_\epsilon|^{-1/2}exp\left\{-\frac{1}{2}(\mathbf{Y}_i^{com} - \mathbf{X}_{1i}\beta - \mathbf{Z}_{1i}\mathbf{b}_i)^T \Sigma_\epsilon^{-1}(\mathbf{Y}_i^{com} - \mathbf{X}_{1i}\beta - \mathbf{Z}_{1i}\mathbf{b}_i)\right\}$$

$$\frac{1}{\sqrt{2\pi}}|\Sigma_b|^{-1/2}exp\left\{-\frac{1}{2}(\mathbf{b}_i - \mathbf{X}'_{3i}\gamma)^T \Sigma_b^{-1}(\mathbf{b}_i - \mathbf{X}'_{3i}\gamma)\right\} \frac{1}{\sqrt{2\pi\sigma_u^2}}exp\left\{-\frac{u_i^2}{2\sigma_u^2}\right\}$$

$$\left\{\prod_{j=1}^{J}\left(\frac{exp(X_{2i}\alpha + Z_{2i}u_i)}{1 + exp(X_{2i}\alpha + Z_{2i}u_i)}\right)^{r_{ij}}\left(1 - \frac{exp(X_{2i}\alpha + Z_{2i}u_i)}{1 + exp(X_{2i}\alpha + Z_{2i}u_i)}\right)^{1-r_{ij}}\right\} du_i d\mathbf{b}_i d\mathbf{Y}_i^{mis}$$

$$(7)$$

where $\mathbf{Y}_i^{com} = (\mathbf{Y}_i^{obs}, \mathbf{Y}_i^{mis})$, $\Sigma_b = \sigma_u^2\gamma\gamma^T + \Psi$. As discussed above, the E-step involves complicated, intractable and high dimension integrations. Hence, the Monte Carlo EM algorithm is applied to obtain ML estimates. Detail of the technique for MCEM will be given in the following section.

3.1 Monte Carlo EM

Inspired by the key idea of the EM algorithm, we will treat $\mathbf{d}_i$ as missing data and implement the expectation and maximization (EM) algorithm for maximizing (7). Since it is difficult to maximize the observed data likelihood L_o directly, we construct the complete-data likelihood and apply the EM algorithm on the augmented log-likelihood $ln\, L_c(\mathbf{W},\mathbf{d}|\theta)$ to obtain the MLE of θ over the observed likelihood function $L_o(\mathbf{Y}^{\mathbf{obs}},\mathbf{R}|\theta)$ where it is assumed that $L_o(\mathbf{Y}^{\mathbf{obs}},\mathbf{R}|\theta) = \int L_c(\mathbf{W},\mathbf{d}|\theta)d\mathbf{d}$. [$\mathbf{W}$ and $\mathbf{d}$ are ensemble matrices for vectors $\mathbf{W}_i$ and $\mathbf{d}_i$ defined in (6)]. In detail, the EM algorithm iterates between a computation of the expected complete-data likelihood

$$Q(\theta|\hat{\theta}^{(r)}) = E_{\hat{\theta}^{(r)}}\{ln\, L_c(\mathbf{W},\mathbf{d}|\theta)|\mathbf{Y}^{obs},\mathbf{R}\} \qquad (8)$$

and the maximization of $Q(\theta|\hat{\theta}^{(r)})$ over θ, where the maximum value of θ at the $(r+1)$th iteration is denoted by $\hat{\theta}^{(r+1)}$ and $\hat{\theta}^{(r)}$ denotes the maximum value of θ evaluated at the rth iteration. Specifically, r represents the EM iteration. Under regularity conditions the sequence of values $\{\hat{\theta}^{(r)}\}$ converges to the MLE $\hat{\theta}$. (See Wu (1983).)

As discussed above, the E-step in our case is analytically intractable, so we may estimate the quantity (8) from Monte Carlo simulations. One could notice that the expectation in (8) is over the latent variables $\mathbf{d}$. In particular,

$$E_{\hat{\theta}^{(r)}}\{ln\,L_c(\mathbf{W}, \mathbf{d}|\boldsymbol{\theta})|\mathbf{Y}^{obs}, \mathbf{R}\} = \int ln\,L_c(\mathbf{W}, \mathbf{d}|\boldsymbol{\theta})g(\mathbf{d}|\mathbf{Y}^{obs}, \mathbf{R}; \hat{\theta}^{(r)})d\mathbf{d}$$

where $g(\mathbf{d}|\mathbf{Y}^{obs}, \mathbf{R}; \hat{\theta}^{(r)})$ is the joint conditional distribution of the latent variables given the observed data and $\boldsymbol{\theta}$. A hybrid algorithm that combines the Gibbs sampler and the MH algorithm is developed to obtain Monte Carlo samples from the above conditional distribution. Once we draw a sample $\mathbf{d}_1^{(r)}, \ldots, \mathbf{d}_T^{(r)}$ from the distribution $g(\mathbf{d}|\mathbf{Y}^{obs}, \mathbf{R}; \hat{\theta}^{(r)})$, this expectation can be estimated by the Monte Carlo average

$$Q_T(\boldsymbol{\theta}|\hat{\theta}^{(r)}) = \frac{1}{T}\sum_{t=1}^{T} ln\,L_c(\mathbf{W}, \mathbf{d}_t^{(r)}|\boldsymbol{\theta}) \qquad (9)$$

where T is the MC sample size and also denotes the dependence of current estimator on the MC sample size. By the law of large numbers, the estimator given in (9) converges to the theoretical expectation in (8). Thus the classic EM algorithm can be modified into an MCEM where the E-step is replaced by the estimated quantity from (9). The M-step maximizes (9) over $\boldsymbol{\theta}$.

3.2 Execution of the E-Step via the Hybrid Algorithm

Let $h(\mathbf{Y}^{mis}, \mathbf{b}, \mathbf{u})$ be a general function of $\mathbf{Y}^{mis}$, $\mathbf{b}$ and $\mathbf{u}$ that are involved in $Q(\boldsymbol{\theta}|\hat{\theta}^{(r)})$, then the corresponding conditional expectation given $\mathbf{Y}^{mis}$, $\mathbf{b}$ and $\mathbf{u}$ is approximated by

$$\hat{E}\{h(\mathbf{Y}^{mis}, \mathbf{b}, \mathbf{u})|\mathbf{Y}^{obs}, \mathbf{R}; \boldsymbol{\theta}\} = \frac{1}{T}\sum_{t=1}^{T} h(\mathbf{Y}^{mis(t)}, \mathbf{b}^{(t)}, \mathbf{u}^{(t)}) \qquad (10)$$

where $\{(\mathbf{Y}^{mis(t)}, \mathbf{b}^{(t)}, \mathbf{u}^{(t)})\}$, $t = 1, \ldots, T$, is a sufficiently large sample simulated from the joint conditional distribution $g(\mathbf{Y}^{mis}, \mathbf{b}, \mathbf{u}|\mathbf{Y}^{obs}, \mathbf{R}; \boldsymbol{\theta})$. We apply the following three-stage Gibbs sampler to sample these observations. At the tth iteration with current values $\mathbf{Y}^{mis(t)}, \mathbf{b}^{(t)}$ and $\mathbf{u}^{(t)}$, (t represents Gibbs sampling iteration) Step I: Generate $\mathbf{Y}^{mis(t+1)}$ from $f(\mathbf{Y}^{mis}|\mathbf{Y}^{obs}, \mathbf{R}, \mathbf{b}^{(t)}, \mathbf{u}^{(t)}; \boldsymbol{\theta})$, Step II: Generate $\mathbf{b}^{(t+1)}$ from $f(\mathbf{b}|\mathbf{Y}^{obs}, \mathbf{R}, \mathbf{Y}^{mis(t+1)}, \mathbf{u}^{(t)}; \boldsymbol{\theta})$, Step III: Generate $\mathbf{u}^{(t+1)}$ from $f(\mathbf{u}|\mathbf{Y}^{obs}, \mathbf{R}, \mathbf{Y}^{mis(t+1)}, \mathbf{b}^{(t+1)}; \boldsymbol{\theta})$, where function $f(\cdot|\cdot)$ specifies full conditionals that are applied for each step of Gibbs sampler. The full conditional for $\mathbf{Y}^{mis}$ is easily specified due to the conditional independence assumptions between $\mathbf{Y}$ and $\mathbf{R}$, $\mathbf{u}$, given $\mathbf{b}$. Hence, the full conditional for $\mathbf{Y}^{mis}$ can be simplified as

$f(\mathbf{Y}^{mis}|\mathbf{Y}^{obs}, \mathbf{b}; \boldsymbol{\theta})$ which is again another normal distribution from the property of conditional distribution of multivariate normal. This conditional can be further simplified in our case due to the assumption that the variance–covariance matrix Σ_ϵ in model (2) is diagonal. In detail, for subject $i = 1, \ldots, n$, since $\mathbf{Y}_i$ are mutually independent given $\mathbf{b}_i$, $\mathbf{Y}_i^{mis}$ are also mutually independent given $\mathbf{b}_i$. Since Σ_ϵ is diagonal, $\mathbf{Y}_i^{mis}$ is conditionally independent with $\mathbf{Y}_i^{obs}$ given $\mathbf{b}_i$. Hence, it follows from model (2) that:

$$f(\mathbf{Y}^{mis}|\mathbf{Y}^{obs}, \mathbf{b}; \boldsymbol{\theta}) = \prod_{i=1}^{n} f(\mathbf{Y}_i^{mis}|\mathbf{b}_i; \boldsymbol{\theta})$$

and

$$(\mathbf{Y}_i^{mis}|\mathbf{b}_i; \boldsymbol{\theta}) \sim MVN(\mathbf{X}_{1i}^{mis}\boldsymbol{\beta} + \mathbf{Z}_{1i}^{mis}\mathbf{b}_i, \ \Sigma_{\epsilon,i}^{mis})$$

where $\mathbf{X}_{1i}^{mis}$ and $\mathbf{Z}_i^{mis}$ are submatrices of $\mathbf{X}_{1i}$ and $\mathbf{Z}_i$ with rows corresponding to observed components deleted, and Σ_ϵ^{mis} is a submatrix of Σ_ϵ with the appropriate rows and columns deleted. In fact, the structure of $\mathbf{Y}^{mis}$ may be very complicated with a large number of missing patterns, however, the corresponding conditional distribution only involves a product of relatively simple normal distributions. Hence, the computational cost for simulating $\mathbf{Y}^{mis}$ is low. Due to the hierarchical structure for the model (2)–(4), the joint distribution that is required in full conditionals for $\mathbf{b}$ and $\mathbf{u}$ can be obtained by multiplying the corresponding densities together, and on the basis of the definition of the model and its assumptions, the following set of full conditionals for $\mathbf{b}$ and $\mathbf{u}$ can be derived: (see Robert and Casella 2010, Chapter 7)

$$\mathbf{b}_i|\mathbf{Y}_i^{com}, \mathbf{R}_i, u_i; \boldsymbol{\theta} \propto exp\left\{-\frac{1}{2}(\mathbf{Y}_i^{com} - \mathbf{X}_{1i}\boldsymbol{\beta} - \mathbf{Z}_{1i}\mathbf{b}_i)^T \Sigma_\epsilon^{-1}(\mathbf{Y}_i^{com} - \mathbf{X}_{1i}\boldsymbol{\beta} - \mathbf{Z}_{1i}\mathbf{b}_i)\right.$$

$$\left. -\frac{1}{2}(\mathbf{b}_i - \mathbf{X}'_{3i}\boldsymbol{\gamma})^T \Psi^{-1}(\mathbf{b}_i - \mathbf{X}'_{3i}\boldsymbol{\gamma})\right\}$$

$$u_i|\mathbf{Y}_i^{com}, \mathbf{R}_i, \mathbf{b}_i; \boldsymbol{\theta} \propto exp\left\{-\frac{u_i^2}{2\sigma_u^2} - \frac{1}{2}(\mathbf{b}_i - \mathbf{X}'_{3i}\boldsymbol{\gamma})^T \Psi^{-1}(\mathbf{b}_i - \mathbf{X}'_{3i}\boldsymbol{\gamma})\right\}$$

$$\prod_{j=1}^{J}\left(\frac{exp(X_{2i}\alpha + Z_{2i}u_i)}{1 + exp(X_{2i}\alpha + Z_{2i}u_i)}\right)^{r_{ij}}\left(1 - \frac{exp(X_{2i}\alpha + Z_{2i}u_i)}{1 + exp(X_{2i}\alpha + Z_{2i}u_i)}\right)^{1-r_{ij}}$$

$$(11)$$

Based on expressions (11), it is shown that the associated full conditional distributions for $\mathbf{b}$ and $\mathbf{u}$ are not standard and are relatively complex. Hence we choose to apply the M-H algorithm for simulating observations efficiently. The M-H algorithm is one of the classic MCMC methods that has been widely used for obtaining random samples from a target density via the help of a proposed distribution when direct sampling is difficult. Here $p_1(\mathbf{b}_i|\mathbf{Y}_i^{com}, \mathbf{R}_i, u_i; \boldsymbol{\theta})$ and $p_2(u_i|\mathbf{Y}_i^{com}, \mathbf{R}_i, \mathbf{b}_i; \boldsymbol{\theta})$ are treated as the target densities. Based on the discussion given in Robert and

Casella (2010), it is convenient and natural to choose $N(\cdot, \sigma^2 \Omega)$ as the proposed distributions, where σ^2 is a chosen value to control the acceptance rate of the M-H algorithm, and $\Omega_1^{-1} = \Sigma_b^{-1} + \mathbf{Z}_i^T \Sigma_\epsilon^{-1} \mathbf{Z}_i$ for $\mathbf{b}_i$ and $\Omega_2^{-1} = (\sigma_u^2)^{-1} + \Sigma_b^{-1}$ for u_i. The implementation of M-H algorithm is as follows: at the tth iteration with current value $\mathbf{b}_i^{(t)}$ and $u_i^{(t)}$, new candidates $\mathbf{b}_i^*$ and u_i^* are generated from $N(\mathbf{b}_i^{(t)}, \sigma^2 \Omega_1)$ and $N(u_i^{(t)}, \sigma^2 \Omega_2)$, respectively. The acceptance of new candidates is decided by the following probabilities:

$$min \left\{ 1, \frac{p_1(\mathbf{b}_i^* | \mathbf{Y}_i^{com}, \mathbf{R}_i, u_i; \boldsymbol{\theta})}{p_1(\mathbf{b}_i^{(t)} | \mathbf{Y}_i^{com}, \mathbf{R}_i, u_i; \boldsymbol{\theta})} \right\} \quad , \quad min \left\{ 1, \frac{p_2(u_i^* | \mathbf{Y}_i^{com}, \mathbf{R}_i, \mathbf{b}_i; \boldsymbol{\theta})}{p_2(u_i^{(t)} | \mathbf{Y}_i^{com}, \mathbf{R}_i, \mathbf{b}_i; \boldsymbol{\theta})} \right\}$$

where $p_1(\cdot)$ and $p_2(\cdot)$ are calculated from Eq. (11). The quantity σ^2 can be chosen such that the average acceptance rate is approximately 1/4, as suggested by Robert and Casella (2010).

Instead of allowing the candidate distributions for $\mathbf{b}$ and $\mathbf{u}$ to depend on the present state of the chain, an attractive alternative is choosing proposed distributions to be independent of this present state, then we get a special case which is named Independent Metropolis-Hastings. To implement this method, we generate candidate for $\mathbf{b}_i$ at step t, $\mathbf{b}_i^*$, from a multivariate normal distribution with mean vector $\mathbf{0}$ and variance covariance Σ_b (denote as the function $h_1(\cdot)$); generate candidate for $\mathbf{u}_i$ at step t, $\mathbf{u}_i^*$, from a univariate normal distribution with mean 0 and variance σ_u^2 (denote as the function $h_2(\cdot)$). The acceptance probability for proposed distributions of $\mathbf{b}_i^{(t+1)}$ and $\mathbf{u}_i^{(t+1)}$ ($i = 1, 2, \ldots, n$) can be obtained by

$$min \left\{ 1, \frac{p_1(\mathbf{b}_i^* | \mathbf{Y}_i^{com}, \mathbf{R}_i, u_i; \boldsymbol{\theta}) \, h_1(\mathbf{b}_i^{(t)})}{p_1(\mathbf{b}_i^{(t)} | \mathbf{Y}_i^{com}, \mathbf{R}_i, u_i; \boldsymbol{\theta}) \, h_1(\mathbf{b}_i^*)} \right\} \quad , \quad min \left\{ 1, \frac{p_2(u_i^* | \mathbf{Y}_i^{com}, \mathbf{R}_i, \mathbf{b}_i; \boldsymbol{\theta}) \, h_2(u_i^{(t)})}{p_2(u_i^{(t)} | \mathbf{Y}_i^{com}, \mathbf{R}_i, \mathbf{b}_i; \boldsymbol{\theta}) \, h_2(u_i^*)} \right\}$$

Let $(\mathbf{Y}_i^{mis(t)}, \mathbf{b}_i^{(t)}, u_i^{(t)})$; $t = 1, \ldots, T$; $i = 1, \ldots, n$ be the random samples generated by the proposed hybrid algorithm from the joint conditionals $(\mathbf{Y}^{mis}, \mathbf{b}, \mathbf{u} | \mathbf{Y}^{obs}, \mathbf{R}; \boldsymbol{\theta})$. Conditional expectations of the complete data sufficient statistics required to evaluate the E-step can be approximated via these random samples as follows: let $\mathbf{Y}_i = (\mathbf{Y}_i^{obs}, \mathbf{Y}_i^{mis})$, and define $Y_i^{(t)} = (Y_i^{obs(t)}, Y_i^{mis(t)})$, where $Y_i^{obs(t)}$ is sampled with replacement from Y_i^{obs},

$$E[\mathbf{Y}_i - \mathbf{Z}_{1i}\mathbf{b}_i | \mathbf{Y}_i^{obs}, \mathbf{R}_i; \boldsymbol{\theta}] = T^{-1} \sum_{t=1}^{T} (Y_i^{(t)} - \mathbf{Z}_{1i}\mathbf{b}_i^{(t)})$$

$$E[\boldsymbol{\epsilon}_i \boldsymbol{\epsilon}_i' | \mathbf{Y}_i^{obs}, \mathbf{R}_i; \boldsymbol{\theta}] = T^{-1} \sum_{t=1}^{T} (Y_i^{(t)} - \mathbf{X}_{1i}\boldsymbol{\beta} - \mathbf{Z}_{1i}\mathbf{b}_i^{(t)})(Y_i^{(t)} - \mathbf{X}_{1i}\boldsymbol{\beta} - \mathbf{Z}_{1i}\mathbf{b}_i^{(t)})'$$

$$E[\mathbf{b}_i | \mathbf{Y}_i^{obs}, \mathbf{R}_i; \boldsymbol{\theta}] = T^{-1} \sum_{t=1}^{T} \mathbf{b}_i^{(t)}$$

$$E[\psi_i \psi_i' | \mathbf{Y}_i^{obs}, \mathbf{R}_i; \boldsymbol{\theta}] = T^{-1} \sum_{t=1}^{T} (\mathbf{b}_i^{(t)} - \mathbf{X}_{3i}'^{(t)} \boldsymbol{\gamma})(\mathbf{b}_i^{(t)} - \mathbf{X}_{3i}'^{(t)} \boldsymbol{\gamma})'$$

$$E[u_i | \mathbf{Y}_i^{obs}, \mathbf{R}_i; \boldsymbol{\theta}] = T^{-1} \sum_{t=1}^{T} u_i^{(t)}, \quad E[u_i u_i' | \mathbf{Y}_i^{obs}, \mathbf{R}_i; \boldsymbol{\theta}] = T^{-1} \sum_{t=1}^{T} u_i^{(t)} u_i'^{(t)} \quad (12)$$

where $\mathbf{X}_{3i}'^{(t)} = [\mathbf{X}_{3i} \ u_i^{(t)}]$.

3.3   Maximization Step

At the M-step we need to maximize $Q(\boldsymbol{\theta} | \boldsymbol{\theta}^{(r)})$ with respect to $\boldsymbol{\theta}$. In other words, the following systems are needed to be solved:

$$\frac{\partial Q(\boldsymbol{\theta} | \boldsymbol{\theta}^{(r)})}{\partial \boldsymbol{\theta}} = E\{\frac{\partial}{\partial \boldsymbol{\theta}} ln L_c(\mathbf{W}, \mathbf{d} | \boldsymbol{\theta}) | \mathbf{Y}^{obs}, \mathbf{R}; \boldsymbol{\theta}^{(r)}\} = 0 \quad (13)$$

It can be shown that

$$\frac{\partial ln L_c(\mathbf{W}, \mathbf{d} | \boldsymbol{\theta})}{\partial \boldsymbol{\beta}} = \sum_{i=1}^{n} \mathbf{X}_i^T \Sigma_\epsilon^{-1} (\mathbf{Y}_i - \mathbf{Z}_{1i} \mathbf{b}_i - \mathbf{X}_{1i} \boldsymbol{\beta})$$

$$\frac{\partial ln L_c(\mathbf{W}, \mathbf{d} | \boldsymbol{\theta})}{\partial \Sigma_\epsilon} = \frac{1}{2} \Sigma_\epsilon^{-1} \sum_{i=1}^{n} \left[(\mathbf{Y}_i - \mathbf{X}_{1i} \boldsymbol{\beta} - \mathbf{Z}_{1i} \mathbf{b}_i)(\mathbf{Y}_i - \mathbf{X}_{1i} \boldsymbol{\beta} - \mathbf{Z}_{1i} \mathbf{b}_i)^T - \Sigma_\epsilon \right] \Sigma_\epsilon^{-1}$$

$$\frac{\partial ln L_c(\mathbf{W}, \mathbf{d} | \boldsymbol{\theta})}{\partial \boldsymbol{\gamma}} = \sum_{i=1}^{n} u_i \Psi^{-1} (\mathbf{b}_i - \mathbf{X}_{3i}' \boldsymbol{\gamma})$$

$$\frac{\partial ln L_c(\mathbf{W}, \mathbf{d} | \boldsymbol{\theta})}{\partial \Psi} = \frac{1}{2} \Psi^{-1} \sum_{i=1}^{n} \left[(\mathbf{b}_i - \mathbf{X}_{3i}' \boldsymbol{\gamma})(\mathbf{b}_i - \mathbf{X}_{3i}' \boldsymbol{\gamma})^T - \Psi \right] \Psi^{-1}$$

$$\frac{\partial ln L_c(\mathbf{W}, \mathbf{d} | \boldsymbol{\theta})}{\partial \boldsymbol{\alpha}} = \sum_{i=1}^{n} \sum_{j=1}^{J} \left\{ r_{ij} X_{2ij} - \frac{exp(X_{2ij} \boldsymbol{\alpha} + Z_{2ij} u_i)}{1 + exp(X_{2ij} \boldsymbol{\alpha} + Z_{2ij} u_i)} \cdot X_{2ij} \right\}$$

$$(14)$$

Due to distinctness of parameters in the model, the ML estimates can be obtained separately: for $\boldsymbol{\beta}$ and Σ_ϵ in the linear mixed model, as well as $\boldsymbol{\gamma}$ and Ψ in latent variable regression model, the corresponding ML estimates can be obtained from sufficient statistics in the E-step, which is given in (12); to estimate $\boldsymbol{\alpha}$, we will implement a quasi-Newton method because of no closed expression; the estimates of Σ_b and σ_u can be obtained from simulated random samples by applying law of total variance.

With the assumption that the missing mechanism is ignorable given latent factors $\mathbf{u}$, and $\mathbf{b}$, the computation of proposed MCEM algorithm can be further reduced.

That is, the ML estimates can be obtained from observed components in $\mathbf{Y}$, given information of $\mathbf{u}$, and $\mathbf{b}$. Specifically, the dimension of integration in E-step will reduce to two, instead of three.

3.4 Monitor Convergence of MCEM via Bridge Sampling

In order to obtain valid ML estimates, one needs to investigate the convergence of the EM algorithm. However, in our case, determining the convergence of the MCEM algorithm is not straightforward. Meng and Schilling (1996) pointed out that the log-likelihood function can "zigzag" along the iterates even without implementation or numerical errors, due to the variability introduced by simulation at the E-step. Further to evaluate the observed-data log-likelihood function, some numerical method has to be used because a closed forms is lacking. In the absence of accurate evaluation of the observed-data log-likelihood function, we could not judge whether any large fluctuation is due to the implementation errors, to the numerical errors in computing the log-likelihood values, or to non-convergence of the MCEM algorithm. We will implement bridge sampling to solve this problem, as suggested by Meng and Schilling (1996).

In the determination of the convergence of a likelihood function, only the evaluation changes in likelihood are of interest, and these changes can be expressed by the logarithm of the ratio of two consecutive likelihood values. In our case, the ratio is given by

$$K(\boldsymbol{\theta}^{(r+1)}, \boldsymbol{\theta}^{(r)}) = log \frac{L_o(\mathbf{Y}^{obs}, \mathbf{R}|\boldsymbol{\theta}^{(r+1)})}{L_o(\mathbf{Y}^{obs}, \mathbf{R}|\boldsymbol{\theta}^{(r)})}$$

Due to the complexity of the observed likelihood function, the accurate value of $K(\boldsymbol{\theta}^{(r+1)}, \boldsymbol{\theta}^{(r)})$ is difficult to obtain. However, as pointed out by Meng and Schilling (1996), it can be approximated by

$$\hat{K}(\boldsymbol{\theta}^{(r+1)}, \boldsymbol{\theta}^{(r)}) = log \left\{ \sum_{t=1}^{T} \left[\frac{L_c(\mathbf{W}, \mathbf{d}^{r,(t)}|\boldsymbol{\theta}^{(r+1)})}{L_c(\mathbf{W}, \mathbf{d}^{r,(t)}|\boldsymbol{\theta}^{(r)})} \right]^{\frac{1}{2}} \right\}$$
$$-log \left\{ \sum_{t=1}^{T} \left[\frac{L_c(\mathbf{W}, \mathbf{d}^{r+1,(t)}|\boldsymbol{\theta}^{(r)})}{L_c(\mathbf{W}, \mathbf{d}^{r+1,(t)}|\boldsymbol{\theta}^{(r+1)})} \right]^{\frac{1}{2}} \right\}$$

(15)

where $\mathbf{d}^{r,(t)}$, $t = 1, \ldots, T$ are random samples generated from $g(\mathbf{d}|\mathbf{W}, \boldsymbol{\theta}^{(r)})$ by the hybrid algorithm. In determining the convergence of the MCEM algorithm, we plot $\hat{K}(\boldsymbol{\theta}^{(r+1)}, \boldsymbol{\theta}^{(r)})$ against iteration index r. Approximate convergence is claimed to be achieved if the plot shows a curve converging to zero.

3.5 Standard Error Estimates

Standard error estimates of the ML estimates can be obtained by inverting the Hessian matrix or the information matrix of the log-likelihood function based on observed data $\mathbf{Y}^{obs}$ and missing pattern matrix $\mathbf{R}$. Unfortunately, these matrices do not have closed forms. Thus, we apply the formula by Louis (1982) with random samples generated from $g(\mathbf{Y}^{mis}, \mathbf{b}, \mathbf{u} | \mathbf{Y}^{obs}, \mathbf{R}, \boldsymbol{\theta})$ via the hybrid algorithm to obtain standard error estimates. From Louis (1982) we have

$$
-\frac{\partial^2 L_o(\mathbf{Y}^{obs}, \mathbf{R} | \boldsymbol{\theta})}{\partial \boldsymbol{\theta} \, \partial \boldsymbol{\theta}^T} = E \left\{ -\frac{\partial^2 L_c(\mathbf{Y}^{obs}, \mathbf{R}, \mathbf{Y}^{mis}, \mathbf{b}, \mathbf{u} | \boldsymbol{\theta})}{\partial \boldsymbol{\theta} \, \partial \boldsymbol{\theta}^T} \right\}
$$
$$
- Var \left\{ \frac{\partial L_c(\mathbf{Y}^{obs}, \mathbf{R}, \mathbf{Y}^{mis}, \mathbf{b}, \mathbf{u} | \boldsymbol{\theta})}{\partial \boldsymbol{\theta}} \right\} \tag{16}
$$

The above expectation involved calculations of expectation and variance with respect to the conditional distribution of $(\mathbf{Y}^{mis}, \mathbf{b}, \mathbf{u})$ given $\mathbf{Y}^{obs}$, $\mathbf{R}$ and $\boldsymbol{\theta}$, and the whole expression is evaluated at $\hat{\boldsymbol{\theta}}$. Again, it is difficult to evaluate the above expression in closed forms; however, they can be approximated by the sample mean and sample variance–covariance matrix of the distinct random sample $\{(\mathbf{Y}^{mis(t)}, \mathbf{b}^{(t)}, \mathbf{u}^{(t)}); \ t = 1, \dots, T_1\}$ generated separately from $g(\mathbf{Y}^{mis}, \mathbf{b}, \mathbf{u} | \mathbf{Y}^{obs}, \mathbf{R}, \hat{\boldsymbol{\theta}})$ using the hybrid algorithm. Let $\mathbf{W} = (\mathbf{Y}^{obs}, \mathbf{R})$ and $\mathbf{d} = (\mathbf{Y}^{mis}, \mathbf{b}, \mathbf{u})$, we have

$$
-\frac{\partial^2 L_o(\mathbf{Y}^{obs}, \mathbf{R} | \boldsymbol{\theta})}{\partial \boldsymbol{\theta} \, \partial \boldsymbol{\theta}^T} = T_1^{-2} \left(\sum_{t=1}^{T_1} \frac{\partial L_c(\mathbf{W}, \mathbf{d}^{(t)} | \boldsymbol{\theta})}{\partial \boldsymbol{\theta}} \right) \left(\sum_{t=1}^{T_1} \frac{\partial L_c(\mathbf{W}, \mathbf{d}^{(t)} | \boldsymbol{\theta})}{\partial \boldsymbol{\theta}} \right)^T \Bigg|_{\boldsymbol{\theta} = \hat{\boldsymbol{\theta}}}
$$
$$
+ T_1^{-1} \sum_{t=1}^{T_1} \left\{ -\frac{\partial^2 L_c(\mathbf{W}, \mathbf{d}^{(t)} | \boldsymbol{\theta})}{\partial \boldsymbol{\theta} \, \partial \boldsymbol{\theta}^T} - \left(\frac{\partial L_c(\mathbf{W}, \mathbf{d}^{(t)} | \boldsymbol{\theta})}{\partial \boldsymbol{\theta}} \right) \left(\frac{\partial L_c(\mathbf{W}, \mathbf{d}^{(t)} | \boldsymbol{\theta})}{\partial \boldsymbol{\theta}} \right)^T \right\} \Bigg|_{\boldsymbol{\theta} = \hat{\boldsymbol{\theta}}} \tag{17}
$$

Finally, the standard errors are obtained from the diagonal elements of inverse Hessian matrix $-\partial^2 L_o(\mathbf{Y}^{obs}, \mathbf{R} | \boldsymbol{\theta}) / \partial \boldsymbol{\theta} \, \partial \boldsymbol{\theta}^T$, evaluated at $\hat{\boldsymbol{\theta}}$.

4   Application: Randomized Study of Dual or Triple Combinations of HIV-1 Reverse Transcriptase Inhibitors

In this section, we present an application using a data set that has appeared previously in the literature. We illustrate the application of CLFM by using data from a randomized, double-blind, study of AIDS patients with advanced immune suppression, which is measured as CD4 counts ≤ 50 cells/ mm^3 (Henry et al. 1998).

4.1 Description of Study

Patients in an AIDS Clinical Trial Group (ACTG) Study 193 A were randomized to dual or triple combinations of HIV-1 reverse transcriptase inhibitors. Specifically, HIV patients were randomized to one of four daily regimens containing 600 mg of zidovudine: zidovudine plus 2.25 mg of zalcitabine; zidovudine plus 400 mg of didanosine; zidovudine alternating monthly with 400 mg didanosine; or zidovudine plus 400 mg of didanosine plus 400 mg of nevirapine (triple therapy). In this study, we focus on the comparison of the first three treatment regimens (dual therapy) with the forth (triple therapy) as described in Fitzmaurice's work (Fitzmaurice et al. 2004).

Measurements of CD4 counts were scheduled to be collected at baseline and at 8-week intervals during follow-up. However, the CD4 count data are unbalanced due to unequal measurements and also CD4 counts have missing data that were caused by skipped visits and dropout. Table 1 presents four randomly selected subjects. The number of measurements of CD4 counts during the first 40 weeks of follow-up varied from 1 to 9, with a median of 4, based on the available data. The goal in this study is to compare the dual and triple therapy groups in terms of short-term changes in CD4 counts from baseline to week 40. The responses of interest are based on log transformation CD4 counts, log(CD4 counts + 1), available on 1,309 patients.

Table 1 Data example on log CD4 counts for four randomly selected subjects from ACTG study 193A

Subject ID	Group	Time	log(CD4 + 1)
56	0	0.0	1.7047
56	0	8.1	1.7981
56	0	16.1	0.6932
56	0	25.4	1.0986
56	0	33.4	0.6932
56	0	39.1	0.6932
529	1	0.0	4.0073
529	1	7.4	3.7136
529	1	16.4	3.5264
529	1	25.4	3.1781
529	1	33.6	3.6636
763	0	0.0	2.8622
763	0	8.0	1.9459
763	0	14.9	1.6094
763	0	21.9	1.7917
777	1	0.0	2.3979
777	1	8.4	1.7918
777	1	10.4	3.0445
777	1	25.3	3.0445

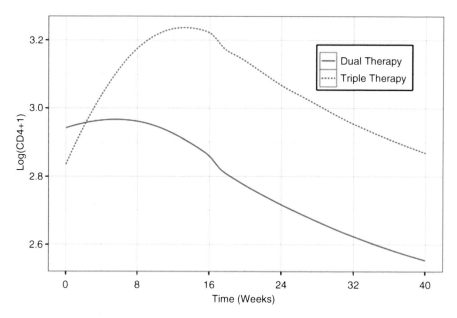

Fig. 3 Lowess smoothed curves of log(CD4 + 1) against time (in weeks), for subject in the dual and triple therapy groups in ACTG study 193A

Figure 3 describes the trend in the mean response in the dual and triple therapy groups via lowess smoothed curves on observed data. The curves reveal a modest decline in the mean response during the first 16 weeks for the dual therapy group, followed by a steeper decline from week 16 to week 40. By comparison, the mean response increases during the first 16 weeks and declines after for the triple therapy group. The rate of decline from week 16 to week 40 appears to be similar for the two groups. However, one has to notice that there is a substantial amount of missing data in the study, therefore the plot of the mean response over time can be potentially misleading, unless the data are missing completely at random (MCAR). Moreover, based on a small random sample of individuals, we observed that those with drop-out tend to have large CD4 counts. In other words, there is a trend that a patient in the study tended to skip a visit due to a large magnitude of current CD4 count. That is, a patient tends to skip a visit because of no treatment benefits or side effects. When data are missing due to this reason, a plot of the mean response over time can be deceptive. Figure 4 describes observed responses at different visit points in each group. Almost all patients from both groups are treated at baseline and their CD4 count data are collected. There are two sharp decreases in response rate, one is from week 0 to week 8 and the other is from week 32 to week 40. Approaching to the end of the study, most patients are dropping out from study, and response

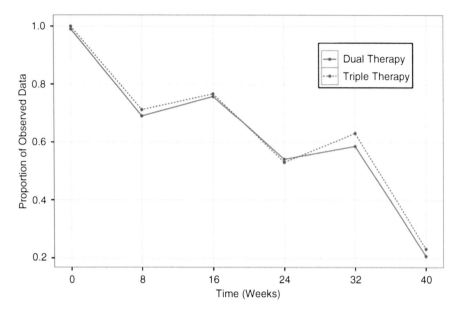

Fig. 4 Proportions of observed responses in the dual and triple therapy groups in ACTG study 193A

rates at week 40 are close to 20% for both treatments. The missing information can substantially influence the analysis and even bias our findings. In the example, we will implement CLFM which assumes missing data are not ignorable, and compare with the conventional model that ignores missingness. We also compare the maximum likelihood CLFM results to results from Roy's (2003) latent class model and to results from a Bayesian method given in Zhang (2014).

In the following we describe a model for the mean response that enables the rates of change before and after week 16 to differ within and between groups, and this model was also been adopted by Fitzmaurice et al. (2004) in their work. Specifically, one could assume that each patient has a piecewise linear spline with a knot at week 16. That is, the response trajectory of each patient can be described with an intercept and two slopes—one slope for the changes in response before week 16, another slope for the changes in response after week 16. Further, we assume the average slopes for changes in response before and after week 16 are allowed to vary by group. Because this is a randomized study, the mean response at baseline is assumed to be the same in the two groups, as supported in Fig. 3. Hence instead of the conventional growth curve model, we applied a special growth curve model to capture changing trends of responses on CD4 counts.

4.2   Model Specification

Let t_{ij} denote the time since baseline for the jth measurement on the ith subject with $t_{ij} = 0$ at baseline, we consider the following linear mixed effects model:

$$E(Y_{ij}|b_i) = \beta_1 + \beta_2 t_{ij} + \beta_3(t_{ij} - 16)_+ + \beta_4 Group_i \times t_{ij} + \beta_5 Group_i \times (t_{ij} - 16)_+$$
$$+ b_{1i} + b_{2i} t_{ij} + b_{3i}(t_{ij} - 16)_+$$

where $Group_i = 1$ if the ith subject is randomized to triple therapy, and $Group_i = 0$ otherwise; $(t_{ij} - 16)_+ = t_{ij} - 16$ if $t_{ij} > 16$ and $(t_{ij} - 16)_+ = 0$ if $t_{ij} \leq 16$; b_{1i}, b_{2i}, and b_{3i} are random effects in this splined growth curve model. In this model, $(\beta_1 + b_{1i})$ is the intercept for the ith subject and has an interpretation as the true log CD4 count as baseline, i.e. when $t_{ij} = 0$. Similarly, $\beta_2 + b_{2i}$ is the ith subject's slope, or rate of change in log CD4 counts from baseline to week 16, if this patient is randomized to dual therapy; $(\beta_2 + \beta_4 + b_{2i})$ is the ith subject's slope if randomized to triple therapy. Finally, the ith subject's slope from week 16 to week 40 is given by $\{(\beta_2 + \beta_3) + (b_{2i} + b_{3i})\}$ if randomized to dual therapy and $\{(\beta_2 + \beta_3 + \beta_4 + \beta_5) + (b_{2i} + b_{3i})\}$ if randomized to triple therapy. The model described above will be fitted without incorporating missing data. In order to fit CLFM, one has to specify the model for the missing part. Assume that $\mathbf{R}$ is a missing indicator matrix where its (i, j)th element $r_{ij} = 1$ if Y_{ij} is missing and $r_{ij} = 0$ if it is observed. Within a framework of CLFM, we incorporate information on missing values through modeling the missing information matrix $\mathbf{R}$ with time location parameters, and a continuous latent factor $\mathbf{u}$. Further, there are strong indications which support an application of this model. Based on Fig. 4 one can see that the response variable tends to be missing over time. In other words, time locations are good indicators for explaining missing data. From Fig. 4 one might also notice that the two therapies have identical missing proportions which suggests a group effect for therapies is not necessary in modeling $\mathbf{R}$. The continuous latent factor $\mathbf{u}$ is used to describe individuals' variability in missingness, and two regression parameters γ_1 and γ_2 are specified to provide information on random intercept $\mathbf{b}_0$ and slope $\mathbf{b}_1$, in order to correct estimation bias. A third regression parameter was also explored which links $\mathbf{u}$ with $\mathbf{b}_3$, but analysis results showed that this parameter is not significant. Hence we exclude this parameter in the final results. To estimate CLFM, we adopt two approaches: MCEM to obtain ML estimates and full Bayesian estimates with specified conjugate priors. Point estimates and corresponding standard errors from a Bayesian perspective are summarized by posterior mean and standard deviation. Roy's model is also implemented by summarized missing patterns from $\mathbf{R}$ into three latent classes. (The number of latent classes for Roy's model is determined by information criteria)

Table 2 Estimated regression coefficients (fixed effects) and variance components (random effects) for the log CD4 counts from a MAR model, Roy's model and CLFM in both approaches

Variables	MAR Estimate	SE	Roy Estimate	SE	MCEM Estimate	SE	Bayesian Estimate	SE
Intercept	2.9415	0.0256	2.9223	0.0374	2.9300	0.0250	2.9320	0.0262
t_{ij}	−0.0073	0.0020	−0.0051	0.0056	−0.0040	0.0052	−0.0047	0.0058
$(t_{ij} - 16)_+$	−0.0120	0.0032	−0.0201	0.0052	−0.0221	0.0090	−0.0223	0.0092
$Group_i \times t_{ij}$	0.0269	0.0039	0.0271	0.0062	0.0272	0.0105	0.0273	0.0109
$Group_i \times (t_{ij} - 16)_+$	−0.0277	0.0062	−0.0240	0.0102	−0.0243	0.0169	−0.0243	0.0177
$Var(b_{1i}) = g_{11}$	585.742	34.754	364.000	49.000	630.050	32.430	640.600	34.7300
$Var(b_{2i}) = g_{22}$	0.923	0.160	1.000	0.500	2.3190	0.9990	2.3230	1.0050
$Var(b_{3i}) = g_{33}$	1.240	0.395	2.000	1.013	37.640	1.9503	38.8600	2.0840
$Cov(b_{1i}, b_{2i}) = g_{12}$	7.254	1.805	−7.106	3.001	−8.6240	3.0500	−8.5240	4.0760
$Cov(b_{1i}, b_{3i}) = g_{13}$	−12.348	2.730	−1.500	3.120	−2.5150	5.3000	−2.5220	6.5000
$Cov(b_{2i}, b_{3i}) = g_{23}$	−0.919	0.236	−6.405	0.892	−7.0130	0.9980	−7.1530	1.0070
$Var(e_i) = \sigma^2$	306.163	10.074	412.000	36.000	500.6300	6.7390	515.3000	9.3570

4.3 Summary of Analyses Under MAR and MNAR

In this study, one research question of interest is treatment effects in the changes in log CD4 counts. The null hypothesis of no treatment group differences can be expressed as $H_0 : \beta_4 = \beta_5 = 0$. The ML estimates on fixed effects from three models are given in Table 2, including the conventional model with a MAR assumption, Roy's model that handles non-ignorable missing data from pattern-mixture modeling and CLFM. The Bayesian estimates for CLFM are also displayed in Table 2. For the likelihood approach with MAR assumptions, a test of $H_0 : \beta_4 = \beta_5 = 0$ yields a Wald statistic, $W^2 = 59.12$, with 2 degrees of freedom, and corresponding p-value is less than 0.0001. For the full Bayesian approach, we compute Deviance information criterion (DIC) to compare two models: one assumes no treatment effects by excluding interaction terms between treatment groups and study time; the other assumes treatment effects are significant. DIC for a model with embracing treatment effects is 15, 792.7, which is less than the one from the model with no groups effects, 18, 076.5. Based on the criteria, "the smaller the better," there is evidence to support the fact that treatment group differences in changes in log CD4 counts are significant. The tests from Roy's model and MCEM approach on CLFM also support this group variety, with p-values for both less than 0.0001. Based on the magnitude of the estimate of β_4, and its standard error from all approaches, there is a significant group difference in the rates of change from baseline to week 16. The estimated response curves for two groups are displayed in Fig. 5. In this figure, dashed lines represent the response curve from CLFM, dotted lines correspond to results from Roy's model, while solid lines are results from the MAR approach. In the dual therapy group, there is a significant decrease in the mean of the log CD4 counts from baseline to week 16, based on the ignorable likelihood approach. The estimated change during the first 16 weeks is -0.12, which can be obtained from 16×-0.0073. On the untransformed scale, this corresponds to an approximate 10 % decrease in CD4 counts. However, CLFM which assumes missing data are not ignorable suggests that this decrease is not significant, since the 95 % credible interval for β_2 covers zero ($[-0.01638, 0.006517]$). Further, Roy's model also confirms this finding with the 95 % confidence interval $[-0.016076, 0.005876]$. By observing missingness from baseline to week 16, subjects with higher log CD4 counts tend to be missing. CLFM involves non-ignorable missing data in the analysis, and the average of log CD4 counts tend to recover to a higher value. Hence, the decrease in the mean of the log CD4 counts from baseline to week 16 is not significant, when non-ignorable missing data are considered. By comparison, in the triple therapy group, there is a significant increase in the mean response. Based on the ignorable approach, the estimated change during the first 16 weeks in the triple therapy group is 0.31, ($16 \times (-0.0073 + 0.0269)$); the estimated slope for the triple therapy group is 0.0196 with a standard error 0.0033. In terms of the untransformed scale, it corresponds to an approximate 35 % increase in CD4 counts. In CLFM, a similar estimate is obtained: the corresponding estimated change is 0.36. ($16 \times (-0.0047 + 0.0273)$); the estimated slope for the triple therapy group is 0.0226, and it corresponds to an approximate 40 % increase in CD4 counts.

The loess curves in Fig. 3 suggest that the rate of decline from week 16 to week 40 is similar for the two groups. The null hypothesis of no treatment group difference in the rates of change in log CD4 counts from week 16 to week 40 can be expressed as $H_0 : \beta_4 + \beta_5 = 0$. The estimates of β_4 and β_5 from all approaches appear to support the null hypothesis since they are of similar magnitude but with opposite signs. In the work of Fitzmaurice et al. (2004), a test of the null hypothesis, $H_0 : \beta_4 + \beta_5 = 0$, is given and a Wald statistic is yielded with $W^2 = 0.07$, with 1 degree of freedom. The corresponding p value is greater than 0.75 based on the ignorable likelihood approach. DIC comparison for the Bayesian version of CLFM also suggests that two groups have similar rate of decline from week 16 to week 40. The Wald tests for Roy's model and MCEM version of CLFM further indicate this parallel change profiles after week 16, with both p-values are greater than 0.6.

The estimated variances of the random effects in Table 2 indicate that there is substantial individual variability in baseline CD4 counts and the rates of change in CD4 counts. For instance, in the triple therapy group, many patients show increases in CD4 counts during the first 16 weeks, but some patients have declining CD4 counts. Specifically, approximately 95 % of patients are expected to have changes in log CD4 counts from baseline to week 16 between -0.64 and 1.27. Hence, there are approximately 26 % of patients who are expected to have decreases in CD4 counts during the first 16 weeks of triple therapy, based on the ignorable likelihood approach; by comparison, a larger variability from patient to patient is indicated by CLFM. 95 % of patients are expected to have changes in log CD4 counts from baseline to week 16 between -1.15 and 1.87, and correspondingly approximately 30 % of patients are expected to decrease CD4 counts from CLFM. Substantial

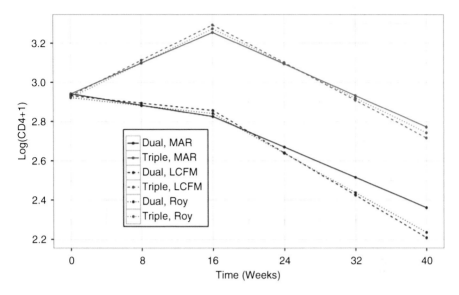

Fig. 5 Fitted response curve in the dual and triple therapy groups in ACTG study 193A

components of variability due to measurement error are also suggested from all models (Table 2).

4.4   Distributions on Latent Factor

In this study, we have explored under the assumption of a normal distribution on the proposed latent factor **u**. The normal distribution is a natural starting point for this CLFM, but it also has limitations. The normal distribution implies non-skewed spread on proposed latent factor which may be too simplistic. In this section, we will extend the distribution of latent factor u to more general distribution. Specifically, we will give an example of logistic distribution on **b** and compare the estimating results, to demonstrate the flexibility of proposed model, as well as the estimating scheme from Bayesian perspective.

As we described earlier, a latent factor **u** is proposed to summarize missing patterns and will be used to compensate for the missing information in a repeated-measure model. At the beginning of the investigation, it is natural to choose a normal distribution for **u**, which assumes more information is needed to be filled in the middle of the study. However, some longitudinal studies may experience missing values, which will lead to a heavy tail on the distribution of **u**. In order to fit this scenario, a complicate distribution is needed, other than classical normal distribution. Further, the proposed Bayesian estimating scheme allows this extension to be more straightforward. To present this flexibility on specifying

Table 3 Estimated regression coefficients (fixed effects) and variance components (random effects) for the log CD4 counts from CLFM with normal distribution and logistic distribution

Variables	Normal distribution		Logistic distribution	
	Estimate	SE	Estimate	SE
Intercept	2.9320	0.0262	2.9310	0.0258
t_{ij}	−0.0047	0.0058	−0.0048	0.0058
$(t_{ij} - 16)_+$	−0.0223	0.0092	−0.0221	0.0090
$Group_i \times t_{ij}$	0.0273	0.0109	0.0273	0.0111
$Group_i \times (t_{ij} - 16)_+$	−0.0243	0.0177	−0.0241	0.0173
$Var(b_{1i}) = g_{11}$	640.600	34.7300	641.300	35.720
$Var(b_{2i}) = g_{22}$	2.3230	1.0050	2.3210	1.0120
$Var(b_{3i}) = g_{33}$	38.8600	2.0840	38.7900	2.0580
$Cov(b_{1i}, b_{2i}) = g_{12}$	−8.5240	4.0760	−8.5760	4.0790
$Cov(b_{1i}, b_{3i}) = g_{13}$	−2.5220	6.5000	−2.5850	6.4420
$Cov(b_{2i}, b_{3i}) = g_{23}$	−7.1530	1.0070	−7.0980	1.0090
$Var(e_i) = \sigma^2$	515.3000	9.3570	515.2000	9.3880

various distribution of the latent factor **u**, we adopted two distribution forms: normal distribution and logistic distribution. In the specification of parameters in logistic distribution, we choose so that the logistic distribution has similar shape with the normal distribution, in order to achieve comparability. Estimation procedure was performed within the full Bayesian framework, and the estimation results of parameters including point estimates and standard errors in the linear mixed model are given in Table 3. The routine experienced longer time to obtain stable mixed Markov chains when a logistic distribution was used. In detail, we extended the burn-in iterations to $20,000$ and started another $30,000$ iterations to obtain posterior estimates, with thinning size 10. From Table 3 one can observe that two distributions produced identical results, due to specified similar distribution shapes. Furthermore, one advantage should be mentioned is that the proposed Bayesian estimating scheme is more flexible in extending distribution of repeated-measures, other than stating different distribution shapes on the latent factor **u**.

In this study, missing data are potentially not ignorable with analyzing a random selected subsample, especially for the first 16 weeks. To evaluate effectiveness of treatment therapies, we compared three approaches, including the ignorable model which assumes missing data are MAR, Roy's model that handles non-ignorable missing data from pattern-mixture perspective, and CLFM with NMAR assumption. Controversial results on change rates of log CD4 counts at dual therapy group during first 16 weeks were obtained, that is, ignorable suggested there is a significant decrease in log CD4 counts, whereas both Roy's model and CLFM indicated this decrease is not substantial. This disagreement is due to those potential non-ignorable missing values. However, all approaches supported that triple therapy has similar change rate on log CD4 counts from week 16 to week 40, compare with dual therapy group. Further, with incorporating missing values, efficacy for both therapy groups is shown to be more substantial from CLFM, which can be seen from the log CD4 counts at week 40. Compared with Roy's model, the proposed CLFM is more flexible in extending the model with a more general distribution.

5   Conclusion and Discussion

In a longitudinal study, an incomplete dataset does not contain information that enables us to identify underlying a missing mechanism, unless extra unverifiable assumptions can be made. In the last two decades, researchers have investigated the implications of NMAR missing data by fitting selection models and pattern-mixture models. However, these models include difficulties to implement in a real case. Selection models make unverifiable assumptions for the missing mechanism, while pattern-mixture models tend to have over-parameterization issues, as well as conditional independence assumptions. In this thesis, we developed a non-ignorable model based on the idea of continuous latent factor of response behavior (missing behavior), and argue that this model excludes most implementing difficulties and is a useful alternative to a standard analysis with MAR assumption.

We believe that this new approach will avoid untestable missing mechanism assumptions from selection models and also believe that the new model will be more appealing to social behavioral and clinical researchers than pattern-mixture models because the new model eliminates over-parameterization issues. Further, the continuous latent factor provides an intuitive description of the response patterns in the study, and offers a feasible way to test conditional independence assumptions. For researchers who are interested in implementing CLFM model, we encourage them to compare latent factor models on missing indicator matrix with either constant slope or heterogeneous slopes and choose the one with better fitting in CLFM based on information criteria or the likelihood ratio test. Lastly, CLFM is more feasible for small samples. With the truth that the underlying missing mechanism for missing data is unknown, (that is whether missingness is due to MAR or NMAR), we take this new method primarily as a tool for sensitivity analysis. In the case that a researcher cannot determine the distribution of missing data, the most responsible and objective approach to proceed is to explore and present alternative results from different plausible models.

In this paper, we have explored the proposed CLFM under the assumption of a multivariate normal distribution for the complete data. The normal model is an intuitive and natural starting point for this method, but it also has limitations. Many longitudinal studies will have discrete responses, such as measuring the total number of bleeding counts in a Hemophilia study; or even binary responses. In the future, we will be extending our method to more flexible models for multivariate discrete responses. One promising approach is the Bayesian estimation approach which allows these extensions to be more straightforward.

To achieve an in-depth understanding of our method's properties, it is desirable to perform more simulation studies to compare this method to existing MAR and

NMAR alternatives under a variety of missing data mechanisms. Some might regard them as artificial, because in each realistic example the true mechanism is unknown. Nevertheless, it would be interesting to explore whether the proposed model performs better or worse than other methods when its assumptions are violated.

In proposing CLFM, we have a fundamental assumption which is conditional independence. Unlike models that belong to pattern mixture family, this assumption is feasible to be tested in CLFM. As another future work, we will explore the assessment on this assumed conditional independence in the CLFM from the fitted residuals. One approach is to calculate the residual from both the longitudinal and missing pattern models. When these residuals can be treated as approximately *iid* normal, a correlation coefficient close to 0 will indicate the conditional independence. For a more complicated distribution, some graphical approaches may be useful and could be applied as auxiliary tools.

References

Adams, R.J., Wilson, M., Wu, M.: Multilevel item response models: An approach to errors in variables regression. J. Educ. Behav. Stat. **22**, 47–76 (1997)

Birch, M.W.: A new proof of the Pearson-Fisher theorem. Ann. Math. Stat. **35**, 818–824 (1964)

Bock, R.D., Aitkin, M.: Marginal maximum likelihood estimation of item parameters: application of an em algorithm. Psychometrika **46**, 443–458 (1981)

Diggle, P., Kenward, M.G.: Informative drop-out in longitudinal data analysis. Appl. Stat. **43**, 49–73 (1994)

Diggle, P., Liang, K.Y., Zeger, S.L.: Analysis of Longitudinal Data. Oxford University Press, Oxford (1994)

Embretson, S.E., Reise, S.P.: Item Response Theory for Psychologists. Erlbaum, Mahwah (2000)

Fitzmaurice, G.M., Laird, N.M., Ware, J.H.: Applied Longitudinal Analysis. Wiley, New York (2004)

Geman, S., Geman, D.: Stochastic relaxation, gibbs distributions, and the bayesian restoration of images. IEEE Trans. Pattern Anal. Mach. Intell. **6**, 721–741 (1984)

Guo, W., Ratcliffe, S.J., Ten Have, T.R.: A random pattern-mixture model for longitudinal data with dropouts. J. Am. Stat. Assoc. **99**(468), 929–937 (2004)

Hastings, W.K.: Monte carlo sampling methods using markov chains and their application. Biometrika **57**, 97–109 (1970)

Henry, K., Erice, A., Tierney, C., Balfour, H.H. Jr., Fischl, M.A., Kmack, A., Liou, S.H., Kenton, A., Hirsch, M.S., Phair, J., Martinez, A., Kahn, J.O.: A randomized, controlled, double-blind study comparing the survival benefit of four different reverse transcriptase inhibitor therapies for the treatment of advanced aids. J. Acquir. Immune Defic. Syndr. Hum. Retrovirol. **19**(3), 339–349 (1998)

Jung, H., Schafer, J.L., Seo, B.: A latent class selection model for nonignorably missing data. Comput. Stat. Data Anal. **55**(1), 802–812 (2011)

Laird, M.M., Ware, J.H.: Random-effects models for longitudinal data. Biometrics **38**(4), 963–974 (1982)

Lin, H., McCulloch, C.E., Rosenheck, R.A.: Latent pattern mixture models for informative intermittent missing data in longitudinal studies. Biometrics **60**(2), 295–305 (2004)

Little, R.J.A.: Pattern-mixture models for multivariate incomplete data. J. Am. Stat. Assoc. **88**, 125–134 (1993)

Little, R.J.A., Rubin, D.B.: Statistical Analysis with Missing Data. Wiley Series in Probability and Statistics. Wiley, New York (2002)

Lord, F.: A Theory of Test Scores (Psychometric Monograph No. 7). Psychometric Corporation, Richmond (1952)

Lord, F.M.: The relation of test score to the trait underlying the test. Educ. Psychol. Meas. **13**, 517–548 (1953)

Lord, F.M.: Applications of Item Response Theory to Practical Testing Problems. Erlbaum, Hillsdale (1989).

Louis, T.A.: Finding the observed information matrix when using the em algorithm. J. R. Stat. Soc. Ser. B. **44**, 226–233 (1982).

McCulloch, C.E., Searle, S.R.: Generalized, Linear, and Mixed Models. Wiley, New York (2001)

Meng, X.L., Schilling, S.: Fitting full-information item factor models and an empirical investigation of bridge sampling. J. Am. Stat. Assoc. **91**, 1254–1267 (1996)

Muthén, B.: Contributions to factor analysis of dichotomous variables. Psychometrika **43**, 551–560 (1978)

Muthén, B., Jo, B., Brown, C.H.: Principal stratification approach to broken randomized experiments: A case study of school choice vouchers in new york city [with comment]. J. Am. Stat. Assoc. **98**(462), 311–314 (2003)

Pirie, P.L., Murray, D.M., Luepker, R.V.: Smoking prevalence in a cohort of adolescents, including absentees, dropouts, and transfers. Am. J. Public Health **78**, 176–178 (1988)

Rasch, G.: Probabilistic Models for Some Intelligence and Attainment Tests. University of Chicago Press, Chicago (1960)

Raudenbush, S.W., Johnson, C., Sampson, R.: A multivariate, multilevel rasch model with applications to self-reported criminal behavior. Sociol. Methodol. **33**, 169–211 (2003)

Rijmen, F., Tuerlinckx, F., De Boeck, P., Kuppens, P.: A nonlinear mixed model framework for item response theory. Psychol. Methods **8**, 185–205 (2003)

Robert, C.P., Casella, G.: Introducing Monte Carlo Methods with R. Springer, New York (2010)

Roy, J.: Modeling longitudinal data with nonignorable dropouts using a latent dropout class model. Biometrics **59**(4), 829–836 (2003)

Schafer, J.L.: Analysis of Incomplete Multivariate Data. Chapman and Hall, New York (1997)

Takane, Y., de Leeuw, J.: On the relationship between item response theory and factor analysis of discretized variables. Psychometrica **52**, 393–408 (1987)

Verbeke, G., Molenberghs, G.: Linear Mixed Models for Longitudinal Data. Springer, New York (2000)

Wei, G.C., Tanner, M.A.: A monte carlo implementation of the em algorithm and the poor man's data augmentation algorithms. J. Am. Stat. Assoc. **85**, 699–704 (1990)

Wu, C.F.J.: On the convergence of properties of the em algorithm. Ann. Stat. **11**, 95–103 (1983)

Zhang, J.: A continuous latent factor model for non-ignorable missing data in longitudinal studies. Unpublished doctoral dissertation, Arizona State Univeristy (2014).

Zhang, J., Reiser, M.: Simulation study on selection of latent class models with missing data. In: JSM Proceedings, Biometrics Section, pp. 98–111. American Statistical Association, Alexandria (2012)

Part III
Healthcare Research Models

Health Surveillance

Steven E. Rigdon and Ronald D. Fricker, Jr.

Abstract This chapter describes the application of statistical methods for health surveillance, including those for health care quality monitoring and those for disease surveillance. The former includes adverse event surveillance as well as the monitoring of non-disease health outcomes, such as rates of caesarean section or hospital readmission rates. The latter includes various types of disease surveillance, including traditional surveillance as well as syndromic surveillance. The methods described are drawn from the industrial quality control and monitoring literature where they are frequently referred to as "control charts." The chapter includes a detailed background of that literature as well as a discussion of the criteria and metrics used to assess the performance of methods of health surveillance methods.

1 Introduction

Health surveillance shares many characteristics with industrial process monitoring. In both cases, the goal is to appropriately manage a process—whether it is, for example, a surgical process or some industrial fabrication process—and it is desirable to detect degradations in process quality as quickly as possible. For this reason, many of the same techniques are used, including the Shewhart control chart, and other types of charts based on accumulating information such as the cumulative sum (CUSUM) chart and the exponentially weighted moving average (EWMA) chart.

However, there are differences between health surveillance and industrial process monitoring that must be taken into account. For example, when an industrial quality control chart raises a signal, the process is usually stopped while an investigation is made into the cause. In contrast, health monitoring, particularly disease surveillance, continues throughout an investigation. Another difference is that a typical disease

S.E. Rigdon (✉)
Department of Biostatistics, Saint Louis University, Saint Louis, MO, USA
e-mail: srigdon@slu.edu

R.D. Fricker, Jr.
Virginia Tech., Blacksburg, VA, USA
e-mail: rf@vt.edu

© Springer International Publishing Switzerland 2015
D.-G. Chen, J. Wilson (eds.), *Innovative Statistical Methods for Public Health Data,*
ICSA Book Series in Statistics, DOI 10.1007/978-3-319-18536-1_10

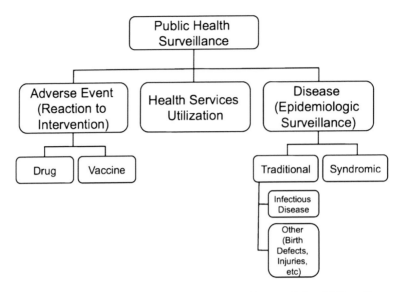

Fig. 1 A taxonomy of public health surveillance activities. *Source*: Fricker (2013, p. 6)

outbreak will naturally grow and recede even when no action is taken to mitigate the outbreak while in the industrial case process degradations typically persist until the cause is detected and corrected.

Figure 1, taken from Fricker (2013, p. 6), is a basic taxonomy of public health surveillance, which includes the surveillance of adverse reactions to medical interventions (particularly drugs and vaccines) and how health services are used, as well as disease (epidemiologic) surveillance. Brookmeyer and Stroup (2004, p. 1) quote Thacker (2000) in defining public health surveillance as "the ongoing systematic collection, analysis, interpretation, and dissemination of health data for the purpose of preventing and controlling disease, injury, and other health problems."

In this chapter, we describe the application of industrial process monitoring (also referred to as statistical process control) methods to health care, where we bifurcate the various health surveillance activities shown in Fig. 1 into those for health care quality monitoring and those for disease surveillance. The former includes adverse event surveillance, such as death following surgery, as well as the monitoring of non-disease health outcomes, such as rates of caesarean section or hospital readmission rates. The latter includes various types of disease surveillance, including traditional surveillance as well as syndromic surveillance. In so doing, we also discuss the criteria and metrics used to assess the performance of methods of health surveillance methods.

2 Background on Industrial Process Monitoring

In any system, there is a certain amount of noise that is present that cannot be reduced without fundamentally changing the system. Occasionally, however, some change is introduced into the system resulting in a change to the output. This change could affect the mean response, the variability of the response, or it could influence the process output in some other way. Monitoring industrial processes via control charts dates back to the 1920s when Walter Shewhart suggested that there is a distinction between *common* causes of variability, the inherent noise in the system, and *special* causes of variability, those sources which induce a change in the system (Shewhart 1931).

Shewhart's insight was to plot quality measures of the output, and to specify upper limit and lower limits that within which the plotted measure is likely to be if the process is *in-control*, that is, producing output with the same mean and variance. Points outside these *control limits* would then be taken to indicate that the process has changed. Often the control limits are placed three standards above and below the process mean, since the probability of a random variable being beyond three standard deviations is very small (e.g., the probability is 0.0027 if the normal distribution is an accurate model for the outcomes).

The kind of chart that is used to monitor the process depends on the type of data collected. These are discussed in the next few subsections.

2.1 Monitoring Continuous Outcomes

When the outcome is the measurement of some quantity, such as length, weight, time, density, etc., then the data are said to be continuous. The quality control literature often uses the term *variables data* for continuous measures.

For continuous data, the typical procedure is to take subgroups of size n (often $n = 3$ to 5) and from each subgroup compute the average $\bar{x}$ and some measure of the variability, such as the range ($R = x_{max} - x_{min}$) or the sample standard deviation s. These statistics, $\bar{x}_1, \bar{x}_2, \bar{x}_3, \ldots$ and either $R_1, R_2, R_3, \ldots$ or $s_1, s_2, s_3, \ldots$, are then plotted in time order in order to monitor the mean and variance of the process.

If the process is normally distributed with a mean of μ_0 and standard deviation of σ_0 when the process is in control, then the *upper control limit* (UCL) and the *lower control limit* (LCL) for the "$\bar{X}$-chart" are:

$$\text{UCL}_{\bar{X}} = \mu_0 + 3\frac{\sigma_0}{\sqrt{n}}$$

$$\text{LCL}_{\bar{X}} = \mu_0 - 3\frac{\sigma_0}{\sqrt{n}}.$$

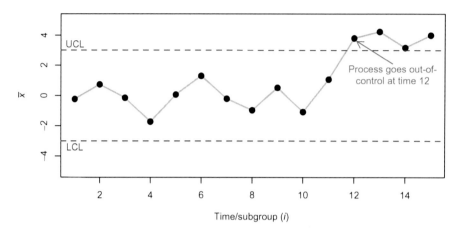

Fig. 2 An illustrative $\bar{X}$-chart where the process goes out of control at time 12

The control limits for the "R-chart" are $\mathrm{UCL}_R = D_2\sigma_0$ and $\mathrm{LCL}_R = D_1\sigma_0$, while for the "$s$-chart" they are $\mathrm{UCL}_s = B_6\sigma_0$ and $\mathrm{LCL}_s = B_5\sigma_0$. The constants D_1, D_2, B_5, and B_6 are functions of the subgroup size n, and are tabulated in most books on statistical quality control (e.g., see Montgomery 2009, Appendix VI, p. 702).

The basic idea of a control chart is to then monitor future observations. Those that fall within the LCL and UCL are determined to have only common variability and thus the process is assumed to be behaving normally. However, if one or more points fall outside of the control limits, that is an indication that one or more special causes of variability are present, and thus the process is not behaving normally. Under these conditions, the control chart is said to *signal* and the process should be investigated and the special causes of variability identified and rectified. Figure 2 is an example of an $\bar{X}$-chart with "3-sigma" control limits where the control chart signals an out-of-control condition at time $i = 12$.

In practice, of course, the parameters μ_0 and σ_0 are unknown and must be estimated from data taken when the process is in control. The iterative process of collecting data, estimating parameters, discarding data for which there is an explainable cause, re-estimating the parameters is called *Phase 1*. This process is often more difficult than it might sound; see Jordan and Benneyan (2012) for a description of the issues involved when health care data are being monitored.

The usual estimate for μ_0 is the grand average of the subgroup means for data taken when the process is in control. That is, for m subgroups,

$$\bar{\bar{x}} = \frac{1}{m}\sum_{i=1}^{m} \bar{x}_i.$$

The in-control standard deviation σ_0 is estimated by

$$\hat{\sigma}_0 = \bar{R}/d_2,$$

if the R-chart is used to monitor the variability, where $\overline{R}$ is the average of the m range measures, or

$$\hat{\sigma}_0 = \frac{1}{m} \sum_{i=1}^{m} s_i.$$

if the s-chart is used. As with the other constants, the constant d_2 is tabulated in, for example, Montgomery (2009, Appendix VI, p. 702).

Once the process parameters are estimated from historical data with reasonable accuracy, that is, with a sufficiently large number of subgroups, the real-time monitoring of the process begins. This is called *Phase II* and it is the phase that is most often associated with the use of control charts. Recent studies indicate that the needed sample sizes can be much larger than previously thought; see Champ et al. (2005), Jensen et al. (2006), and Champ and Jones-Farmer (2007).

Subgrouping is widely recommended because a sample average is more likely to signal a change (if there is one) than control charts based on individual observations. There are times, however, when each individual data value should be plotted and a decision made about the process. For example, if data points are taken very infrequently, it might be desirable to plot each one. In cases like this, the "individuals chart," or simply the "X-chart" can be applied. If the mean and standard deviation are known, then the control limits for an individuals chart based on 3-sigma limits are simply

$$\text{UCL}_X = \mu_0 + 3\sigma_0$$

$$\text{LCL}_X = \mu_0 - 3\sigma_0.$$

Since the parameters are generally not known in practice, it is necessary to estimate them from the data (when the process is in control). The estimate for μ_0 is $\bar{x}$, the sample average, but there are different approaches to estimating σ_0. One approach is to simply compute the sample standard deviation of the observed data. This, however, will overestimate σ_0 if the process was not completely in-control when the data were collected. Instead, the usual procedure is to first compute the moving ranges

$$MR_i = |x_i - x_{i-1}|, \quad i = 2, 3, \ldots,$$

and then estimate σ_0 as $\hat{\sigma}_0 = \overline{MR}/1.128$. This "short term" estimate of the variability is less likely to overestimate σ_0.

Some authors suggest running an X-chart to monitor the process mean and a chart of the moving ranges to monitor the process dispersion. Rigdon et al. (1994) have shown that the MR-chart is nearly powerless to detect changes in variability. They suggest plotting only an X-chart to monitor both mean and variability.

2.2   Monitoring Discrete Outcomes

Rather than measuring the quality of a unit on a continuous scale, there are cases where each unit can be only be classified as *conforming* or *nonconforming*, where conforming means that the unit meets the requisite quality standards. For example, a requirement that the unit should be free of surface blemishes does not yield a measurement; a unit either has or does not have surface blemishes. A similar type of data occurs when, for example, one is counting the number of scratches in a roll of sheet metal. Data such as these are called *attributes* data in the quality literature and *discrete* data in much of the statistics literature.

In the situation where each unit is either conforming or nonconforming, the usual procedure is to take a subgroup of size n_i at time i and observe the number X_i of nonconforming units. If the units are independent with constant probability (within the subgroup) of being nonconforming, p_i, then X_i has a binomial distribution with parameters n_i and p_i. When the process is in-control, the probability is constant, that is, $p_i = p_0$ for all i. The goal is to detect a change as quickly as possible if the nonconforming probability shifts to p_1, which could be larger or smaller than p_0.

A chart of $\hat{p}_i = x_i/n_i$ against the time index i is called a "p-chart." The mean and variance of $\hat{p}_i$ are $E(\hat{p}_i) = p_0$ and $V(\hat{p}_i) = p_0(1 - p_0)/n_i$ for an in-control process. The control limits are then placed three standard deviations above and below the mean:

$$\mathrm{UCL}_p = p_0 + 3\sqrt{\frac{p_0(1 - p_0)}{n_i}}, \tag{1}$$

$$\mathrm{LCL}_p = \max\left(0, p_0 - 3\sqrt{\frac{p_0(1 - p_0)}{n_i}}\right). \tag{2}$$

The max in the formula for the LCL is needed because the second expression in Eq. (2) can be negative for small values of p_0 or n_i. If the LCL is equal to 0, then no signal can be raised for a decrease in the proportion nonconforming. It is usually desirable to detect a decrease in p for two reasons: first, a low value of $\hat{p}$ could be due to measurement error (e.g., a new employee who misunderstands the criteria for nonconforming), and second, a change in the process that leads to *better* quality is worth knowing so that the change can be made permanent (or more widely implemented).

Often, the subgroup size n_i is constant, in which case the control limits in Eqs. (1) and (2) are constant. However, there are cases where the n_i will vary from subgroup to subgroup. For example, in monitoring surgical outcomes, the time frame might be fixed at one month, and the number of surgeries will vary from month to month. In these types of cases, the control limits will vary.

In practice, the probability that an item is nonconforming is unknown, so its value must be estimated from past data. The usual estimate is to take all values taken from the process when it was in control and compute

$$\bar{p}_0 = \frac{x_1 + x_2 + \cdots + x_m}{n_1 + n_2 + \cdots + n_m}.$$

Of course, if $n_i = n$ for all subgroups, then this estimate of p_0 is simply the average of the $\hat{p}_i$.

Occasionally, the total number of nonconforming units X_i is monitored rather than the proportion. This is called an "np-chart" since $X_i = n_i \hat{p}_i$ when the process is stable. The np-chart is normally used only when the subgroup sizes n_i are constant.

There are situations where the output is a count of the number of nonconformities *per unit*. For example, the measurement might be the number of voids (air pockets) in a plastic molded part; for any unit, there could be 0, or 1, or 2, etc., voids. That is, there can be more than one nonconformity per unit. For count data such as this, the Poisson distribution is often an appropriate model for the number of nonconformities X_i per unit at time i. The Poisson distribution has one parameter λ, which is also the mean and variance of the distribution: $E(X_i) = \lambda$ and $V(X_i) = \lambda$.

A plot of x_i against i is called a "c-chart," and the control limits are

$$\text{UCL}_c = \lambda_0 + 3\sqrt{\lambda_0},$$
$$\text{LCL}_c = \max\left(0, \lambda_0 - 3\sqrt{\lambda_0}\right), \tag{3}$$

where λ_0 is the Poisson distribution parameter when the process is in control. The maximum function is needed in Eq. (3) because $\lambda_0 - 3\sqrt{\lambda_0}$ is negative when $\lambda_0 < 9$. Of course, in practice the value of λ_0 is unknown and must be estimated from prior data,

$$\hat{\lambda}_0 = \frac{1}{m} \sum_{i=1}^{m} x_i,$$

where the estimate is calculated for the m Phase I data periods when the process in control.

The Poisson distribution is often a reasonable model for the number of events that occur in a fixed time interval, or the number of occurrences on a fixed area of the output. There are cases, though, where the variance is larger than the mean. This phenomenon is called *overdispersion*, and if this occurs for some data set, the negative binomial distribution (a two-parameter distribution) is often used in place of the Poisson.

The *c*-chart assumes that the sample consists of a single unit, and the number x_i of nonconformities on that unit is recorded. The sample at each time unit could, however, consist of n_i units, rather than a single unit. The statistic $u_i = x_i/n_i$ is then plotted. A plot of u_i against time i is called a "*u*-chart." The control limits for the *u*-chart are

$$\text{UCL}_u = \lambda_0 + 3\sqrt{\frac{\lambda_0}{n_i}},$$

$$\text{LCL}_u = \max\left(0, \lambda_0 - 3\sqrt{\frac{\lambda_0}{n_i}}\right).$$

All of the charts described in Sects. 2.1 and 2.2 are commonly referred to as Shewhart charts—named after Walter Shewhart, who first used them—and they share the property that the decision made at the current time is based on data collected only at the current time. If, for example, a point is inside the control limits, then the process is deemed to be in-control and when the next data point is collected, this point and all past data points are ignored.[1]

For Shewhart charts, the number of subgroups between signals has a geometric distribution with parameter p which is the probability of being outside of the control limits. The expected number of subgroups between signals is commonly referred to as the *average run length* (or ARL), where ARL= $1/p$, and the ARL is used to quantify and compare the performance of control charts.

For the $\overline{X}$-chart with 3-sigma limits, for example, the probability of signaling when the process is in-control is $p = 0.0027$ and so the *in-control ARL* or ARL(0) is $1/p = 370$. This is the average time until a *false* signal—it is a false signal because the process is in-control—and thus ARL(0) is a measure of how well the control chart performs when the process is in-control.

Now, if a process were to go out-of-control, say with the mean increasing by one standard deviation (i.e., $\mu_1 = \mu_0 + \sigma/\sqrt{n}$), then the probability is $p = 0.0227$ that a subgroup mean will exceed the UCL (and negligible probability that the subgroup mean would fall below the LCL: 0.00003). Under these conditions, the *out-of-control ARL* or ARL(1) is $1/p \approx 44$. (Here, ARL(δ) is the average run length when the process mean shifts by the amount δ standard deviations.) The result is that it can take a Shewhart $\overline{X}$-chart a long time to signal for small to moderate changes in the mean.

---

[1] Sometimes Shewhart charts are used with supplementary runs rules, such as "also signal if there are eight points in a row on the same side of the center line." In these cases, it is no longer true that past data are ignored, but even with the addition of such rules, the charts just described are often referred to as Shewhart charts.

2.3   Control Charts Based on Accumulating Data

In order to improve on the ability to detect small to moderate changes in processes, charts have been developed that accumulate information across time, rather than discarding all in-control past data. This section describes the two most popular: the *cumulative sum* (CUSUM) and the *EWMA* control charts.

2.3.1   CUSUM Charts

The CUSUM chart is based on the sequential probability ratio test of Wald (1945) which is designed to test the simple hypotheses $H_0 : \theta = \theta_0$ and $H_1 : \theta = \theta_1$. The sequential probability ratio test is designed to do this sequentially in time; that is, at each stage, the decision can be to accept H_0, reject H_0, or continue taking data. Wald (1945) showed that the optimal form of the test is to compute the cumulative sum

$$X_i = X_{i-1} + \log \frac{L_{1i}}{L_{0i}},$$

where L_{ji} is the likelihood under H_j, $j = 0, 1$. The sequential probability ratio test terminates when

$$X_i > b = \log \left(\frac{1 - \beta}{\alpha} \right)$$

or when

$$X_i < a = \log \left(\frac{\beta}{1 - \alpha} \right),$$

where α and β are the desired (or target) probabilities of Type I and Type II errors, respectively. (The values given for a and b given above yield values of α and β that are only approximately correct; the true probabilities of Type I or Type II errors will differ slightly from the target.) In the case of process monitoring, whether it be quality or health, there is really never an option to "accept" the null hypothesis, so the lower limit is ignored. Thus, the lower boundary is normally replaced by a reflecting boundary, usually at zero.

Because the null hypothesis is never "accepted" and eventually the statistic X_i will cross its boundary b, the probabilities of Type I and Type II errors are really 1 and 0, respectively. For this reason, the metrics of Type I and Type II errors are never used in process monitoring. Rather, we look at properties of the run length distribution. Since we want to detect quickly a large shift, the run length should be small when the process change is large, and since we don't want false alarms, we want the run length to be large when there is no change. The ARL defined in

Sect. 2.2 is a common metric, especially in the quality monitoring literature, but there are other metrics that can be used. See Fraker et al. (2008) for a discussion of other metrics.

The CUSUM control chart of Page (1954) and Lorden (1971) is a well-known industrial process monitoring methodology. The simplest form involves the sum

$$C_i = \sum_{j=1}^{i} (x_i - \mu_0), \tag{4}$$

where $x_1, x_2, \ldots$ is the process output, μ_0 is the in-control mean, and $C_0 = 0$. The CUSUM expression in Eq. (4) can also be calculated recursively as

$$C_i = C_{i-1} + (x_i - \mu_0).$$

This version of the CUSUM chart involves plotting C_i against the time index i and looking for changes in the *slope* of the data. This is rather difficult to do by eye, so graphical procedures, such as the V-mask (Montgomery 2009, p. 415), have been developed.

An alternative to the V-mask is to accumulate two separate cumulative sums: one to detect upward increases in the mean, and one to detect decreases. Suppose that μ_0 and σ_0 are the process mean and standard deviation when the process is in-control, and suppose it is desirable to detect a change of k standard deviations in the mean, i.e., a shift from μ_0 to $\mu_1 = \mu_0 + k\sigma_0/\sqrt{n}$ if subgroups of size n are used. The two CUSUMs are defined by

$$C_0^+ = 0$$

$$C_i^+ = \max\left(0, C_{i-1}^+ + \frac{x_i - \mu_0}{\sigma_0} - k\right) \tag{5}$$

and

$$C_0^- = 0$$

$$C_i^- = \min\left(0, C_{i-1}^- + \frac{x_i - \mu_0}{\sigma_0} + k\right). \tag{6}$$

The CUSUM chart raises a signal when $C_i^+ > h$ or $C_i^- < -h$. Since in some cases it is more desirable to detect quickly an increase in the mean than a decrease (or vice-versa), it is possible to use different values of k and h for the upper and lower CUSUMs.

For small to moderate shifts, the CUSUM chart will signal a change with a shorter ARL than the Shewhart chart when the two charts have the same in-control ARL. For example, the CUSUM chart with $k = 0.5$ and $h = 5$ yields

$$ARL_{CUSUM}(0) = 465$$

$$ARL_{CUSUM}(1) = 10.4$$

whereas the Shewhart chart with 3.069σ limits has

$$ARL_{Shewhart}(0) = 465$$

$$ARL_{Shewhart}(1) = 52.0.$$

Thus, the CUSUM will catch a one standard deviation shift in the mean, on average, in one-fifth the time as the Shewhart chart with the same ARL(0) performance. Although the CUSUM will catch small to moderate shifts much quicker than the Shewhart, the reverse is true when there is a very large shift. For example, $ARL_{CUSUM}(4) = 2.0$ whereas $ARL_{Shewhart}(4) = 1.2$. For this reason, the CUSUM and the Shewhart charts are often used in tandem, often with limits of ± 3.5 standard deviations or higher on the Shewhart chart.

The CUSUM can also be used to monitor process variability. For example, to monitor an increase in process variability, following Hawkins and Olwell (1998, p. 67), use the CUSUM recursion

$$V_i = \max[0, V_{i-1} + y_i - k],$$

where

$$y_i = \frac{\sqrt{|x_i|} - 0.822}{0.394}.$$

As recommended by Hawkins and Olwell, the same value for k should be used in these CUSUMs for monitoring variability as in the CUSUMs for the mean.

2.3.2 The Exponentially Weighted Moving Average Chart

The EWMA chart of Roberts (1959) calculates weighted averages of the current data value (x_i) and the previous EWMA statistic (z_{i-1}),

$$z_i = \lambda x_i + (1 - \lambda)z_{i-1}, \tag{7}$$

where λ is a smoothing constant between 0 and 1 and typically $z_0 = \mu_0$. The statistic z_i can be written in terms of all previous x_i values as

$$z_i = \lambda x_i + \lambda(1 - \lambda)x_{i-1} + \lambda(1 - \lambda)^2 x_{i-2} + \cdots + \lambda(1 - \lambda)^{i-1}x_1 + (1 - \lambda)^i \mu_0.$$

The weights on past data values decrease exponentially, hence the name of the control chart.

When the process is in-control

$$E(z_i) = \mu_0$$

and

$$V(z_i) = \frac{\lambda}{2-\lambda}\left[1 - (1-\lambda)^{2i}\right]\sigma_0^2.$$

The quantity $\left[1 - (1-\lambda)^{2i}\right]$ approaches 1 as $i \to \infty$; this gives the asymptotic variance as

$$V(z_i) \approx \frac{\lambda}{2-\lambda}\sigma_0^2.$$

The exact control limits for the EWMA chart are therefore

$$\text{UCL}_{\text{EWMA}} = \mu_0 + L\sigma_0\sqrt{\frac{\lambda}{2-\lambda}\left[1 - (1-\lambda)^{2i}\right]},$$

$$\text{LCL}_{\text{EWMA}} = \mu_0 - L\sigma_0\sqrt{\frac{\lambda}{2-\lambda}\left[1 - (1-\lambda)^{2i}\right]},$$

while the asymptotic control limits are

$$\text{UCL}_{\text{EWMA}} = \mu_0 + L\sigma_0\sqrt{\frac{\lambda}{2-\lambda}},$$

$$\text{LCL}_{\text{EWMA}} = \mu_0 - L\sigma_0\sqrt{\frac{\lambda}{2-\lambda}}.$$

The values of λ and L are chosen to give the desired in-control and out-of-control ARLs. The EWMA chart has properties much like the CUSUM chart. ARLs for small to moderate shifts are much smaller for the EWMA or CUSUM chart than for the Shewhart chart. For example, with $\lambda = 0.1$ and $L = 2.79$:

$$\text{ARL}_{\text{EWMA}}(0) = 468$$

$$\text{ARL}_{\text{EWMA}}(1) = 10.2$$

$$\text{ARL}_{\text{EWMA}}(4) = 2.2.$$

Comparing these numbers to those of the CUSUM chart, note that the EWMA and CUSUM charts have similar ARL properties.

Very small values of λ, such as $\lambda = 0.05$, for example, produce a nearly uniform weighting of past observations, with very little weight on the current data value. As a result, similar to the CUSUM, large shifts are difficult to detect quickly with the EWMA chart.

2.4   Multivariate Control Charts

In even the simplest process there is frequently more than one quality characteristic to be monitored and these quality characteristics are often correlated. For example, in industrial process monitoring, measurements of dimensions on a plastic part are generally affected by the pressure and length of time that the plastic was intruded into the mold. If the time and pressure are both high, then all dimensions of the part will tend to be on the high side. Similar issues arise in health and monitoring; for example, when monitoring systolic and diastolic blood pressure.

Assuming the quality measures have a multivariate, specifically a p-variate, normal distribution with mean vector μ_0 and covariance matrix Σ, so that $\mathbf{x} \sim N_p(\mu_0, \Sigma)$, then the Mahalonobis distance

$$T^2 = (\mathbf{x} - \mu_0)' \, \Sigma^{-1} \, (\mathbf{x} - \mu_0) \tag{8}$$

is the distance from $\mathbf{x}$ to the distribution's mean μ_0, taking into account the covariance. Two points with the same Mahalonobis distance will have equal probability density height. Note that observations of the multiple quality characteristics within a single unit are correlated, but successive random vectors are independent.

A chart based on the T^2 statistic is called the Hotelling T^2 chart (Hotelling 1947). If subgroups of size n are used, then the sample mean $\bar{\mathbf{x}}_i$ and is computed for each subgroup and the T^2 statistic becomes

$$T_i^2 = n(\bar{\mathbf{x}}_i - \mu_0)' \, \Sigma^{-1} \, (\bar{\mathbf{x}}_i - \mu_0).$$

If the parameters μ_0 and Σ are known (which is unlikely in practice), then T^2 has a $\chi^2(p)$ distribution, so the UCL is

$$\text{UCL}_{T^2} = \chi_\alpha^2(p).$$

Since T^2 measures the distance from the middle of the distribution, there is no LCL. If the parameters are unknown, and estimated by the grand mean

$$\bar{\bar{\mathbf{x}}} = \frac{1}{m} \sum_{j=1}^{m} \bar{\mathbf{x}}_j$$

and

$$\bar{\mathbf{S}} = \frac{1}{m} \sum_{j=1}^{m} \mathbf{S}_j,$$

where $\bar{\mathbf{x}}_j$ and $\mathbf{S}_j$ are the sample mean vector and sample covariance matrix within the jth subgroup, then the T^2 statistic becomes

$$T_i^2 = (\bar{\mathbf{x}}_i - \bar{\bar{\mathbf{x}}})' \, \bar{\mathbf{S}}^{-1} \, (\bar{\mathbf{x}}_i - \bar{\bar{\mathbf{x}}}).$$

The UCL for the Phase II (i.e., prospective monitoring) is then

$$\text{UCL}_{T^2} = \frac{p(m+1)(m-1)}{m(m-p)} F_{\alpha,p,m-p}.$$

Champ et al. (2005) showed that very large sample sizes are needed in order to make the T^2 with estimated parameters behave like the T^2 chart with assumed known parameters.

The T^2 chart is a Shewhart chart in the sense that the decision at time i depends only on data from time i; no accumulation of data is done. It is also directionally invariant, that is, the run length distribution depends only on the magnitude of the shift, measured by the Mahalonobis distance

$$(\mu_1 - \mu_0)' \Sigma^{-1} (\mu_1 - \mu_0),$$

and not on the direction of the shift.

The CUSUM chart from Sect. 2.3.1 has been generalized to the multivariate setting. For example, Crosier (1988) proposed a *multivariate CUSUM* (or MCUSUM) control chart that at each time i calculates the cumulative sum

$$\mathbf{C}_i^* = \mathbf{C}_{i-1} + \mathbf{x}_i - \mu_0$$

and the statistical distance

$$d_i = \sqrt{\mathbf{C}_i^{*'} \Sigma_0^{-1} \mathbf{C}_i^*},$$

where μ_0 is the mean vector and Σ_0 is the variance–covariance matrix when the process is in-control. It then "shrinks" the cumulative sum by

$$\mathbf{C}_i = \begin{cases} \mathbf{C}_i^*(1 - k/d_i), & d_i > k \\ \mathbf{0}, & d_i \leq k \end{cases}, \tag{9}$$

where k is a predetermined statistical distance, and calculates the statistic

$$S_i = \sqrt{\mathbf{C}_i' \Sigma_0^{-1} \mathbf{C}_i}.$$

The control chart starts with $\mathbf{C}_0 = \mathbf{0}$ and it signals a change has occurred when $S_i \geq h$, for some threshold h.

The literature contains a number of other MCUSUM control charts. In fact, Crosier's MCUSUM control chart described above is one of a number of other multivariate CUSUM-like algorithms he proposed, but Crosier generally preferred the above procedure after extensive simulation comparisons. Pignatiello and Runger (1990) proposed other multivariate CUSUM-like algorithms but found that they performed similar to Crosier's. Healy (1987) derived a sequential likelihood ratio test to detect a shift in a mean vector of a multivariate normal distribution. However, while Healy's procedure is more effective when the change is to the precise mean vector to be detected, it is less effective than Crosier's for detecting other types of shifts, including mean shifts that were close to but not precisely the specified mean vector.

As with the CUSUM, the EWMA chart from Sect. 2.3.2 is also easily extended to the multivariate case, and the resulting chart is called the *multivariate EWMA* (or MEWMA) chart (Lowry et al. 1992). Similar to Eq. (7), the MEWMA statistic is defined as

$$\mathbf{z}_0 = \boldsymbol{\mu}_0,$$

$$\mathbf{z}_i = \lambda \mathbf{x}_i + (1 - \lambda)\mathbf{z}_{i-1},$$

where λ is a scalar value, $0 < \lambda \leq 1$. Then at time i, the T^2 statistic is calculated, analogous to Eq. (8), by

$$T_i^2 = n\,(\bar{\mathbf{z}}_i - \boldsymbol{\mu}_0)'\,\Sigma_{z_i}^{-1}\,(\bar{\mathbf{z}}_i - \boldsymbol{\mu}_0) \tag{10}$$

where

$$\Sigma_{z_i} = \frac{\lambda}{2 - \lambda}\left[1 - (1 - \lambda)^{2i}\right]\Sigma.$$

A signal is raised on the MEWMA chart whenever T^2 exceeds the value h. Just as for the univariate EWMA chart, the parameters λ and h are chosen to produce some of the desired ARL properties of the chart. Note that it is possible to use the exact covariance matrix or the asymptotic covariance matrix

$$\Sigma_z \approx \frac{\lambda}{2 - \lambda}\Sigma$$

in the computation of the T^2 statistic in Eq. (10). Thus, there are actually two versions of the MEWMA chart. Tables for choosing λ and h are given in Lowry et al. (1992) and Montgomery (2009).

The MCUSUM and MEWMA can detect small to moderate shifts in the mean more quickly than the Hotelling T^2 chart. For example, when $p = 6$, $\lambda = 0.2$, $h = 17.51$ and the shift is

$$\delta = \left[(\boldsymbol{\mu}_0 - \boldsymbol{\mu}_1)'\,\Sigma^{-1}\,(\boldsymbol{\mu}_0 - \boldsymbol{\mu}_1)\right]^{1/2}$$

the MEWMA ARL is 14.6. In contrast, the Hotelling T^2 chart with UCL $= h = 18.55$ gives an ARL of 74.4 for the same shift. Both control charts have an in-control ARL of 200.

3   Health Care Monitoring

In quality monitoring, it is usually assumed that the input materials are homogeneous, and that the resulting process output has a fixed mean and variance. Health care monitoring of individual patients, on the other hand, must account for differences among patients. This *case mix*, that is, the variability in risk factors among the patients being monitored, must be taken into account. Otherwise, providers who take on patients with high risk factors would be penalized when fewer patients survive.

Thus, the first important difference from industrial process monitoring is that health monitoring data must be *risk-adjusted*, so that comparison among or across providers is done fairly. In this context, risk adjustment means building a model using historical data relating risk factors, such as age, body mass index (BMI), diabetes status, etc., to the outcome variable. What is charted, then, is some statistic that does not depend on the levels of the predictor variable.

3.1   Risk-Adjusted Charts

Before any risk-adjusted chart can be applied, a model must be developed that relates the probability p_i of the adverse outcome for patient i to the predictor variables $x_{i1}, x_{i2}, \ldots, x_{ip}$. A logistic regression model assumes that this relationship is of the form

$$\text{logit}(p_{0i}) = \log \frac{p_{0i}}{1 - p_{0i}} = \beta_{00} + \beta_{01}x_1 + \cdots + \beta_{0p}x_p. \tag{11}$$

The parameters $\beta_{00}, \beta_{01}, \ldots, \beta_{0p}$ must be estimated from some baseline set of data taken when the process is stable. We will look for a change in the parameters from $\beta_{00}, \beta_{01}, \ldots, \beta_{0p}$ to $\beta_{10}, \beta_{11}, \ldots, \beta_{1p}$. If we write $\mathbf{x}_i = \begin{bmatrix} 1, x_{i1}, \ldots, x_{ip} \end{bmatrix}'$ and $\boldsymbol{\beta}_0 = \begin{bmatrix} \beta_{00}, \beta_{01}, \ldots, \beta_{0p} \end{bmatrix}'$, then we can write the logistic model in Eq. (11) as

$$p_{0i} = \frac{\exp\left(\mathbf{x}_i'\boldsymbol{\beta}_0\right)}{1 + \exp\left(\mathbf{x}_i'\boldsymbol{\beta}_0\right)}. \tag{12}$$

Consider, for example, the cardiac survival data from Steiner et al. (2000). The response variable is a dichotomous variable that indicates death within 30 days ($Y = 1$) or survival past 30 days ($Y = 0$).[2] The predictor variable is the Parsonnet score, a

---

[2] Attributes or discrete data are much more common in health care monitoring. In fact, many variables are dichotomized, that is changed from a continuous measurement into a yes/no measurement. Here, for example, the variable of interest is whether or not the patient survived for 30 days, not the actual survival time.

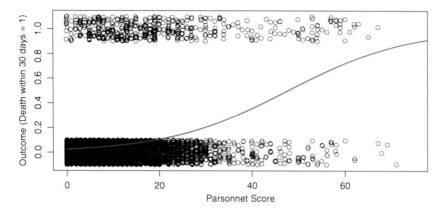

Fig. 3 Outcome (death within 30 days of surgery) versus Parsonnet score. Some "jitter" has been introduced to avoid many overlapping points

measure of a patient's condition. The Parsonnet score is a function of pre-operative measures of the patient's health, and including age and a number of categorical variables such as gender, diabetes status, hypertension status, etc. Higher Parsonnet score is associated with a weaker condition, and a higher chance of dying in the 30-day follow-up period. Generally, the Parsonnet scores vary from 0 to about 60, and follow somewhat closely the exponential distribution with mean 10. See Geissler et al. (2000) for a survey of other risk measures.

Figure 3 shows the Parsonnet score on the x-axis (with some jitter to avoid overlapping points) against the response ($Y = 1$ if the patient died within 30 days, and $Y = 0$ if the patient survived 30 days). The curve in this figure is the logistic fit of $p_i = P(Y_i = 1)$,

$$\text{logit}(\hat{p}_i) = -3.67 + 0.077x_i \tag{13}$$

or, equivalently,

$$\hat{p}_i = \frac{\exp(-3.67 + 0.077x_i)}{1 + \exp(-3.67 + 0.077x_i)}. \tag{14}$$

Once the in-control parameters $\boldsymbol{\beta}_0$ are estimated, we can monitor prospectively the outcomes of patients with varying risk factors. For example, suppose that the risk variables for patient i are contained in the vector $\boldsymbol{x}_i$ and we have estimates $\hat{\boldsymbol{\beta}}_0 = \left[\hat{\beta}_0, \hat{\beta}_1, \ldots, \hat{\beta}_p\right]$. From this, we can estimate from Eq. (12) the probability p_{i0} that patient i will experience the adverse effect (given that the process is in-control). The outcome y_i, where $y_i = 1$ if the adverse outcome occurs, and $y_i = 0$ if it doesn't, is compared to the expected outcome. The various ways this comparison is done, and the statistic that is computed, determines the type of chart.

In industrial process monitoring, the usual procedure is to compare data from a process with past data from that process when it was stable, that is, operating in a state of statistical control. Often in health care monitoring, the process output is compared to an external standard, not past data from the process (hospital, surgeon, etc.). This affects the interpretation of a point outside the control limits. In industrial process monitoring, a point outside the limits is evidence that the process has changed. When data are compared to an external standard, a point outside the limits is evidence that the process is not meeting the standard.

The next subsections cover risk-adjusted p-charts, CUSUM charts, EWMA charts, variable life adjusted display (VLAD) charts, and charts based on the sets method.

3.1.1   Risk-Adjusted p-Charts

One approach to monitoring binary outcomes $y_1, y_2, \ldots$ is to use subgrouping and to compare the observed proportion of adverse outcomes to the expected proportion. When health care monitoring is done using risk adjustment, the successive observations y_i are independent but not identically distributed because of the varying risk factors. (This is in contrast to the quality monitoring situation where successive observations are assumed to be independent and identically distributed.) For patients $i = 1, 2, \ldots$ we have $y_i \sim \text{Bin}(1, p_i)$. The total number of adverse outcomes in the subgroup of n observations $y_1, y_2, \ldots, y_n$ is $\sum_{i=1}^{n} y_i$, which has mean and variance

$$E\left(\sum_{i=1}^{n} y_i\right) = \sum_{i=1}^{n} p_i$$

and

$$V\left(\sum_{i=1}^{n} y_i\right) = \sum_{i=1}^{n} V(y_i) = \sum_{i=1}^{n} p_i(1 - p_i).$$

Because the varying risk factors cause the p_i to vary, the sum $\sum_{i=1}^{n} y_i$ does not have a binomial distribution. For the usual p-chart in industrial monitoring, the Central Limit Theorem is applied to argue that the proportions of nonconforming units in each subgroup is approximately normally distributed, and therefore that three standard deviation limits above and below the mean should include nearly all of the observed proportions. Similar reasoning applies here.

For the risk-adjusted p-chart, the plotted statistic is the proportion of adverse events $\hat{\pi} = \sum_{i=1}^{n} y_i/n$.[3] Since the mean and standard deviation of the plotted

---

[3]We use $\hat{\pi}$ rather than the $\hat{p}$ used in industrial quality monitoring because we reserve p_i to be the (estimated) probability of adverse outcome or patient i.

statistic $\hat{\pi}$ are

$$E(\hat{\pi}) = \frac{1}{n} \sum_{i=1}^{n} p_i$$

and

$$\sqrt{V(\hat{\pi})} = \sqrt{\frac{1}{n^2} \sum_{i=1}^{n} p_i (1 - p_i)} = \frac{1}{n} \sqrt{\sum_{i=1}^{n} p_i (1 - p_i)}$$

the control limits for the risk-adjusted p-chart are thus

$$\text{UCL} = \frac{1}{n} \sum_{i=1}^{n} p_i + \frac{3}{n} \sqrt{\sum_{i=1}^{n} p_i (1 - p_i)},$$

$$\text{LCL} = \frac{1}{n} \sum_{i=1}^{n} p_i - \frac{3}{n} \sqrt{\sum_{i=1}^{n} p_i (1 - p_i)}. \tag{15}$$

Here, the sums are over all of the outcomes in the current subgroup. Often, the LCL is negative, making it impossible for the risk-adjusted p chart to detect a decrease in the probability of an adverse outcome (i.e., an improvement in outcomes). Note that the control limits will vary from one subgroup to the next because of the varying risk factors.

The choice of the subgroup size n involves some trade-offs. If n is large, then there will be a lot of information in each subgroup, making it likely that a shift will be detected on *that* subgroup. Large subgroups, however, mean that data points for the chart will be obtained infrequently (since n patients must be accumulated before a subgroup is completed) making quick detection more difficult. On the other hand, small subgroups mean that the plotted statistics will be obtained more frequently but each will contain less information. See Jordan and Benneyan (2012) for a more detailed description of the issues involved in selecting the subgroup size.

To illustrate the risk-adjusted CUSUM chart, we return to the Steiner et al. (2000) cardiac surgery data and the logistic regression model fit in Eqs. (13) and (14). Now, consider, for illustration, the first patient, who had a Parsonnet score of 19. Using the logistic model from the first two years' worth of data, we would estimate this person's probability of death to be

$$p_{01} = \frac{\exp(-3.67 + 0.077 \times 19)}{1 + \exp(-3.67 + 0.077 \times 19)} = 0.09912$$

assuming, of course, that the process is operating at the standard defined by the logistic regression model in Eq. (13). This patient did survive past 30 days, so $y_1 = 0$.

If we were to use a subgroup size of $n = 20$, then patients 1–20 would be in the first subgroup, patients 21–40 would be in the second subgroup, etc. The number of adverse outcomes in the first 20 patients was one since only patient 12 died within the 30-day window. The proportion of deaths was then $\hat{\pi}_1 = 1/20 = 0.05$. The expected proportion of deaths is equal to the average of the risks

$$\frac{1}{20} \sum_{i=1}^{20} p_i = \frac{1.706}{20} = 0.085.$$

The UCL for the first subgroup is then

$$\mathrm{UCL} = \frac{1}{n} \sum_{i=1}^{20} p_i + \frac{3}{20} \sqrt{\sum_{i=1}^{20} p_i (1 - p_i)}$$

$$= 0.085 + \frac{3}{20} \sqrt{1.396}$$

$$= 0.262$$

and the LCL is zero since the formula for LCL in Eq. (15) yields a negative number. Figure 4 shows the p-chart for the first 40 subgroups. The 27th observation was slightly above the UCL, indicating that the process is not operating according to the standard set by the logistic regression model. This is indicated on the chart by the solid dot.

Figure 5 shows the resulting p-charts for the entire data set for subgroups of size $n = 20, 40, 80$, and 160. Note that the LCLs are zero in most cases for $n \leq 80$. Only for larger subgroup sizes is the risk-adjusted p chart able to detect an improvement in surgical outcomes. Among the four p-charts in Fig. 5 there are five signals (three on the $n = 20$ chart and two on the $n = 80$ chart), which in this case may be false alarms. In all five cases, the plotted point is barely above the UCL, and the signals do

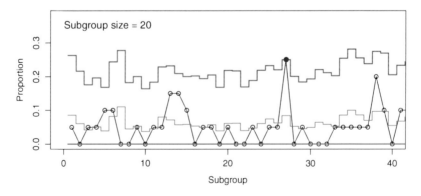

Fig. 4 p-Chart for first 41 subgroups of 20 patients each

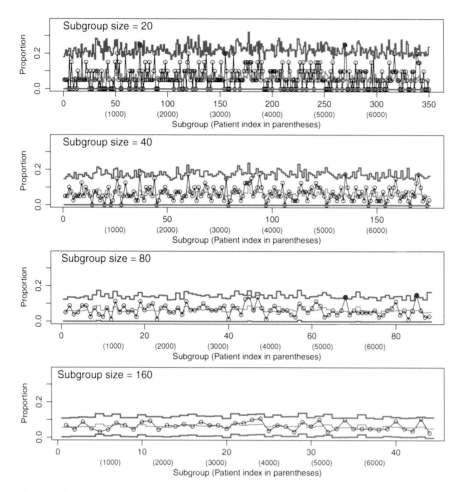

Fig. 5 *p*-Charts for cardiac survival data. Response is whether the patient survived for 30 days. The four plots show the *p*-chart for subgroup sizes of 20, 40, 80, and 160

not match up in chronological time. We would expect more false alarms for smaller sample sizes, such as $n = 20$, simply because there are more plotted points and more opportunities for a false alarm.

3.1.2 Risk-Adjusted CUSUM Charts

We begin by looking at the CUSUM chart for a *constant* probability of an adverse outcome. Suppose that at time i we observe the variable y_i which is equal to 1 if some adverse outcome occurs in the given time window, and 0 if the adverse outcome does not occur. Then, $y_i \sim \text{Bin}(1, p)$, or equivalently, $y_i \sim \text{Bern}(p)$. We would like to test the hypotheses $H_0 : p = p_0$ versus the alternative $H_1 : p = p_1$. If we let

$$R = \frac{p_1/(1-p_1)}{p_0/(1-p_0)} \tag{16}$$

be the odds ratio, then our null and alternative hypotheses for testing whether the odds ratio has changed by a factor of R can be written as

$$H_0 : p = p_0$$

$$H_1 : p = \frac{Rp_0}{1 + (R-1)p_0}$$

in which case the weights W_i will be

$$\begin{aligned}
W_i &= \log \frac{p_1^{y_i}(1-p_1)^{1-y_i}}{p_0^{y_i}(1-p_0)^{1-y_i}} \\
&= \log \left(\frac{R^{y_i}}{1+(R-1)p_0} \right) \\
&= \begin{cases} \log \left(\frac{R}{1+(R-1)p_0} \right), & \text{if } y_i = 1 \\ \log \left(\frac{1}{1+(R-1)p_0} \right), & \text{if } y_i = 0. \end{cases}
\end{aligned} \tag{17}$$

The non-risk-adjusted Bernoulli CUSUM for detecting an increasing in the probability p is then defined by

$$X_0 = 0$$

$$X_i = \max(0, X_{i-1} + W_i) \tag{18}$$

while the CUSUM for detecting a decrease in p is defined as

$$X_0 = 0$$

$$X_i = \min(0, X_{i-1} - W_i) \tag{19}$$

In Eq. (18), $p_1 > p_0$, whereas in Eq. (19), $p_1 < p_0$. For the CUSUM with limit $h = 5$ for the upper chart and $h = -5$ for the lower chart the in-control ARL is approximately 6,939 (estimated by simulation).

Consider now the risk-adjusted CUSUM chart. We assume that a logistic regression model has already been developed that relates the predictor variable(s) to the response and that the model parameters have been estimated. The probability p_i of an adverse outcome, computed from the logistic model, is incorporated into the likelihood ratio. Note that the parameters $\beta_0, \beta_1, \ldots, \beta_p$ in the logistic model are assumed to be known, much as the mean and variance in the $\bar{X}$ and R-charts are assumed known. Note also that $Y_i \sim \text{Bin}(1, p_{0i})$, so that $E(Y_{0i}) = p_{0i}$. The resulting weights W_i are as in Eq. (17), except now the weight for patient i depends on the probability of the adverse event for that patient. Often, the change we would like to detect is expressed in terms of the odds ratio R, rather than in terms of ratio of probabilities p_{1i}/p_{0i} or the difference of probabilities $p_{1i} - p_{0i}$ because

$$
\begin{aligned}
R &= \frac{p_{1i}/(1 - p_{1i})}{p_{0i}/(1 - p_{0i})} \\
&= \exp\left(\log \frac{p_{i1}}{1 - p_i 1} - \log \frac{p_{i0}}{1 - p_i 0}\right) \\
&= \exp\left[(\beta_{10} - \beta_{00}) + (\beta_{11} - \beta_{01})x_{1i} + \cdots + (\beta_{1p} - \beta_{0p})x_{pi}\right].
\end{aligned}
$$

Here β_0 is the parameter vector when the process is in control (or not operating at the standard) and β_1 is the parameter vector when the process is out of control (or not operating at the standard). Thus, R is independent of the levels of the predictor variables x_i if and only if $\beta_{11} = \beta_{01}, \ldots, \beta_{1p} = \beta_{0p}$; in other words, the only change in β is in the constant term β_0 which shifts from β_{00} to β_{10}.

The risk-adjusted CUSUM is then defined the same as in Eqs. (18) and (19), although the weights will differ; in this case, the weights will depend on the patient's condition through the predictor variables.

Consider, for illustration, the cardiac surgery data from Sect. 3.1. If we set up the risk-adjusted CUSUM chart to detect a *doubling* of the odds ratio (that is, $R = 2$), then since the first patient survived for 30 days the weight for patient 1 is

$$
\begin{aligned}
W_1 &= y_1 \log R - \log(1 + (R - 1)p_{01}) \\
&= y_1 \log 2 - \log(1 + p_{01}) \\
&= 0 \times \log 2 - \log(1.09912) \\
&= -0.0945.
\end{aligned}
$$

Note that had this first patient died within the 30-day window, the weight would have been

$$
W_1 = 1 \times \log 2 - \log(1.09912) = 0.9054.
$$

Thus, since the first patient did survive past 30 days, the CUSUM at time $i = 1$ is $\max(0, 0 - 0.0945) = 0$. The second patient had a Parsonnet score of $x_2 = 0$ so the probability of survival was $p_2 = \exp(-3.67)/(1 + \exp(-3.67)) = 0.02484$. This patient, who also survived for 30 days, produces a weight of

$$
W_2 = 0 \times \log 2 - \log(1.02484) = -0.0245.
$$

This weight is less in magnitude than the weight for the first patient who had a higher Parsonnet score. Had the second patient died within the 30-day period, the weight would have been

$$W_2 = 1 \times \log 2 - \log(1.02484) = 0.9754.$$

Thus, the death of a low risk patient contributes more to the upper CUSUM than the death of a higher risk patient. Analogously, the survival of a higher risk patient contributes more in magnitude to the lower CUSUM than the survival of low risk patient.

The lower CUSUM might be set up to detect a halving (i.e., $R = 0.5$) of the odds ratio. In this case, the weight for the first patient would be

$$W_1 = y_1 \log R - \log\left(1 + (R-1)p_{01}\right)$$
$$= y_1 \log 0.5 - \log(1 - 0.5p_{01})$$
$$= 0 \times \log 0.5 - \log(1 - 0.5 \times 0.09912)$$
$$= 0.05083.$$

This lower CUSUM would then be $X_1 = \min(0, 0 - 0.0503) = -0.05083$.

The risk-adjusted CUSUM charts (both the lower and the upper) for the cardiac data are shown in Fig. 6. The control limits of $h = 5$ and $h = -5$ were designed to give an in-control ARL of about 6,700 (determined by simulation). We see in Fig. 6 that just before the 4000th patient, the upper CUSUM exceeds the UCL of $h = 5$, indicating an increase in the probability of death; that is, a lowering of quality. Shortly thereafter, the lower CUSUM begins to pick up steam and eventually (around patient 5,000) drops below the lower limit of $h = -5$, indicating a decrease in the probability of death; that is an improvement of quality.

Woodall et al. (2015) point out that it is often claimed that the risk-adjusted CUSUM is *optimal*, citing Moustakides (1986). The work of Moustakides, however, assumes independent and identically distributed observations. In the case of the risk-adjusted CUSUM, the patients' risk factors vary, which means that the expected values of the y_i vary. The random variables $y_1, y_2, \ldots$ are thus not identically distributed, although they are assumed to be independent.

Loke and Gan (2012) have suggested that the distribution of the patients' risk has an effect on the ARL, particularly the in-control ARL. Zhang and Woodall (2015) propose using dynamic probability control limits with the risk-adjusted CUSUM chart in order to address this issue; their method makes no assumptions about the distribution of patient risk.

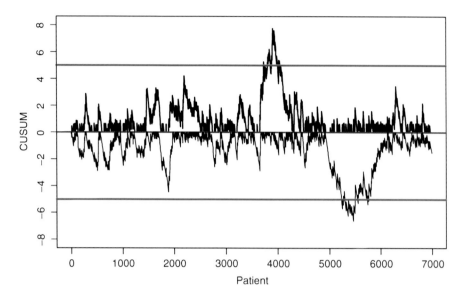

Fig. 6 Risk-adjusted CUSUM of cardiac survival data. Response is whether the patient survived for 30 days

3.1.3 VLAD Charts

If p_i is the probability of the adverse outcome, obtained from some model relating the risk factors $\mathbf{x}_i$ for patient i, then the expected value of y_i is

$$E\left(y_i | \mathbf{x}_i\right) = p_i.$$

Thus, y_i is the observed outcome and p_i is the expected outcome at time i. A plot of the accumulated values of

$$\text{Observed}_i - \text{Expected}_i = O_i - E_i = y_i - p_i$$

on the y-axis and time i on the x-axis is called a variable life adjusted display (VLAD), although it goes by other names, such as the cumulative risk-adjusted mortality (CRAM) chart. The cumulative sum

$$S_i = \sum_{j=1}^{n} (y_i - p_i)$$

represents the difference between the cumulative number of deaths and the expected value of this quantity. For this reason, the cumulative sum can be interpreted as the number of lives lost above that which was expected. The vertical axis is often labeled as "Lives Lost" or "Excess Mortality." If the cumulative sums are formed as

$$S_i = \sum_{j=1}^{i} (p_j - y_j)$$

then the vertical axis is labeled as "Lives Saved."

Control limits can be placed on the VLAD chart, although many authors, such as Winkel and Zhang (2007), recommend against this. The limits are based on the mean and variance of the plotted VLAD statistic, which are

$$E(V_i) = \sum_{j=1}^{i} E(O_j - E_j) = \sum_{j=1}^{i} (p_j - p_j) = 0$$

and

$$\text{Var}(V_i) = \sum_{j=1}^{i} \text{Var}(O_j - E_j) = \sum_{j=1}^{i} \text{Var}(O_j) = \sum_{j=1}^{i} p_j(1 - p_j).$$

The control limits are then

$$\text{UCL} = 3 \sqrt{\sum_{j=1}^{i} p_j(1 - p_j)}$$

$$\text{LCL} = -3 \sqrt{\sum_{j=1}^{i} p_j(1 - p_j)}.$$

When i is large, the variance of V_i is approximately $n\bar{p}(1 - \bar{p})$, so the standard deviation is approximately $\sqrt{n\bar{p}(1 - \bar{p})}$. If the control limits are placed at plus and minus three of these "average" standard deviations, then

$$\text{UCL} = 3\sqrt{n\bar{p}(1 - \bar{p})}$$
$$\text{UCL} = -3\sqrt{n\bar{p}(1 - \bar{p})}.$$

Because these control limits create a convex in-control region opening to the right, they are often called "rocket tails." The reason these limits are not recommended is that if the change occurs when the plotted statistic is currently near the middle or opposite end of the shifted direction, then the chart will take a long time to signal. This phenomenon is called *inertia* in the quality literature.

The VLAD chart for the cardiac surgery data is shown in Fig. 7. There seems to be a decrease in excess mortality starting just before patient 5,000, though it

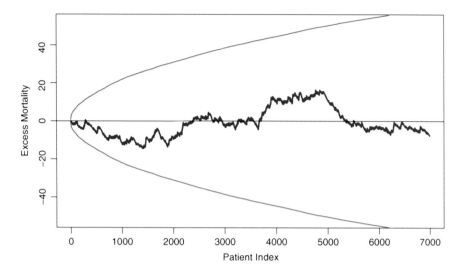

Fig. 7 Variable life adjusted display of cardiac survival data. Response is whether the patient survived for 30 days

is important not to overinterpret the VLAD plot. Figure 8 shows the same VLAD chart as in Fig. 7, with an additional four plots simulated with nothing but noise. Even though there some ups and downs in Fig. 8 that seem to be as distinct as those in Fig. 7, in the last four plots there was no change in either the surgical performance or the distribution of risk factors.

Woodall et al. (2015) suggest that the VLAD chart is easily understood and can serve as a visual aid to get an overall sense of the data. However, since there is no good way for the VLAD to raise an out-of-control signal, the VLAD should be used together with some other method, such as the risk-adjusted CUSUM, that *can* raise a signal.

The weights from the risk-adjusted CUSUM in Eq. (17) can be written as

$$W_i = \log \frac{L_{1i}}{L_{0i}} = y_i \log \frac{p_1/(1-p_1)}{p_0/(1-p_0)} - p_0 \frac{\log\left(\frac{1-p_0}{1-p_1}\right)}{p_0}.$$

Noting that y_i is the observation O_i at time i, and $p_0 = E(y_i) = E_i$, we can write this last expression as a linear combination of O_i and E_i

$$\log \frac{L_{1i}}{L_{0i}} = AO_i - BE_i \tag{20}$$

where

$$A = \log \frac{p_1/(1-p_1)}{p_0/(1-p_0)}$$

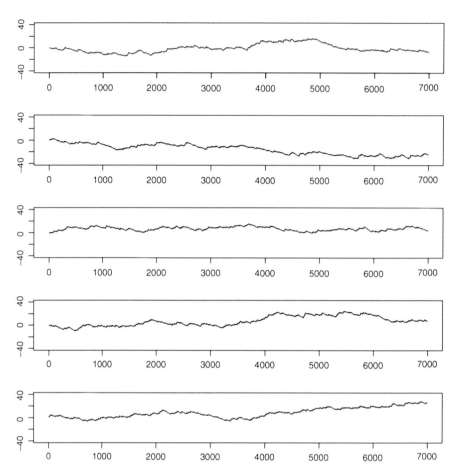

Fig. 8 Variable life adjusted display of cardiac survival data. Response is whether the patient survived for 30 days. The top figure is the cardiac survival data. The other for are simulated from a stable process

and

$$B = \frac{\log \left(\frac{1-p_1}{1-p_0} \right)}{p_0}.$$

The weights from the risk-adjusted CUSUM are given in Eq. (17). Note that there is no value of (p_0, p_1) which makes the coefficients A and B in Eq. (20) both equal to 1, which are the coefficients of O_i and E_i in the VLAD. This implies that the VLAD is never equivalent to the risk-adjusted CUSUM procedure.

3.1.4 The Risk-Adjusted EWMA Chart

The EWMA chart described in Sect. 2 can be applied to risk-adjusted data. One way to do this is to compute the observed statistic $O_i = y_i$ minus the expected statistic $E_i = p_i$, as in the VLAD chart, and to maintain an EWMA statistic on these values. This is the approach described by Steiner (2014). More general approaches are described in Grigg and Spiegelhalter (2007) and Steiner and Jones (2010). The EWMA statistic is computed by

$$z_0 = 0$$

$$z_i = \lambda (y_i - p_i) + (1 - \lambda)z_{i-1}.$$

Since health monitoring involves a fairly substantial amount of data, we usually choose small values of λ. This allows for small changes in the outcome to be detected quickly. It also makes for a nearly uniform weighting of past observations. For example, if $\lambda = 0.02$, then the current observation gets a weight of $\lambda = 0.02$; the previous observation gets a weight of $\lambda(1 - \lambda) = 0.02 \times 0.98 = 0.0196$; the one before that a weight of $\lambda(1 - \lambda)^2 = 0.02 \times 0.98^2 = 0.0192$. The weights do die out exponentially as we move back in time, though. For instance, the observation 50 time units in the past has a weight of $\lambda(1 - \lambda)^{50} = 0.02 \times 0.98^{50} = 0.00728$. Typically, values of λ between 0.01 and 0.10 are used for such an EWMA chart. Figure 9 shows the risk-adjusted EWMA chart for the cardiac data using $\lambda = 0.02$.

Compare the risk-adjusted EWMA chart on $y_i - p_i$ to the VLAD; the VLAD places a uniform weight on the current and all previous observations, whereas the EWMA places weights that decay (albeit slowly when λ is small) back in time. The risk-adjusted EWMA chart can also be based on scores other than the $y_i - p_i$ as suggested here. For example, we could use the scores obtained from the likelihood ratio as given in Eq. (17).

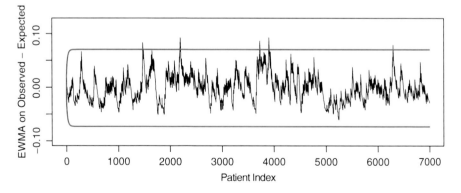

Fig. 9 The risk-adjusted EWMA chart applied to the observed minus expected statistics $y_i - p_i$

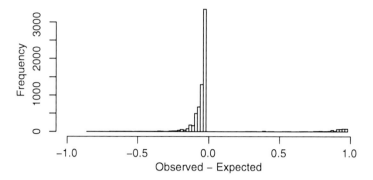

Fig. 10 Histogram of the observed minus expected statistics $y_i - p_i$ showing a highly nonnormal distribution

Although the EWMA chart, as described in the quality monitoring literature, assumes a normally distributed response, such an assumption is not needed. Since we are taking the weighted average of a large number of observations, the sample statistic Z_i will be approximately normally distributed even if the original distribution is not. This is an important characteristic for the risk-adjusted EWMA chart since the distribution of $y_i - p_i$ is distinctly nonnormal. When a patient survives, the statistic is usually just under 0.0, and when a patient dies, the statistic is usually just under 1.0. Figure 10 shows a histogram of $y_i - p_i$ illustrating the extent of the nonnormality.

3.1.5 The Risk-Adjusted Sets Method

Chen (1978) proposed the "Sets" method for surveilling the occurrence of congenital malformations. The idea behind the sets method is to monitor the times between successive events, that is the number of elements in the "set" of patients between events. Normally, the set includes the first patient after the previous event and the next patient who had the event. For the non-risk-adjusted chart, the probability of the event is constant from patient to patient, so the random variable which is equal to the number of patients G in the set has a geometric distribution with probability p_0, where p_0 is the probability of the adverse event when the process is in control. The rule for inferring "out of control" is that n successive G's are less than or equal to the value T. The values chosen for n and T then determine the chart. The sets method was studied further by Gallus et al. (1986). Later Chen (1987) compared the sets method with the risk-adjusted CUSUM chart and found that "The sets technique is ... more efficient than monthly cusum when the number of cases expected in a year is no greater than five, but less efficient otherwise."

Figure 11 shows the sets plot for the first 700 or so patients in the cardiac data set. The plotted statistic increases by one for each additional patient who survives. After each death, the y-coordinate is reset to zero. A plot such as this is called a "grass"

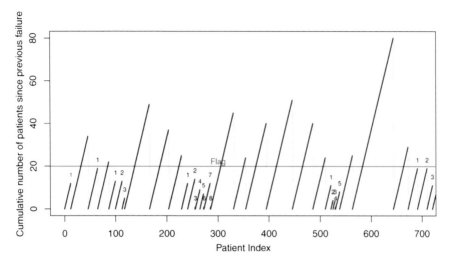

Fig. 11 Grass plot for the unadjusted sets method for the cardiac data

plot, since the plotted lines look like blades of grass. It is helpful to put a horizontal line on the graph at the value of T and to make notes of those cases where the set has size less than or equal to T. If we chose $T = 20$ and $n = 8$, then we would say "out of control" when we get eight straight sets of 20 or fewer patients. In Fig. 11 the out of control flag would be raised at time 286 when eight consecutive sets had 20 or fewer patients.

The risk-adjusted sets method of Grigg and Farewell (2004) involves computing the size of the set beginning with the first patient after the previous event and ending with the patient having the current event. Now, the "size" of the set is defined to be the scaled total risk of this patient pool. More precisely, we define

$$w_i = \frac{p_{0i}}{\bar{p}_0}$$

where p_{0i} is the probability of the adverse event for patient i under the assumption that the process is operating at the standard level. This method of scaling is based on the intuitive assumption that a patient with a high probability of the adverse event who does not experience the event should add more to the risk pool for that set than a patient with a lower probability. This scaling also reduces to the unadjusted sets method because if all patients have the same probability, say p_0, then the expected value of the measure of the set would be

$$E\left(G\frac{p_0}{\bar{p}}\right) = \frac{p_0}{\bar{p}}E(G) = \frac{p_0}{\bar{p}}\frac{1}{p_0} = \frac{1}{\bar{p}}\,.$$

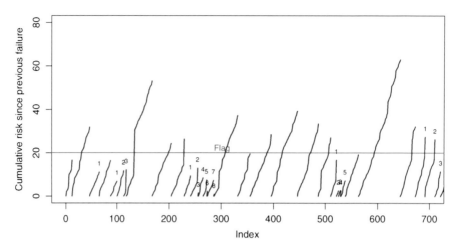

Fig. 12 Grass plot for the adjusted sets method for the cardiac data

The size of the set of patients between adverse events is then

$$S_j = \sum_{i \in \text{Set } j} w_i$$

For the risk-adjusted sets method, a grass plot is defined to be a plot of the accumulated risk between events. The same out of control rule, n consecutive sets whose total risk is T or less, is used here. Figure 12 shows the risk-adjusted grass plot for the cardiac data.

3.2   Other Aspects of Health Care Monitoring

Donabedian (2005, 1988) suggests three categories for assessing the quality of health care: structural, process, and outcomes. The structural category refers to the availability of equipment, nurse-to-bed ratios, etc. The process category involves measurements on variables related to the delivery of health care; for example, lab turnaround time, "door-to-balloon" time (for certain myocardial infarction patients), and hand washing compliance. The outcomes category involves characteristics of the patients after receiving treatment, and includes, for example, 30-day survival after surgery, hospital readmission within 30 days, ventilator-associated pneumonia, etc.

  We will add to this list of categories one which we call *personal*, whereby the health characteristics of a single patient are monitored in much the same way as process or outcomes are monitored. For example, a patient may monitor his blood pressure daily, where any departure from normal could be reported to the physician.

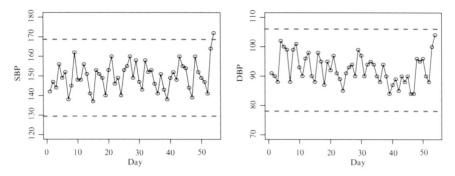

Fig. 13 Individuals charts for systolic blood pressure (SBP) and diastolic blood pressure (DBP)

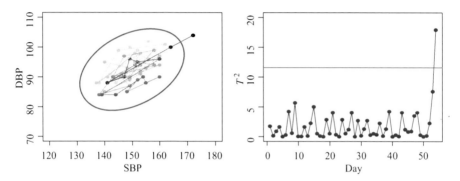

Fig. 14 Hotelling T^2 chart for variables systolic blood pressure (SBP) and diastolic blood pressure

Figure 13 shows individuals charts of systolic and diastolic blood pressures for a hypothetical patient. Values that plot outside the three standard deviation limits above and below the mean would suggest a potential health problem and, in Fig. 13, we see that the last data point on the systolic blood pressure exceeds the UCL, causing a signal that the process has changed.

However, since blood pressure is inherently a two-dimensional process (systolic and diastolic), a multivariate control chart, such as those described in Sect. 2.4, would be appropriate. Figure 14 shows the bivariate plot of systolic and diastolic blood pressure measurements with older observations in a lighter shade of gray. The other part of Fig. 14 shows the Hotelling T^2 chart of

$$T^2 = [x_{\mathrm{SBP}} - \bar{x}_{\mathrm{SBP}}, \ x_{\mathrm{DBP}} - \bar{x}_{\mathrm{DBP}}] \, \mathbf{S}^{-1} \, [x_{\mathrm{SBP}} - \bar{x}_{\mathrm{SBP}}, \ x_{\mathrm{DBP}} - \bar{x}_{\mathrm{DBP}}]'$$

where x_{SBP} and x_{DPB} are the observed systolic and diastolic blood pressures at each time period, while $\bar{x}_{\mathrm{SBP}}$ and $\bar{x}_{\mathrm{DPB}}$ are the mean systolic and diastolic blood pressures and $\mathbf{S}$ is the sample covariance matrix taken when the patient is in his or her normal condition.

In Fig. 14, Hotelling T^2 raises a signal at the very last data point. The ellipse in the first part of Fig. 14 is the "control ellipse" in the sense that a point inside the ellipse will lead to a T^2 value below the UCL, and a point outside the ellipse will lead to a T^2 value above the UCL.

The ease with which personal data can be collected may lead to tremendous opportunities in the monitoring of data on individuals. This can lead to the availability of massive data sets, often called "big data," which have the potential to monitor health to a greater extent. To illustrate one possible use of monitoring personal data, consider the touch sensitive floor called a "magic carpet" that can be installed in the home or in independent or assisted living communities. Baker (2008) described this concept in his book *The Numerati*. This special flooring can record the exact time, location, angle and pressure of every step the person takes. Numerous characteristics about a person's gait can be gleaned from such data. Obviously, the absence of any such data on a given day is cause for alarm (although it could also just indicate the person was on vacation). Data showing slower steps, or uneven steps, could indicate a problem as well. Intel has developed SHIMMER (Sensing Health with Intelligence, Modularity, Mobility and Experimental Reusability) technology (see Boran 2007). These involve wearable Bluetooth devices that can monitor many health characteristics. Large data sets that would be obtained using such devices present challenges for data analysis and opportunities for improving health care while reducing costs.

4 Disease Surveillance

Many of the methods used in disease surveillance have been drawn from or are related to those of industrial process monitoring. However, there are important differences between the typical industrial process monitoring application and disease surveillance, which means that the standard industrial methods described in Sect. 2 usually must be modified before being applied to disease surveillance. In this section, to distinguish between the two different uses, methods designed for or discussed within an industrial context are referred to as control charts while methods designed for or discussed in a disease surveillance context are referred to as *detection methods*.

A key difference in the two applications is the assumption that the observations are *independent and identically distributed* (or *iid*). In industrial process monitoring applications, with appropriate implementation of the procedures, this assumption can often be met with the raw data. But this is often not the case for disease surveillance data. There are two main reasons for the difference.

- First, while industrial process monitoring and disease surveillance are both time series data, in industrial monitoring the process is explicitly controlled and thus the raw data is the noise resulting from the process when it is in-control. As such, the data can reasonably be assumed to be identically distributed.

In contrast, background disease incidence process in disease surveillance is inherently uncontrollable and thus the data itself is usually autocorrelated and so it cannot be identically distributed.

- Second, industrial data are usually samples from a process, and the sampling times are controlled with the data taken far enough apart in time so that the resulting data is at least approximately independent from one sample to the next. In contrast, particularly in the case of biosurveillance, in the interest of making disease detection as fast as possible, all the available data is used so that autocorrelation is virtually unavoidable.

Thus, disease surveillance data generally violates the *iid* assumption underlying the control charts described in Sect. 2. However, it is often reasonable to assume that the residuals from a model that removes the systematic effects from disease surveillance data *are iid*.

The lack of independence between observations is only one way that disease surveillance may differ from the typical industrial process monitoring assumptions. As shown in Table 1, other differences include a lack of time series stationarity, the types of statistics to monitor in order to most effectively detect outbreaks, and how the transient nature of outbreaks affects detection performance. For best performance, detection methods must be designed to accommodate these and other disease surveillance data characteristics.

Table 1 Characteristics of classical industrial process monitoring data compared to disease surveillance data

Classical Control Chart Data Characteristics	Typical Disease Surveillance Data Characteristics
1. The in-control distribution of the data is (or can reasonably be assumed to be) stationary	1. There is little to no control over disease incidence and the disease incidence distribution
2. Observations can be drawn from the process so they are independent (or nearly so)	2. Autocorrelation and the potential need to monitor all the data can result in dependence
3. The asymptotic distributions of the statistics being monitored are known and thus can be used to design control charts	3. Individual observations may be monitored; if so, asymptotic sampling distributions not relevant
4. Monitoring the process mean and standard deviation is usually sufficient	4. Little is known about which statistics are useful; often looking for anything unusual
5. Out-of-control condition remains until it is detected and corrective action is taken	5. Outbreaks are transient, with disease incidence returning to its original state when the outbreak has run its course
6. Temporal detection is the critical problem	6. Detecting both temporal and spatial anomalies are critical

Source: Modified from Fricker (2013, p. 154)

4.1 Modeling Disease Incidence

Disease surveillance data often have systematic effects (i.e., explainable trends and patterns). These can include day-of-the-week effects, where patient health-seeking behavior systematically varies according to the day of the week. It may also include seasonal effects where, for example, influenza-like illness is generally higher in the winter months of the year compared to the summer months.

These trends and patterns can be used to build models and the models can then be used to better understand and characterize historical trends, to assess how the current state compares to historical trends, and to forecast what is likely to occur in the near future. For example, one might use a model f to forecast the disease incidence at time i, $\hat{x}_i$, using past disease incidence $(x_{i-1}, x_{i-2}, x_{i-3}, \ldots)$ as well as other covariates $(y_1, y_2, y_3, \ldots)$:

$$\hat{x}_i = f(x_{i-1}, x_{i-2}, x_{i-3}, \ldots, y_1, y_2, y_3, \ldots).$$

For example, many diseases have a clear seasonal component to their incidence rate. Some diseases such as influenza or pertussis peak in the winter, whereas others such as *E. coli* peak in the summer. Serfling (1963) first considered the use of trigonometric models that account for the seasonality in disease rates. He applied models of the form

$$\mu_i = a_0 \sum_{k=1}^{p} \left(b_k \sin \frac{2k\pi i}{52} + c_k \cos \frac{2k\pi i}{52} \right) \tag{21}$$

for weekly counts of influenza. For his purpose, the counts were large enough that the normal distribution was reasonable. For diseases that are much rarer than influenza, such an assumption is unreasonable. Rigdon et al. (2014) considered the reportable diseases that are monitored by the state of Missouri. For most diseases a first-order model, that is $p = 1$ in Eq. (21), is sufficient, but in some cases a second-order model ($p = 2$) is needed. They assumed Poisson distributed counts for the reportable diseases and constructed control limits that were based on the current estimated mean; thus, the control limits varied in a seasonal fashion along with the estimated disease incidence.

One advantage of modeling the counts directly is that the resulting chart is easily understood. Also, one can see from the plot the current situation along with the past history of the disease. Figure 15 shows the incidence of pertussis in Missouri from 2002 to 2011. From this plot, the years when there was a pertussis outbreak are obvious.

Perhaps most important for this discussion, many of the detection methods discussed in Sect. 2 are most effective when the systematic components of disease surveillance data are removed. This is best accomplished by first modeling the data, where the model is used to estimate the systematic effects, and then using the detection methods on the model *residuals*. The residuals r_i are what remain after

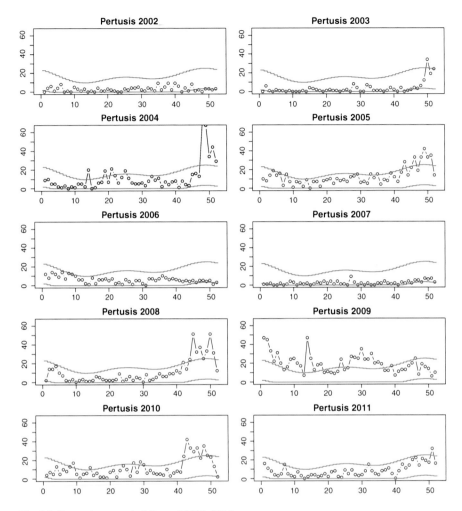

Fig. 15 Pertussis counts in Missouri 2002–2011

the modeled values are subtracted from the raw data, $r_i = x_i - \hat{x}_i$, and thus what is monitored are changes from forecast values. Correctly done, the residuals may then be independent, or nearly so, and then the industrial process monitoring methods of Sect. 2 more appropriately apply. There are also cases where the disease counts are modeled directly. See Fricker (2013, Chap. 5) for a more in-depth discussion about methods for modeling disease incidence data.

4.2 Detection Methods

The *historical limits* method is commonly used by public health practitioners to compare data from a current time period to data from an equivalent historical period or periods. The idea is to assess whether the current observed counts are significantly larger or smaller than equivalent historical totals after accounting for the natural variation inherent in the data.

An example of a system that uses historical limits is the CDC's National Notifiable Diseases Surveillance System (NNDSS). NNDSS aggregates and summarizes data on specific diseases that health care providers are required by state law to report to public health departments. Reportable diseases include anthrax, botulism, plague, and tularemia.[4] Each week the states report counts of cases for each of the reportable diseases to the CDC.

A simple use of comparisons to historical data is the "Notifiable Diseases/Deaths in Selected Cities Weekly Information" report published on-line each week in the CDC's *Morbidity and Mortality Weekly Report* (MMWR). Here the most recent weekly totals for each of the notifiable diseases, $T_{i,j,k}$, for reportable disease i, in week j and year k, are compared to the mean totals from similar weeks over the past five years plus or minus two standard deviations:

$$T_{i,j,k} \geq \hat{\mu}_{i,j,k} + 2\hat{\sigma}_{i,j,k}$$

or

$$T_{i,j,k} \leq \hat{\mu}_{i,j,k} - 2\hat{\sigma}_{i,j,k},$$

where for each disease,

$$\hat{\mu}_{i,j,k} = \frac{1}{15} \sum_{s=1}^{5} \sum_{r=-1}^{1} T_{i,j-r,k-s},$$

and the variance as

$$\hat{\sigma}_{i,j,k}^2 = \frac{1}{14} \sum_{s=1}^{5} \sum_{r=-1}^{1} \left(T_{i,j-r,k-s} - \hat{\mu}_{i,j,k} \right)^2,$$

This is just a specific form of the $\bar{X}$-chart with two standard deviation limits.

Interestingly, rather than plotting the data as a time series on a control chart, the CDC uses a bar plot of the natural log-transformed (4-week) counts. For example, Fig. 16 is Figure I from "Notifiable Diseases/Deaths in Selected Cities Weekly Information" for week 47 of 2009 (CDC 2009), where for this week the mumps count exceeded its historical limits as shown by the crosshatched top of the bar.

---

[4]See www.cdc.gov/ncphi/disss/nndss/phs/infdis.htm for a complete list of reportable diseases.

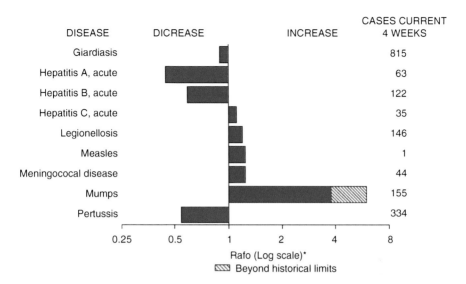

Fig. 16 Figure I from "Notifiable Diseases/Deaths in Selected Cities Weekly Information" for the week 47 of 2009 (CDC 2009). For this week, the mumps count exceeded its historical limits

In the preceding example, a formal model of disease counts was not required as comparisons to historical data were limited to those time periods in previous years expected to be similar to the current period. This too is a model, but an informal one which assumes that counts at the same time of the year are *iid*. For other types of disease surveillance, particularly in biosurveillance, a more formal model may have to be applied. Once done, many of the detection methods of Sect. 2, applied to forecast residuals, are useful for monitoring disease incidence.

Now, for some types of surveillance, only monitoring for increases in disease incidence is of interest. A benefit of so doing is greater detection power for the same rate of false positive signals. In such cases, it is only necessary to use an UCL for Shewhart charts. Similarly, for the CUSUM, one only need calculate C^+, using Eq. (5), and not C^- using Eq. (6), and signal at time i when $C_i^+ > h$. For the EWMA, in addition to only using the UCL, the EWMA can be "reflected" (in the spirit of the CUSUM) to improve its performance in detecting increases (Crowder and Hamilton 1992). To do so, Eq. (7) is modified to:

$$z_i = \max[\mu_0, \lambda x_i + (1 - \lambda)z_{i-1}]. \tag{22}$$

With this modification, the EWMA statistic must always be greater than or equal to μ_0, meaning that it cannot drift too far downwards, and thus it will more readily signal when a positive shift occurs. The method starts at $z_0 = \mu_0$ and a signal is generated as before when $z_i > h$, where the UCL is

$$\text{UCL} = h = \mu_0 + L\hat{\sigma} \sqrt{\frac{\lambda}{2 - \lambda}[1 - (1 - \lambda)^{2i}]}.$$

When run on standardized forecast residuals, so that $\mu_0 = 0$ and $\sigma = 1$, then Eq. (22) becomes

$$z_i = \max[0, \lambda x_i + (1 - \lambda)z_{i-1}]$$

with $z_0 = 0$. The exact UCL is

$$h = L\sqrt{\frac{\lambda}{2 - \lambda}[1 - (1 - \lambda)^{2i}]},$$

and asymptotically it is

$$h = L\sqrt{\frac{\lambda}{2 - \lambda}}.$$

In a similar manner, Joner et al. (2008) propose a reflected multivariate EWMA (MEWMA):

$$\mathbf{z}_i = \begin{cases} \max[\mathbf{0}, \lambda(\mathbf{z}_i - \mu_0) + (1 - \lambda)\mathbf{z}_{i-1}], & \text{for } i > 0 \\ \mathbf{0}, & \text{for } i = 0 \end{cases},$$

where the maximum function is applied component-wise. As with the MEWMA control chart, Σ_z is used to calculate z_i where

$$z_i = \mathbf{z}_i' \Sigma_z^{-1} \mathbf{z}_i.$$

And, as before, the MEWMA detection method signals whenever $z_i > h$.

Variants of the MCUSUM that make it directionally sensitive also exist. And, various multivariate spatio-temporal methods, which are important to disease surveillance, have been proposed. See Chap. 8 of Fricker (2013) for more detail.

4.3 Performance Metrics

Unfortunately, as yet there is no set of performance metrics that are commonly accepted throughout the disease and biosurveillance communities. Furthermore, because of the transient nature of disease outbreaks, the ARL metrics of the industrial process monitoring are insufficient. Fricker (2013) proposes the following metrics:

- *Average time between false signals* (ATFS) is the mean number of time periods it takes for the early event detection (EED) method to re-signal after the method first signals, given there are no outbreaks. Thus, the ATFS is the expected time between false signals.

- *Conditional expected delay* (CED) is the mean number of time periods it takes for the method to first signal, given that an outbreak is occurring *and* that the method signals during the outbreak. Thus, the CED is the expected number of time periods from the start of an outbreak until the first true signal during that outbreak.
- *Probability of successful detection* (PSD) is the probability the method signals during an outbreak, where the probability of detection is both a function of the EED method and the type of outbreak.

The metrics are mathematically defined as follows. Let $\mathscr{S}_t$ denote a generic detection method statistic at time t, where $\mathscr{S}_0$ is the value of the statistic when the detection method is first started. Let h denote the method's threshold, where if $\mathscr{S}_t \geq h$ the method signals at time t. Also, let τ_s denote the first day of a disease outbreak, where the notation $\tau_s = \infty$ means that an outbreak never occurs, and let τ_e denote that last day of an outbreak, where if $\tau_s = \infty$ then by definition $\tau_e = \infty$. Finally, let t^* denote the first time the method signals, $t^* = \min(t : \mathscr{S}_t \geq h)$, and let t^{**} denote the next time the method signals, $t^{**} = \min(t : t > t^* \text{ and } \mathscr{S}_t \geq h)$.
Then

$$\text{ATFS} = E(t^{**} - t^* | \mathscr{S}_{t^*+1} = \mathscr{S}_0 \text{ and } \tau_s = \infty), \tag{23}$$

$$\text{CED} = E(t^* - \tau_s | \tau_s \leq t^* \leq \tau_e), \tag{24}$$

and

$$\text{PSD} = P(\tau_s \leq t^* \leq \tau_e). \tag{25}$$

Mathematically, the ATFS metric as defined in Eq. (23) is the same as the in-control ARL *because* after each signal the method's statistic is re-set to its starting value. However, some disease surveillance practitioners prefer not to re-set after each signal, so in that case,

$$\text{ATFS} = E(t^{**} - t^* | \tau_s = \infty). \tag{26}$$

Note the difference between Eqs. (23) and (26): in the former, the statistic is re-set to its starting value after each time the detection method signals, while in the latter it is not. If the time series of statistics is autocorrelated, then the resulting ATFS performance can be very different since, with autocorrelation, once a signal has occurred in one time period more signals are likely to occur in subsequent periods.

Under the condition that the statistic is not re-set, Fraker et al. (2008) have proposed the *average time between signal events* (ATBSE) metric, where a *signal event* is defined as consecutive time periods during which an EED method signals. Under these conditions, the ATBSE may be a more informative measure, since it quantifies the length of time between groups of signals, but it may not provide sufficient information about the number of false positive signals that will occur.

The CED is conceptually similar to the out-of-control ARL in industrial process monitoring, but in that application when a process goes out of control it stays out of control so that the out-of-control ARL $= E(t^* - \tau_s | t^* \geq \tau_s)$. Since outbreaks are transient in disease surveillance the definition differs because it must incorporate the idea that a signal is only useful if it occurs sometime during the outbreak.

PSD does not have an analogue in the industrial process monitoring literature. As defined above, it is the probability of detecting an outbreak at any time during the outbreak. For longer outbreaks this definition may be too loose, meaning that detection later in the outbreak may not be medically useful. If that is the case, the definition by Sonesson and Bock (2003) may be more operationally relevant:

$$\text{PSD} = P(t^* - \tau_s \leq d | \tau_s \leq t^* \leq \tau_l),$$

where d is the maximum delay required for a successful detection, and where "successful detection" means early enough in the outbreak that an intervention is medically effective.

4.3.1 Alternative Metrics

Fraker et al. (2008) note that "Substantially more metrics have been proposed in the public health surveillance literature than in the industrial monitoring literature." These include run length and time to signal based metrics such as the ARL and *average time to signal* (ATS). However, these metrics fail both to account for the transient nature of disease outbreaks and that detection method statistics are often not re-set after they signal. In comparison, when an industrial process goes out-of-control it stays in that condition until the control chart signals and the cause is identified and corrected. Thus, in industrial process monitoring, once a process goes out of control any signal is a true signal, and so the probability of signaling during an out-of-control condition is always 1. This is not the case in disease surveillance where outbreaks are transient and after some period of time disappear. In this situation, it is possible for a detection method to fail to signal during an outbreak, after which a signal is a false signal.

To overcome the issues associated with applying the control chart ARL metrics to disease surveillance, various modifications have been proposed. For example, in addition to the ATBSE Franker et al. (2008) also define the *average signal event length* (ASEL) as how long, on average, a detection method signals over consecutive time periods. The ATBSE and ASEL metrics are designed for how disease surveillance systems are often currently operated, where the detection methods are not re-set after they signal. In this situation, disease surveillance system operators allow the detection methods to continue to run after they signal and interpret the resulting sequence of signals (or lack thereof) as additional information about a potential outbreak. Under these conditions, the ATBSE maybe preferred to the ATFS metric. See Fricker (2013, Chap. 6) for a more in-depth discussion of these and other metrics.

4.4   Detecting Seasonal Outbreaks: An Example

Consider the problem of detecting seasonal flu outbreaks. Figure 18 is a plot of 2.5 years of gastrointestinal (GI) syndrome data, a useful surrogate for the flu, for one hospital. Note how, in retrospect, three episodes of seasonal increases in GI are visually obvious. To illustrate prospectively detecting seasonal increases, we turn the clock back to day 400 in order to define the parameters of the detection methods, and then run the methods forward from day 401 to day 980.

So, given the historical data from days 1 to 400, one might decide that days 200 to 400, delineated by the dotted lines in Fig. 17, best characterize normal (i.e., non-seasonal outbreak) disease incidence. For this period, the mean incidence is estimated as

$$\hat{\mu}_0 = \frac{1}{201} \sum_{i=200}^{400} x_i = 13.6$$

per day with an estimated standard deviation of

$$\hat{\sigma}_0 = \sqrt{\frac{1}{200} \sum_{i=200}^{400} (x_i - \hat{\mu}_0)^2} = 4.5.$$

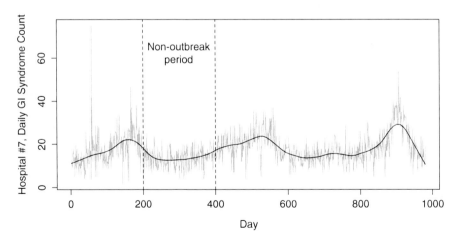

Fig. 17 Plot of 2-1/2 years of GI syndrome data from a hospital. The dotted lines indicate a period of "normal" (i.e., non-seasonal outbreak) disease incidence from days 220 to 400

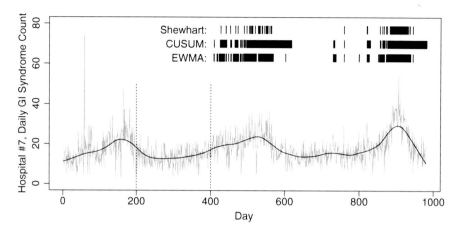

Fig. 18 Plot of the hospital GI syndrome data with signal times, where the Shewhart, CUSUM and EWMA detection method signaling times are indicated with the vertical lines. Thresholds were set with an ATFS of 365 days and the methods are not re-set after signals

Ignoring day and other systematic effects potentially present in the data, one approach is to simply standardize future observations with

$$y_i = \frac{x_i - \hat{\mu}_0}{\hat{\sigma}_0} = \frac{x_i - 13.6}{4.5}, i = 401, 402, \ldots$$

and apply the Shewhart, CUSUM, and EWMA detection methods to the y_i (without re-setting after signals). For an ATFS of 365 days, assuming the standardized values are approximately normally distributed (which a Q-Q plot shows is reasonable) set $h = 2.7775$ for the Shewhart, $h = 1.35$ and $k = 1.5$ for the CUSUM, and $L = 2.815$ and $\lambda = 0.3$ for the EWMA.

The results are shown at the top of Fig. 18, where the signaling times for each detection method are indicated by the short vertical lines. The figure shows that all three detection methods clearly indicate the two large seasonal increases (after day 400) in GI. However, there are some differences in how they indicate the duration of the outbreaks and, because the methods are not re-set, the CUSUM's and EWMA's signals are more persistent.

In particular, note how the CUSUM continues to signal well after the two seasonal increases have subsided. In addition, the EWMA and CUSUM detection methods tend to signal earlier because of the gradual increase in GI counts at the start of the outbreaks. Finally, note that there are a couple of smaller potential outbreaks in between the two larger outbreaks that are more obvious given the signals. See Chap. 9 of Fricker (2013) for additional detail and further development of this example.

5   Summary

Many of the methods of industrial quality control can be used directly, or adapted, in order to monitor health data. Monitoring of patient outcomes can be done so long as the patients' risk is taken into account. It is also possible to monitor process variables, such as laboratory times, using methods such as control charts. Public health can be studied by monitoring the rates of disease. Methods of plotting that are related to control charts can provide information about disease outbreaks so that practitioners can take action.

6   Further Reading

6.1   Industrial Process Monitoring

1. Montgomery, D.C. (2009). *Introduction to Statistical Quality Control,* John Wiley & Sons.

6.2   Health Care Monitoring

1. Faltin, F., Kenett, R., and Ruggeri, F., editors (2012) *Statistical Methods in Healthcare,* Wiley, West Sussex, UK.
2. Winkel, P. and Zhang, N. F. (2007) *Statistical Development of Quality in Medicine,* Wiley, West Sussex, UK.

6.3   Disease Surveillance

1. Brookmeyer, R. and D.F. Stroup, eds. (2004). *Monitoring the Health of Populations: Statistical Principles and Methods for Public Health Surveillance,* Oxford University Press.
2. Fricker, Jr., R.D. (2013). *Introduction to Statistical Methods for Biosurveillance: With an Emphasis on Syndromic Surveillance,* Cambridge University Press.
3. Lombardo, J.S., and D.L. Buckeridge, eds. (2007). *Disease Surveillance: A Public Health Informatics Approach,* Wiley-Interscience.

References

Baker, S.: The Numerati. Mariner, Boston (2008)

Boran, M.: Age Beautifully with Intel (2007). Accessed on-line at Business Technology website www.independent.ie/business/technology/age-beautifully-with-intel-26302591.html on 24 December 2014

Brookmeyer, R., Stroup, D.F. (eds.): Monitoring the Health of Populations: Statistical Principles and Methods for Public Health Surveillance. Oxford University Press, Oxford (2004)

CDC. Notifiable diseases/deaths in selected cities weekly information. Morb. Mortal. Wkly Rep. **58**(46), 1304–1315 (2009)

Champ, C.W., Jones-Farmer, L.A.: Properties of multivariate control charts with estimated parameters. Seq. Anal. **26**, 153–169 (2007)

Champ, C.W., Jones-Farmer, L.A., Rigdon, S.E.: Properties of the T^2 control chart when parameters are estimated. Technometrics **47**, 437–445 (2005)

Chen, R.: A surveillance system for congenital malformations. J. Am. Stat. Assoc. **73**, 323–327 (1978)

Chen, R.: The relative efficiency of the sets and CUSUM techniques in monitoring the occurrence of a rare event. Stat. Med. **6**, 517–525 (1987)

Crosier, R.B.: Multivariate generalizations of cumulative sum quality control schemes. Technometrics **30**, 291–303 (1988)

Crowder, S.V., Hamilton, M.D.: An EWMA for monitoring a process standard deviation. J. Qual. Technol. **24**, 12–21 (1992)

Donabedian, A.: The quality of care: how can it be assessed? J. Am. Med. Assoc. **121**, 1145–1150 (1988). Doi:10.1001/jama.1988.03410120089033

Donabedian, A.: Evaluating the quality of medical care. Milbank Mem. Fund Q. (Pt. 2) **83**, 691–725 (2005). Doi:10.1111/j.1468-0009.2005.00397.x

Fraker, S.E., Woodall, W.H., Mousavi, S.: Performance metrics for surveillance schemes. Qual. Eng. **20**, 451–464 (2008)

Fricker, R.D. Jr.: Introduction to Statistical Methods in Biosurveillance. Cambridge University Press, Cambridge (2013)

Gallus, G., Mandelli, C., Marchi, M., Radaelli, G.: On surveillance methods for congenital malformations. Stat. Med. **5**, 565–571 (1986)

Geissler, H.J., Hölzl, P., Marohl, S., Kuhn-Régnier, F., Mehlhorn, U., Südkamp, M., Rainer de Vivie, V.: Risk stratification in heart surgery: comparison of six score systems. Eur. J. Cardiothorac. Surg. **17**, 400–406 (2000)

Grigg, O.A., Farewell, V.T.: A risk-adjusted sets method for monitoring adverse medical outcomes. Stat. Med. **23**, 1593–1602 (2004)

Grigg, O., Spiegelhalter, D.: A simple risk-adjusted exponentially weighted moving average. J. Am. Stat. Assoc. **102**, 140–152 (2007)

Hawkins, D.M., Olwell, D.H. (eds.): Cumulative Sum Charts and Charting for Quality Improvement. Springer, Berlin (1998)

Healy, J.D.: A note on multivariate CUSUM procedures. Technometrics **29**, 409–412 (1987)

Hotelling, H.: Multivariate quality control illustrated by air testing of sample bombsights. In: Eisenhart, C., Hastay, M.W., Wallis, W.A. (eds.) Selected Techniques of Statistical Analysis. McGraw-Hill, New York (1947)

Jensen, W.A., Jones-Farmer, L.A., Champ, C.W.: Effects of parameter estimation on control chart properties: a literature review. J. Qual. Technol. **38**, 349–362 (2006)

Joner, M.D. Jr., Woodall, W.H., Reynolds, M.R. Jr., Fricker, R.D. Jr.: A one-sided MEWMA chart for health surveillance. Qual. Reliab. Eng. Int. **24**, 503–519 (2008)

Jordan, V., Benneyan, J.C.: Common challenges and pitfalls using SPC in Healthcare. In: Faltin, F.W., Kenett, R.S., Ruggeri, F. (eds.) Statistical Methods in Healthcare, chap. 15. Wiley, London (2012)

Loke, C.K., Gan, F.F.: Joint monitoring scheme for clinical failures and predisposed risk. Qual. Technol. Quant. Manag. **9**, 3–21 (2012)

Lorden, G.: Procedures for reacting to a change in distribution. Ann. Math. Stat. **42**, 1897–1908 (1971)

Lowry, C.A., Woodall, W.H., Champ, C.W., Rigdon, S.E.: A multivariate exponentially weighted moving average control chart. Technometrics **34**, 46–53 (1992)

Montgomery, D.C.: Introduction to Statistical Quality Control, 6th edn. Wiley, London (2009)

Moustakides, G.V.: Optimal stopping times for detecting a change in distribution. Technometrics **14**, 1379–1388 (1986)

Page, E.S.: Continuous inspection schemes. Biometrika **41**, 100–115 (1954)

Pignatiello, J.J. Jr., Runger, G.C.: Comparisons of multivariate CUSUM charts. J. Qual. Technol. **3**, 173–186 (1990)

Rigdon, S.E., Cruthis, E.N., Champ, C.W.: Design strategies for individuals and moving range control charts. J. Qual. Technol. **26**, 274–287 (1994)

Rigdon, S.E., Turabelidze, G., Jahanpour, E.: Trigonometric regression for analysis of public health surveillance data. J. Appl. Math. **2014** (2014)

Roberts, S.W.: Control chart tests based on geometric moving averages. Technometrics **1**, 239–250 (1959)

Serfling, R.E.: Methods for current statistical analysis of excess pneumonia-influenza deaths. Public Health Rep. **78**, 494–506 (1963)

Shewhart, W.A. (ed.): Economic Control of Quality of Manufactured Product. D. van Nostrand Company, New York (1931)

Sonesson, C., Bock, D.: A review and discussion of prospective statistical surveillance in public health. J. R. Stat. Soc. Ser. A **166**, 5–21 (2003)

Steiner, S.H.: Risk-adjusted monitoring of outcomes in health care. In: Lawless, J.F. (ed.) Statistics in Action: A Canadian Outlook, pp. 225–241. CRC/Chapman Hall, Boca Raton/London (2014)

Steiner, S.H., Jones, M.: Risk-adjusted survival time monitoring with an updating exponentially weighted moving average (EWMA) control chart. Stat. Med. **29**, 444–454 (2010)

Steiner, S.H., Cook, R., Farewll, V.T., Treasure, T.: Monitoring surgical performance using risk-adjusted cumulative sum charts. Biostatistics **1**, 441–452 (2000)

Thacker, S.B.: Historical development. In: Teutsh, S.M., Churchill, R.E. (eds.) Principles and Practices of Public Health Surveillance, pp. 1–16. Oxford University Press, Oxford (2000)

Wald, A.: Sequential tests of statistical hypotheses. Ann. Math. Stat. **16**, 117–186 (1945)

Winkel, P., Zhang, N.F.: Statistical Development of Quality in Medicine. Wiley, London (2007)

Woodall, W.H., Fogel, S.L., Steiner, S.H.: The monitoring and improvement of surgical outcome quality. J. Qual. Technol. (2015, To appear)

Zhang, X., Woodall, W.H.: Dynamic probability control limits for risk-adjusted Bernoulli CUSUM charts. Stat. Med. (2015, to appear)

Standardization and Decomposition Analysis: A Useful Analytical Method for Outcome Difference, Inequality and Disparity Studies

Jichuan Wang

Abstract Standardization and decomposition analysis (SDA) is a traditional demographic analytical method that is widely used for comparing rates between populations with difference in composition. The method can be readily applied to many other research fields. SDA decomposes the observed outcome difference between populations into component effects that are attributed to: (1) the "real" outcome difference; and (2) compositional difference of specific confounding factors between populations. The results of SDA are easy to interpret and understand, and it can be readily applied not only to cross-sectional outcome comparisons, but also to studying outcome changes in longitudinal studies. Importantly, SDA does not need the assumptions that are usually required for statistical analysis. Traditionally SDA has no statistical significance testing for component effects. However, the author of this chapter has developed a Windows-based computer program that employs bootstrapping techniques to estimate standard errors of the component effects, thus significance testing for component effects becomes possible in SDA.

1 Introduction

Standardization and decomposition analysis (SDA) is a well-established demographic analytical method for comparing rates between populations when difference in rate of some phenomena is confounded by difference in population composition. It is well-known that what appears to be a difference in the observed rate (crude rate) between populations may be due to difference in the compositions of confounding factors between populations (Kitagawa 1955, 1964). For example, it is possible for a population to have a crude death rate (the number of deaths occurring in a given year divided by the total population) that is lower than another's when the first population actually has a higher mortality or higher age-specific death rates

J. Wang (✉)
Department of Epidemiology and Biostatistics, The George Washington University School of Medicine, Children's National Medical Center, 111 Michigan Avenue Northwest, Washington, DC 20010, USA
e-mail: jiwang@gwu.edu; jiwang@cnmc.org

© Springer International Publishing Switzerland 2015
D.-G. Chen, J. Wilson (eds.), *Innovative Statistical Methods for Public Health Data*,
ICSA Book Series in Statistics, DOI 10.1007/978-3-319-18536-1_11

(i.e., the death rates for specific age groups). This paradox is often a result of the fact that the first population has a considerably larger proportion of its population in age groups (e.g., age 5–44) that are subject to lower mortality. In this death rate example, the observed difference in crude death rate between the two populations is confounded by difference in composition of a confounding factor (i.e., age structure) between the two populations. Once the composition of the confounding factor (i.e., age structure) is standardized across the two populations, the adjusted death rate of the first population would be certainly higher than that of the second population.

SDA is a useful analytical method for studying outcome difference, inequality or disparity between populations. The technique of standardization is used to adjust or purge the confounding effects on observed (crude) rate of some phenomena in two or more populations. Decomposition takes standardization a step further by revealing the relative contributions of various confounding factors in explaining the observed outcome difference, inequality or disparity. Its results tell how much of the difference in the crude rate between populations is "real" rate difference that is attributed to different factor-specific rates; and what factors significantly confound the crude rate difference, and how much of the observed rate difference is attributed to each specific confounding factor (Kitagawa 1955, 1964; Pullum 1978; United Nations 1979). Returning to the death rate comparison example, based on the results of standardization, the difference in crude death rate between the two populations can be decomposed into two additive component effects: (1) the rate effect attributed to the difference in the age-specific death rates; and (2) the factor component effect attributed to the difference in age structure between the two populations. The former is the "real" rate difference, and the latter is the observed rate difference due to confounding effects (i.e., difference in age structure in this example). If another confounding factor (e.g., ethnicity) were taken into account, the difference in the crude death rate would be decomposed into three component effects: (1) the rate effect due to the difference in the factor specific (i.e., age-ethnicity specific) death rates; (2) factor-1 component effect due to the difference in age structure; and (3) factor-2 component effect due to the difference in ethnic composition.

SDA can be readily applied to outcome comparison in various research fields. For example, suppose we would like to study difference, inequality or disparity in health and health care outcomes (e.g., prevalence of HIV, cancer, asthma, diabetes, hypertension, obesity, mental disorder, likelihood of health service utilization, etc.) between Black and White populations, application of SDA would tell how much of the observed outcome difference could be the "real" difference in the outcome measure between the populations; and how much would be attributed to compositional differences of specific confounding factors (e.g., age, gender, education, family income, location, immigrant status, etc.) in the populations.

The advantages of SDA include but not limited to: (1) its results can be presented in a manner that is initiatively understandable, like presenting a decomposition of the observed rate difference into different component effects and the relative contributions of the component effects sum up to 100 %. (2) SDA is based on algebraic calculation, it, therefore, has no constraints on the specification of relationship (e.g., linearity), the nature of the variables (e.g., random), the form of variable distributions (e.g., normality), and observation independence that are usual assumptions for statistical analyses. (3) SDA can be used to study a wide range of outcome measures such as rate, percentage, proportion, ratio, and arithmetic mean. And (4) SDA can also be readily applied to analyze outcome change and confounding effects on the change in longitudinal studies.

Various SDA methods have been developed by demographers. In general, the methods of standardization and decomposition are grouped into two broad categories (Das Gupta 1991; Das et al. 1993). In the first category, a crude rate is expressed as a function of one or several factors (Bongaarts 1978; Pullum et al. 1989; Nathanson and Kim 1989; Wojtkiewicz et al. 1990). In the second and more common category standardization and decomposition are performed on cross-classified or contingency table data (Kitagawa 1955, 1964; Das Gupta 1991; Das et al. 1993; Cho and Retherford 1973; Kim and Strobino 1984; Liao 1989). In both categories, standardization and decomposition are all performed based on algebraic calculation rather than statistical modeling. In a series of papers, Clogg and his colleagues (Clogg and Eliason 1988; Clogg et al. 1990) have developed a statistical model—the Clogg Model—to standardize rates. Based on log-linear models, the Clogg Model centers around the idea of purging the effects of confounding factors. However, the Clogg model is not designed for, and can't be applied directly to, decomposition analysis. Liao (1989) has developed a method which applies the results of the Clogg models to decompose the difference in crude rates into component effects representing compositional effects, rate effect, and possible interactions between the two.

The choice of a standardization and decomposition method first depends on the type of data (aggregate data, contingency table, or individual data) available for analysis; second, the choice of a method is a matter of personal preference. Nonetheless, the Das Gupta's method is more preferable because its symmetric approach integrates factor interactions into additive main effects (Das Gupta 1991; Das et al. 1993). As such, multiple factors can be easily included and the result interpretation becomes much easier. Unfortunately, none of the existing SDA methods can take sampling variability into account when survey data are analyzed because they are all based on algebraic calculation. Although Liao's (1989) method is based on the results of statistical modeling (i.e., the Clogg purging model) (Clogg and Eliason 1988; Clogg et al. 1990), the actual calculation of the component effects in decomposition analysis is still based on algebraic equations. Therefore, like the other methods, it does not provide statistical significance testing for component effects neither. Wang and colleagues (2000) have developed a Windows-based computer program, DECOMP, that employs bootstrapping techniques (Efron 1979, 1981) to estimate standard errors of SDA component effects, therefore, significance testing for component effects becomes possible in SDA.

SDA is an important demographical analytical method that has been widely used to compare birth rates, death rates, unemployment rates, etc. between different populations/groups in population studies. It has also been increasingly applied to study outcomes difference, inequality or disparity in many other research fields. Wang et al. (2000) applied the computer program DECOMP to conduct SDA to compare gender difference with regard to HIV seropositive rate among injection drug users (IDUs) in the U.S. A sample of 7,378 IDUs (1,745 females and 5,633 males) was obtained from the National Institute on Drug Abuse's National AIDS Demonstration Research (NADR) project (Brown and Beschner 1993) for the study. Their findings show that the HIV seropositive rate among the IDUs was high (overall 36.73 %) in the U.S. IDU population. The corresponding rates for the male and female IDUs were 37.39 % and 34.60 %, respectively, and the gender difference (about 2.79 %) is statistically significant ($t = 2.10$, d.f. $= 7,376$, $p = 0.0358$). In addition, the age structure and ethnic composition were significantly different between the gender populations. To evaluate the difference in HIV seropositive rate between the gender populations, age structure and ethnic composition were standardized across the two populations. And then, the observed difference in HIV seropositive rate between the two populations was decomposed into three components: (1) the rate effect attributed to difference in factor-specific rates; (2) factor-1 component effect attributed to difference in age structures; and (3) factor-2 component effect attributed to difference in ethnic composition between the populations. Once age structure and ethnic composition were standardized, gender difference in HIV seropositive rate disappeared, indicating that the observed gender difference was simply because of compositional difference between the two populations. However, only age structure shows a significant confounding effect on the observed difference in HIV seropositive rate between the gender IDU populations. Similar studies were conducted to assess difference in HIV prevalence rate in different regions in the U.S., such as high HIV prevalence region vs. low HIV prevalence region (Wang 2003), and between four different geographic regions (Wang and Kelly 2014). Their results show that ethnicity and education are important confounding factors in HIV prevalence comparison among IDUs across different U.S. regions.

The SDA was also applied to compare drug abuse among rural stimulant drug users in three geographically distinct areas of the U.S. (Arkansas, Kentucky, and Ohio) (Wang et al. 2007). The findings show that the observed rate of "ever used" methamphetamine and the frequency of methamphetamine use in the past 30 days were much higher on average in Kentucky than in the other two states. However, after the compositions of socio-demographic confounding factors (e.g., gender, ethnicity, age, and education) were standardized across the populations, the two measures of methamphetamine use ranked highest in Arkansas, followed by Kentucky, and then Ohio. Different confounding factors contributed in various dimensions to the differences in the observed measures of methamphetamine use between the geographical drug injection populations. Differential ethnic compositions in the populations largely accounted for the observed difference in both ever used methamphetamine and frequency of using methamphetamine in the past 30 days between Arkansas and other project sites. Since non-Whites were found to be less likely to report methamphetamine use than Whites, regardless of location, and the much higher proportion of non-Whites in Arkansas made the observed measures of methamphetamine use substantially lower than the real level.

Recently, SDA has been successfully applied to study health disparity in nursing research (Yuan et al. 2014). The authors examined disparity in self-efficacy related cancer care behaviors among four groups of cancer patients with different socioeconomic status ("Lower SES Group," "Retiree Group," "Higher Education Group," and "Government Employee Group") in China. The findings show that the compositions of the confounding factors affect self-efficacy difference between SES groups in different ways. The most important confounding factor is social support. Once the composition of social support factor was standardized across SES groups, difference in self-efficacy between SEM groups substantially declined. The findings provide important information on development of tailored interventions of promoting the level of self-efficacy for disadvantaged and underserved population of cancer survivors.

In this chapter, the author will first briefly introduce SDA method, and then demonstrate the application of SDA using DECOMP with real research data.

2 Method

2.1 Algebraic Expression of SDA

For two-population comparison with only one confounding factor, the algebraic expression of SDA can be shown as follows (Das Gupta 1991; Das et al. 1993):

$$R_1 = \sum_{j=1}^{J} \frac{N_{1j}R_{1j}}{N_1} = \sum_{j=1}^{J} F_{1j}R_{1j} \tag{1}$$

$$R_2 = \sum_{j=1}^{J} \frac{N_{2j}R_{2j}}{N_2} = \sum_{j=1}^{J} F_{2j}R_{2j} \tag{2}$$

where R_1 denotes the observed rate (or mean if the outcome is a continuous measure) for Population 1; R_{1j} the observed factor-specific rate in the jth category of the confounding factor with J categories ($j = 1, 2, \ldots J$) in Population 1; N_1 is the total number of cases in Population 1; N_{1j} specifies the number of cases in the jth category of the confounding factor in Population 1; and $F_{1j} = N_{1j}/N_1$ represents the proportion or relative frequency of the Population 1 members who fall into the jth category of the confounder, and $\sum F_{1j} = 1$. R_2, R_{2j}, N_2, N_{2j}, and F_{2j} are the equivalent notations for Population 2. In both Eqs. (1) and (2), the observed rate is expressed as a summation of weighted factor-specific rates: for instance, the weight is $F_{1j} = N_{1j}/N_1$ for Population 1, and $F_{2j} = N_{2j}/N_2$ for Population 2, which are the compositions of the confounder in the respective populations. The rate difference between Populations 1 and 2 can be expressed accordingly:

$$R_1. - R_2. = \sum_{j=1}^{J} \frac{F_{1j} + F_{2j}}{2} \left(R_{1j} - R_{2j}\right) + \sum_{j=1}^{J} \frac{R_{1j} + R_{2j}}{2} \left(F_{1j} - F_{2j}\right) \tag{3}$$

Equation (3) shows that the difference between the two observed rates, $(R_1. - R_2.)$, can be decomposed into two components: a rate effect (i.e., the first term on the right side of the equation) and a factor component effect (i.e., the second term on the right side of the equation). As shown in the first term, the composition of the confounding factor is standardized across populations; thus, the observed rate difference contained in this term can be considered having resulted from differential factor-specific rates between the populations under study. Therefore, we called it *rate effect*. In contrast, the second term on right side of Eq. (3), where the factor-specific rate is standardized, represents the component in the crude rate difference that is attributed to differential factor compositions between the two populations. We call this term *factor component effect*, which describes the effect of the factor composition on the observed rate difference.

The traditional SDA could only deal with two confounding factors and compare two populations (Kitagawa 1955, 1964). When multiple confounding factors are involved, the decomposition equations become progressively more complex because of the proliferation of relationships between variables. In addition, when multiple populations are involved in SDA, naive pairwise comparisons are usually conducted separately, which is inappropriate because the results of pairwise comparisons may lack internal consistency (Das Gupta 1991; Das et al. 1993). As a result, the estimate of a standardized rate for each population may not be consistent in different pairwise comparisons. For example, when comparing three populations, the difference in the estimated standardized rates between Population 1 and Population 2 plus the difference between Population 2 and Population 3 may not equal the difference between Population 1 and Population 3. The same problem remains when studying temporal outcome changes in a single population at multiple time-points. The SDA was generalized by Das Gupta (1991) and Das et al. (1993) for multiple population comparisons with multiple confounding factors. In theory, the generalized SDA does not have a limit on the number of populations to compare and number of confounding factors to analyze. The formulas for comparing Populations 1 and 2 in the presence of Populations 3, 4, ..., and K are described as the following (Das Gupta 1991; Das et al. 1993):

$$A_{1.23...K} = \frac{\sum_{j=2}^{K} A_{1.j}}{(K-1)} + \frac{\sum_{i=2}^{K} \left(\sum_{j\neq 1,i}^{K} A_{i,j} - (K-2) A_{i.1}\right)}{K(K-1)} \tag{4}$$

$$A_{12.3...K} = A_{12} + \frac{\sum_{i=3}^{K} \left(A_{12} + A_{2j} - A_{1j}\right)}{K} \tag{5}$$

where $A_{1.23...K}$ and $A_{12.3...K}$ are the standardized rate in Population 1 and the component effect of factor A, respectively, standardizing all other factors but A, when Populations 1 and 2 are compared in presence of Populations 3, 4, ..., K. When Populations 2 and 3 are compared in presence of Populations 1, 4, ..., K, the corresponding standardized rate in Population 2 and the effect of factor A would be $A_{2.31 \ldots K}$ and $A_{23.14 \ldots K}$, respectively. As a result, each population will have a consistent estimate of standardized rate when standardization is conducted with respect to the same set of factors no matter which population it is compared with. It, therefore, solves the problem of internal inconsistency in component effect estimation in multiple population comparisons. The standardized rates and factor component effects with respect to other factors can be calculated in the same way. That is, the same formulas apply to other factors regardless of how many factors are involved in the SDA (Das Gupta 1991; Das et al. 1993).

2.2 Statistical Significance Testing for Component Effect

SDA is traditionally implemented using aggregated population data based on algebraic calculation, thus no significance testing is available. When survey data are used for analysis, sampling variation must be taken into account. In order to make statistical inference from survey data, significance testing for the component effects is needed in SDA. This challenge is completed by the author of the present chapter by applying the bootstrapping techniques in the computer program DECOMP (Wang et al. 2000). As noted by Chevan and Sutherland: "Wang et al. (2000) contributed to the enhancement of decomposition methods stemming from Das Gupta's work by developing tests of significance for decomposed rates using bootstrapping techniques to estimate standard errors"(2009, p. 430).

Bootstrap is a data-based simulation method for statistical inference in situations where it is difficult or impossible to derive the standard error of a statistic in the usual way (Efron 1979, 1981). Bootstrap uses a computer to draw a large number of "resamples" randomly from the original sample with replacement and with the same size of the original sample. Rather than having analytic formulas with distribution assumptions, bootstrapping generates an empirical sampling distribution of a statistic of interest from all the resamples. Then the standard error and the confidence interval of the statistic can be estimated from the empirical sampling distribution and used to make statistical significance test. Suppose that one is to infer population characteristic θ from $\widehat{\theta}$, a total of B resamples are drawn randomly from the original sample with replacement. Since each resample yields a $\widehat{\theta}_b$, which is an empirical estimate of $\widehat{\theta}$, there would be a total of B $\widehat{\theta}_b$s estimated from all the resamples. Thus, the standard error of $\widehat{\theta}$ can be estimated as:

$$\widehat{\sigma}_{\widehat{\theta}} = \left\{ \frac{\sum \left(\widehat{\theta}_b - \widehat{\theta}_{(.)} \right)^2}{(B-1)} \right\}^{1/2} \tag{6}$$

where $\widehat{\theta}_{(.)} = \sum_{b=1}^{B} \widehat{\theta}_b/B$. When bootstrapping option is specified in the computer program DECOMP, B resamples will be generated and each of them will be used to generate a contingency table for SDA. Component effects will be estimated separately from each of the B bootstrap resamples, and the empirical distributions of the component effect estimates will be used to estimate the standard error of each component effect. The distribution normality of the component effects estimated from bootstrapping with various numbers of resamples was tested in the author's previous study, using Q–Q normal probability plots (Wang et al. 2000). The results show that the plot points cluster around a straight line, indicating that the bootstrapping estimated values of component effects display a normal distribution when a moderately large number (e.g., 200) of bootstrap resamples were used. However, statisticians recommend that 800 or more bootstrap resamples are needed to estimate the standard error of $\widehat{\theta}$ (Booth and Sarkar 1998). It is remindful that bootstrapping is conducted using raw (individual) survey data. In case that only grouped survey data (contingency table) are available, a utility function built in DECOMP will allow one to convert the grouped data into raw (individual) data if the outcome is a rate, percentage, proportion, or ratio (Wang et al. 2000).

2.3   Computer Program for SDA

SDA is usually implemented using grouped data or contingency tables in data spreadsheet programs. In late 1980s, Dr. Ruggles (1986–1989) developed a computer program, for SDA (http://www.hist.umn.edu/~ruggles/DECOMP.html). The program was written for DOS, and has not been upgraded to Windows version since then. The first Windows-based computer program for SDA, which is still the only Windows-based SDA program to the best of my knowledge, was developed by the author of this chapter and his colleagues in late 1990s (Wang et al. 2000). Interesting, the two programs were both named "DECOMP" coincidently. However, in addition to its user-friendly interface, the Windows version DECOMP has a unique feature, that is, it allows one, for the first time, to conduct statistical significance testing for component effects in SDA, using bootstrapping to estimate the standard errors of the component effects. Both grouped data and individual data can be used for SDA in the Windows version DECOMP. When individual data are analyzed, the outcome measure could be either a dichotomous or a continuous variable; when analyzing grouped data, the outcome measure could be a rate, proportion, percentage, ratio, or arithmetic mean. The program allows an unlimited number of populations/samples for multiple population SDA; however, the number of confounding factors is limited up to 10. If significance testing for component effects needs to be conducted, individual data must be used for bootstrapping.

   Although the mathematical formulas expressed in Eqs. (4) and (5) for multi-population and multi-factor SDA are complicated, they can be easily implemented in the Windows version DECOMP and results are interpreted in the similar way as two-population SDA (Wang and Kelly 2014; Wang et al. 2007). All populations will be compared in a pairwise way, adjusting for internal inconsistence.

Application of the Windows version DECOMP is straightforward (Wang et al. 2000). What one needs to do are: (1) open the program in Windows and input data file with text or ASCII format; (2) specify the population variable (a categorical variable that has as many categories as the number of populations); (3) specify the outcome variable and select the confounding factors; (4) specify the number of bootstrapping resamples if significance testing is preferred; and then (5) click the Run button. The results of SDA can be saved in different formats (e.g., pdf, MS Word). The program is freely available to download online (www.wright.edu/~jichuan.wang/).

2.4   Example of Application

This chapter demonstrates how to apply SDA in real research. The example of application assesses regional difference in the HIV prevalence rate among IDUs in the U.S. A total of 9,824 IDUs located in three geographic regions (e.g., Northeast, Midwest, and West) were retrieved from the large national database of *the National Institute on Drug Abuse's Cooperative Agreement for AIDS Community-Based Outreach/Intervention Research Program (COOP)* (Needle et al. 1995) for the purpose of demonstration. In the SDA, differences in the observed regional HIV prevalence rate were decomposed into component effects, such as "real" difference in HIV prevalence that is attributed to difference in factor-specific rates; and factor component effects that are attributed to compositional differences of specific confounding factors. The outcome is a dichotomous variable at individual level (1-HIV positive; 0-HIV negative); thus, the mean of the outcome in a regional population is an estimated HIV prevalence rate in the regional target population. The confounding factors included in the analysis are: Ethnicity (0-Nonwhite; 1-White), gender (0-Female; 1-Male), age group (1: <30; 2: 30–39; 3: 40+), and education level (1: <High school; 2: High school; 3: College+). The Windows version DECOMP was used to implement the multi-population SDA with multiple confounding factors.

3   Results

The sample descriptive statistics and the estimates of HIV prevalence rates among IDUs are shown by region in Table 1. The HIV prevalence rate was high in the Northeast (17.52 %), moderate in the West (8.04 %), and low in the Midwest (4.56 %). The HIV prevalence rate was higher among Black IDUs than among White IDUs across the regions. Age and education are significantly associated with HIV prevalence rate only in the West. Gender is not significantly associated with

Table 1 Socio-demographic compositions and HIV prevalence rate by region ($N^a = 6,985$)

| Variable | Region | | | | | |
| | Northeast | | Midwest | | West | |
	n (%)	HIV[b]	n (%)	HIV[b]	n (%)	HIV[b]
Ethnicity						
Black	630 (76.64)	18.73	1,670 (80.10)	5.57	1,923 (47.16)	14.09
White	192 (23.36)	13.54	415 (19.90)	0.48	2,155 (52.84)	2.65
($\chi^2 p$-value)	(0.0978)		(<0.0001)		(<0.0001)	
Gender						
Female	174 (21.17)	16.67	508 (24.36)	6.10	1,182 (28.98)	8.12
Male	648 (78.83)	17.75	1,577 (75.64)	4.06	2,896 (71.02)	8.01
($\chi^2 p$-value)	(0.7393)		(0.0547)		(0.9061)	
Age						
<30	77 (9.37)	15.58	98 (4.70)	1.02	469 (11.50)	4.05
30–39	337 (41.00)	20.77	749 (35.92)	5.47	1,590 (38.99)	7.74
40+	408 (49.64)	15.20	1,238 (59.38)	4.28	2,019 (49.51)	9.21
($\chi^2 p$-value)	(0.1230)		(0.1014)		(0.0009)	
Education						
<High School	337 (41.00)	18.69	735 (35.25)	4.08	1,191 (29.21)	8.98
High School	337 (41.00)	18.40	808 (38.75)	4.70	1,758 (43.11)	8.59
College+	148 (18.00)	12.84	542 (26.00)	4.98	1,129 (27.69)	6.20
($\chi^2 p$-value)	(0.2533)		(0.7239)		(0.0257)	
Overall	822	17.52	2,085	4.56	4,078	8.04

[a] Number of IDUs who took voluntary and confidential HIV antibody tests at the baseline interview
[b] The percentage of HIV positives among the IDUs in each sample was used as an estimate of HIV prevalence rate for that sample

HIV prevalence rate in all the regions. Notably, the compositions of the socio-demographic factors, ethnicity in particular, vary across regions. For example, only 47.16 % of the IDUs in the West were Blacks, while the corresponding figures were 76.64 % in the Northeast, and 80.10 % in the Midwest, respectively.

The results of SDA are shown in Table 2. The upper panel of the table shows the results comparing HIV prevalence rates between the Northeast and Midwest regions. The observed HIV prevalence rate was about 12.91 % higher in the Northeast than in the Midwest. Significance testing for the rate difference was conducted using t-test, where the standard error of the difference was estimated based on 1,000 bootstrap resamples. Only education shows significant confounding effect (t-ratio = 0.0027/0.0011 = 2.45) on the regional difference in HIV prevalence rate. Nonetheless, the factor component effect is very small, contributing only 2.09 % to the observed rate difference. Other socio-demographic factors do not significantly confound the regional difference of HIV prevalence rates. As such, the regional rate difference (12.81 %) remains almost unchanged after adjusting for confounding effects.

Table 2 Results of multi-population standardization and decomposition analysis based on 1,000 bootstrap resamples

| | Standardization | | Decomposition | | |
| | | | Difference | | |
	Northeast	Midwest	Diff	S.E.	Percent distribution of effect (%)
Ethnicity	0.1112	0.1131	−0.0019	0.0015	−1.4722
Gender	0.1069	0.1067	0.0002	0.0009	0.1550
Age	0.1078	0.1077	0.0001	0.0011	0.0775
Education	0.1090	0.1063	0.0027*	0.0011	2.0920
Adjusted rate	0.1697	0.0416	0.1281*	0.0094	99.2549
Observed rate	0.1752	0.0462	0.1291*	0.0096	100.0297

| | Standardization | | Decomposition | | |
| | | | Difference | | |
	Northeast	West	Diff	S.E.	Percent distribution of effect (%)
Ethnicity	0.1112	0.0855	0.0257*	0.0028	27.1254
Gender	0.1069	0.1076	−0.0007	0.0011	−0.7388
Age	0.1078	0.1063	0.0015	0.0009	1.5832
Education	0.1090	0.1057	0.0033*	0.0012	3.4830
Adjusted rate	0.1697	0.1046	0.0651*	0.0092	68.7107
Observed rate	0.1752	0.0805	0.0947*	0.0094	99.9524

| | Standardization | | Decomposition | | |
| | | | Difference | | |
	Midwest	West	Diff	S.E.	Percent distribution of effect (%)
Ethnicity	0.1131	0.0855	0.0276*	0.0020	−80.4277
Gender	0.1067	0.1076	−0.0009	0.0006	2.6226
Age	0.1077	0.1063	0.0014	0.0008	−4.0797
Education	0.1063	0.1057	0.0006	0.0009	−1.7484
Adjusted rate	0.0416	0.1046	−0.0630*	0.0059	183.5849
Observed rate	0.0462	0.0805	−0.0343*	0.0057	99.9518

*Statistically significant at $\alpha = 0.05$

The HIV prevalence difference between the Northeast and the West decreased from 9.47 to 6.51 % after adjusting for the confounding factors (see the middle panel of Table 2). That is, adjusting for socio-demographic compositions, the regional difference in HIV prevalence rate would be about 31.26 % smaller. The adjusted prevalence difference reflects the factor-specific rate difference, which accounts for about 68.71 % of the observed regional prevalence difference (see the last column of the panel in Table 2). Ethnic composition had a significantly confounding effect (t-ratio = 0.0257/0.0028 = 9.18), accounting for about 27.13 % of the observed HIV prevalence difference. Education had a significant confounding effect (t-ratio = 0.0033/0.0012 = 2.75), but its contributions to the regional difference in HIV prevalence rate were limited, accounting for only 3.48 %. Gender (t-ratio = −0.0007/0.0011 = 0.64) and age (t-ratio = −0.0015/0.0009 = 1.67) had no significant confounding effects. In comparison between the Midwest and the West, only ethnicity had a significant confounding effect (t-ratio = 0.0276/0.0020 = 13.80) (see the lower panel of Table 2).

Notice that the confounding effect of ethnicity is positive sometimes (e.g., Northeast vs. West; Midwest vs. West), but negative sometimes (e.g., Northeast vs. Midwest though not statistically significant). A positive confounding effect means that the rate difference between populations would be enlarged if the confounding effect were not controlled; on the contrary, a negative confounding effect indicates the extent to which the rate difference would be narrowed if the confounding effect were not controlled.

4 Discussion

This chapter briefly introduces SDA and demonstrates its application using real research data. The results of the example SDA show that ethnicity and education, particularly ethnicity, are important confounding factors in comparison of HIV prevalence among IDUs between the U.S. geographic regions. Gender and age had no significantly confounding effects on regional HIV prevalence difference because age structure and gender compositions do not vary much between the regions (see Table 1). It is remindful that decomposition of outcome differences using SDA is not equivalent to analyzing variation of a dependent variable in a regression model or ANOVA. A variable may significantly explain the variation of a dependent variable in regression, but may not have a significant confounding effect in SDA. For example, both binary and multivariate statistics may show a significant relationship between a variable and an outcome measure of interest; however, the variable would have no significant confounding effect on outcome difference between populations if its composition does not vary much across the populations under study. In the example demonstrated in this chapter, ethnicity shows significant confounding effect when comparing the West region with the Northeast and Midwest regions. However, such a confounding effect was not statistically significant (t-ratio = 0.0019/0.0015 = 1.26) when comparing the Northeast and Midwest regions because ethnic composition was similar in the two regions (see Table 1). That is, although ethnicity is significantly related to HIV seropositive status, its confounding effect on regional difference of HIV prevalence rate depends on the regional ethnic composition.

In many research fields, such as epidemiology, health and health care studies, and behavior research, outcome difference, inequality or disparity is often a significant concern. An observed outcome measure (e.g., crude death rate, prevalence of a specific disease, adverse event or symptom, average medical expenses, average cost of medical insurance, school dropout rate, crime rate, etc.) depends not just on the level of the outcome, but also the composition of the underlying population. That is, the observed outcome measure for a population depends on a number of confounding factors that need to be taken into account when comparing outcome measures across populations. SDA is a useful analytical method for such outcome comparison. It enables to evaluate what factors contribute, and how, to the observed outcome difference, inequality or disparity between populations. It provides not only an opportunity of viewing and interpreting outcome difference, inequality or disparity from a different perspective, but also important policy implications with regard to intervention efforts that are tailored to meet the needs of the populations.

References

Bongaarts, J.: A framework for analyzing the proximate determinants of fertility. Popul. Dev. Rev. **4**, 105–132 (1978)

Booth, J.G., Sarkar, S.: Monte Carlo approximation of bootstrap variances. Am. Stat. **52**, 354–357 (1998)

Brown, B.S., Beschner, G.M.: Handbook on Risk of AIDS: Injection Drug Users and Sexual Partners. Greenwood Press, Westport (1993)

Chevan, A., Sutherland, M.: Revisiting Das Gupta: refinement and extension of standardization and decomposition. Demography **46**, 429–449 (2009)

Cho, L.J., Retherford, R.D.: Comparative analysis of recent fertility trends in East Asia. Proc. IUSSP Int. Popul. Conf. **2**, 163–181 (1973)

Clogg, C.C., Eliason, S.R.: A flexible procedure for adjusting rates and proportions, including statistical method for group comparisons. Am. Sociol. Rev. **53**, 267–283 (1988)

Clogg, C.C., Shockey, J.W., Eliason, S.R.: A general statistical framework for adjustment of rates. Sociol. Methods Res. **19**, 156–195 (1990)

Das Gupta, P.: Decomposition of the difference between two rates and its consistency when more than two populations are involved. Math. Popul. Stud. **3**, 105–125 (1991)

Das Gupta, P.: Standardization and Decomposition of Rates: A User's Manual. U.S. Bureau of the Census, Current Population Reports, Series P23-186. U.S. Government Printing Office, Washington, DC (1993)

Efron, B.: Bootstrap methods: another look at the Jackknife. Ann. Stat. **7**, 1–26 (1979)

Efron, B.: Nonparametric standard errors and confidence intervals (with discussion). Can. J. Stat. **9**, 139–172 (1981)

Kim, Y.J., Strobino, D.M.: Decomposition of the difference between two rates with hierarchical factors. Demography **15**, 99–112 (1984)

Kitagawa, E.M.: Components of a difference between two rates. J. Am. Stat. Assoc. **50**, 1168–1194 (1955)

Kitagawa, E.M.: Standardized comparisons in population research. Demography **1**, 296–315 (1964)

Liao, T.F.: A flexible approach for the decomposition of rate differences. Demography **26**, 717–726 (1989)

Nathanson, C.A., Kim, Y.J.: Components of change in adolescent fertility. Demography **26**, 85–98 (1989)

Needle, R., Fisher, D.G., Weatherby, N., Chitwood, D., Brown, B., Cesari, H., et al.: Reliability of self-reported HIV risk behaviors of drug users. Psychol. Addict. Behav. **9**, 242–250 (1995)

Pullum, T.W.: Standardization (World Fertility Survey Technical Bulletins, No. 597). International Statistical Institute, Voorburg (1978)

Pullum, T.W., Tedrow, L.M., Herting, J.R.: Measuring change and continuity in parity distributions. Demography **26**, 485–498 (1989)

Ruggles, S.: Software for Multiple Standardization and Demographic Decomposition. http://www. hist.umn.edu/~ruggles/DECOMP.html (1986–1989)

United Nations: The Methodology of Measuring the Impact of Family Planning Programs, Manual IX, Population Studies, No. 66. U.N., New York (1979)

Wang, J.: Components of difference in HIV seropositivity rate among injection drug users between low and high HIV prevalence regions. AIDS Behav. **7**, 1–8 (2003)

Wang, J., Kelly, B.: Gauging regional differences in the hiv prevalence rate among injection drug users in the U.S. Open Addict. J. **7**, 1–7 (2014)

Wang, J., Rahman, A., Siegal, H.A., Fisher, J.H.: Standardization and decomposition of rates: useful analytic techniques for behavior and health studies. Behav. Res. Methods Instrum. Comput. **32**, 357–366 (2000)

Wang, J., Carlson, R.G., Falck, R.S., Leukefeld, C., Booth, B.M.: Multiple sample standardization and decomposition analysis: an application to comparisons of methamphetamine use among rural drug users in three American states. Stat. Med. **26**, 3612–3623 (2007)

Wojtkiewicz, R.A., Mclanahan, S.S., Garfinkel, I.: The growth of families headed by women: 1950–1980. Demography **27**, 19–30 (1990)

Yuan, C., Wei, C., Wang, J., Qian, H., Ye, X., Liu, Y., Hinds, P.S.: Self-efficacy difference among patients with cancer with different socioeconomic status: application of latent class analysis and standardization and decomposition analysis. Cancer Epidemiol. **38**, 298–306 (2014)

Cusp Catastrophe Modeling in Medical and Health Research

Xinguang (Jim) Chen and Ding-Geng Chen

Abstract Further advancement in medical and health research calls for analytical paradigm shifting from linear and continuous approach to nonlinear and discrete approach. In response to this need, we introduced the cusp catastrophe modeling method, including the general principle and two analytical approaches to statistically solving the model for actual data analysis: (1) the polynomial regression method and (2) the likelihood estimation method, with the former for analyzing longitudinal data and the later for cross-sectional data. The polynomial regression method can be conducted using most software packages, including SAS, SPSS, and R. A special R-based package "cusp" is needed to run the likelihood method for data analysis. To assist researchers interested in using the method, two examples with empirical data analyses are included, including R codes for the "cusp" package.

Keywords Cusp catastrophe modeling • Likelihood estimation • Polynomial regression • Analytical paradigm • Clinical epidemiology • Behavioral epidemiology

1 Linear and Continuous Paradigm

A primary goal of quantitative and statistical analysis is to extract information from data supporting causal conclusions in etiological, intervention and evaluation research. An analytical conceptual framework that dominates the modern scientific research is the *linear and continuous* (LC) *paradigm*. The most commonly used analytical and statistical methods under the LC paradigm include, from simple comparative analysis of student t-test to more complex variance and covariance

X. (Jim) Chen (✉)
Department of Epidemiology, University of Florida, 2004 Mowry Road, CTRB #4228, Gainesville, FL 32610, USA
e-mail: jimax.chen@phhp.ufl.edu

D.-G. Chen
School of Social Work, University of North Carolina, Chapel Hill, NC, 27599 USA
e-mail: dinchen@email.unc.edu

© Springer International Publishing Switzerland 2015   265
D.-G. Chen, J. Wilson (eds.), *Innovative Statistical Methods for Public Health Data*, ICSA Book Series in Statistics, DOI 10.1007/978-3-319-18536-1_12

analysis, correlation, interaction, regression, path analysis, and structural equation modeling. The LC paradigm can be mathematically described as:

$$y = f_{lc}(x, c) \tag{1}$$

where x is a vector of independent variables, y the dependent variable, c a set of covariates, and f_{lc} is a linear and continuous function.

Figure 1 depicts the analytical feature of the LC paradigm. Understanding the characteristics of LC paradigm is of great significance to consider the application of various analytical methodologies in research. Three key characteristics of the LC paradigm are summarized below.

Fig. 1 Linear continuous paradigm

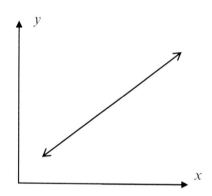

1. Under the LC paradigm, the relationship between x and y is determined by a linear relations. Corresponding to each value of x, there is one and only one value of y. If there are multiple values of y, a mean structure of these multiple values is modeled with an appropriate "error" structure as commonly seen in linear regression analysis. With this paradigm, error-prone analytical result cannot be ruled out if multiple y values are true at a given x. For example, in etiological research, we often observe the phenomenon of the same level of blood pressure or blood lipids in patients, but only some suffer from heart attack and the rest are not. In clinical research, given the same dosage of a medicine to patients suffering from the same disease, some respond positively while others do not. In behavioral studies, given the same level of motivation to engage in HIV protective behaviors (e.g., use a condom during sexual intercourse), only some use protection while others do not.

2. Uni-directional or single path is another characteristic of the LC paradigm. Under the LC paradigm, changes in the dependent variable y always follow the same path along with changes in the independent variable x, no matter the x increases or declines. This paradigm may be true in physics, chemistry, engineering, but may not always be true in medical, health and behavioral sciences. It is well established that the process of disease occurrence and recovery follows different

paths; the development of a drug addiction and the recovery from the addiction treatment also follow different paths. The limitation is obvious if methods based on the LC paradigm are used to quantify a condition with multiple progression paths.

3. LC paradigm assumes that changes in y are continuous in response to changes in x. However, in medical and behavioral research, non-continuous changes are not uncommon. Typical examples in medicine include the occurrence of heart attack, stroke, asthma, and fatigue; and in health behaviors include injury and accidents, use of drugs and substance, sexual debut, and condom use during sex. In these cases, analytical methods based on LC paradigm are inadequate to quantify the process, including the overall trends and the threshold in x for the sudden change in y.

2   Nonlinear and Continuous Paradigm

To deal with the categorical variables that are neither continuous nor linear, the likelihood approach is adopted capitalizing on the linear and continuous paradigm. The most typical example is the logistic regression model established for binary dependent variable to regress all independent variable x (can be continuous such as age, blood pressure) in predicting the likelihood (e.g., the odds ratio or other similar measures) of the occurrence of the dependent variable y (e.g., a disease or death). With this approach, the predicted likelihood/probability is nonlinear to the linear independent variables. This approach extends the LC paradigm and it can be more generally termed as *nonlinear continuous* (NLC) paradigm. Mathematically, an NLC paradigm can be expressed as:

$$y = f_{nlc}(x, t, c) \qquad (2)$$

where x is the independent variable that can be continuous or categorical, the dependent variable y is categorical, t is the threshold in x, c is a set of covariates, and f_{nlc} is a nonlinear and continuous (typically likelihood) function characterize the relationship between x and y. Often the function f_{nlc} can be converted into linear for statistical solutions capitalizing on the achievements in solving LC paradigm-based statistical models.

Figure 2 depicts this NLC paradigm. As the predict variable x increases, the likelihood for y to increase slowly at the beginning; when x approaches a threshold t, the likelihood surges; with further increases in x, the likelihood for y to increases slows down and gradually levels off. In addition to logistic regression, a number of other analytical and statistical methods belong to this family, including Poisson regression, or the family of generalized linear models. A feature common to these methods is the application of a logarithm or similar link function to convert this non-linear relation into a linear relation to solve the model; and odds ratio is thus estimated by a reverse computing.

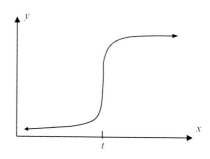

Fig. 2 Nonlinear continuous paradigm

Compared to the linear and continuous paradigm as depicted in Fig. 1, analytical methods under the NLC paradigm is the adaptation of threshold t in the independent variable x to accommodate sudden changes in the dependent variable y, although this threshold has rarely been quantified and used in medical and health research. The advantages of the NLC model have not been fully explored. Analytical methods guided by this paradigm such as logistic regression, Poisson regression, and Cox regression have gained wide acceptance in medical and health research to investigate categorical variables; however, methods directly quantifying the nonlinear change rather than the likelihood of change have not been well developed. The group-based developmental trajectory analysis methods by Nagin and Jones (Nagin 2005; Jones and Nagin 2007) and Muthen (Muthen and Muthen 2000) are some examples. These methods are commonly used in psychology, sociology, and criminology; they began to gain popularity in medical and health research in recent years to study developmental trajectories of overweight, obesity (Barnes et al. 2011; Chen and Brogan 2012; Wong et al. 2012), and substance use behaviors (Chen and Jacques-Tiura 2014).

3   Nonlinear and Discrete Paradigm

One of the most innovations of the nonlinear continuous paradigm described in the previous section is the creative application of the linear approach in solving a nonlinear and non-continuous system as measured by the dependent variable y. However, methods based on the nonlinear continuous paradigm will not be efficient in quantifying a phenomenon characterized by the dynamic pattern depicted in Fig. 3.

The conceptual framework depicted in the figure assumes two separate processes governing the relationship between x and y with two different thresholds d and u. When the independent variable x increases from left to right, the dependent variable y increases gradually first following a nonlinear path; when x passes the threshold u (u for upward change), y increases suddenly, showing a phase change just like a person from healthy to suddenly being sick (e.g., heart attack, stroke). As x further increases, y experiences no substantial change and maintains at the high levels.

```
> # combine results from M imputed data sets
> analysis←summary(pool(fit, method="small sample"))
> # view results
> analysis
```

The results from complete case analysis, multiple imputation with norm, and multiple imputation with mice are compared to the original complete data in Table 1. The most important variable in the original analysis by Cain et al. (2012) was the significance and magnitude of the SHEBEEN variable. In the original complete data, the variable SHEBEEN was significant. However, in CCA, this significance is not

Table 1 HIV risk behavior example: linear model estimates with original complete data, complete case analysis, multiple imputation—norm (M=300), multiple imputation—mice (M=300)

Coefficients	Estimate	SE	Confidence interval	$\hat{\gamma}$
Original complete data				
(Intercept)	1.554	0.290	(0.986, 2.122)	
GENDER	−0.017	0.093	(−0.200, 0.166)	
AGE	0.003	0.005	(−0.007, 0.012)	
UNEMP	−0.291	0.084	(−0.456, −0.126)	
ALC	0.011	0.003	(0.005, 0.017)	
SHEBEEN	0.506	0.506	(0.259, 0.754)	
Complete case analysis				
(Intercept)	1.685	0.531	(0.640, 2.730)	
GENDER	−0.142	0.170	(−0.476, 0.193)	
AGE	0.008	0.009	(−0.009, 0.026)	
UNEMP	−0.332	0.153	(−0.634, −0.031)	
ALC	0.021	0.006	(0.009, 0.034)	
SHEBEEN	0.283	0.219	(−0.147, 0.714)	
Multiple imputation—norm (M=300)				
(Intercept)	1.355	0.426	(0.517, 2.194)	0.552
GENDER	−0.054	0.126	(−0.302, 0.194)	0.482
AGE	0.016	0.008	(0.001, 0.0316)	0.641
UNEMP	−0.382	0.119	(−0.615, −0.149)	0.525
ALC	0.018	0.006	(0.006, 0.029)	0.711
SHEBEEN	0.356	0.170	(0.021, 0.690)	0.479
Multiple imputation—mice (M=300)				
(Intercept)	1.429	0.438	(0.569, 2.291)	0.574
GENDER	−0.074	0.131	(−0.332, 0.184)	0.520
AGE	0.014	0.008	(−0.002, 0.030)	0.654
UNEMP	−0.369	0.113	(−0.592, −0.147)	0.479
ALC	0.016	0.006	(0.005, 0.027)	0.684
SHEBEEN	0.373	0.171	(0.037, 0.710)	0.484

captured. Both mice and norm provide similar results to one another. While there is negative bias of the coefficient of SHEBEEN, the bias is far less extreme than it is with CCA. Additionally, both multiple imputation methods find SHEBEEN to be significant. In terms of bias, the chained equations approach outperformed the joint model approach where we assumed multivariate normality—this may be due to the inadequacy of the multivariate normal model for this data. For all other coefficients, multiple imputation consistently provided narrower interval estimates than complete case analysis. The rates of missing information are relatively high, which implies the missing values have substantial impact on the coefficients we estimated.

6 Concluding Remarks

The problem of missing data is one which researchers encounter regularly. Visualizing the missing data is one important first step in understanding how much of a problem it may be and also may help support what missingness mechanisms may exist in your data. Expert knowledge and unverifiable assumptions accompany any missing data method, so assumptions should be made cautiously. While there are several principled and established methods for dealing with missing data, multiple imputation provides flexibility in terms of analysis capabilities and is readily available to implement in many statistical software programs.

Acknowledgements The authors wish to thank Dr. Seth Kalichman for generously sharing his data. This project was supported in part by the National Institute of Mental Health, Award Number K01MH087219. The content is solely the responsibility of the authors, and it does not represent the official views of the National Institute of Mental Health or the National Institutes of Health.

References

Barnard, J., Rubin, D.B.: Small-sample degrees of freedom with multiple imputation. Biometrika **86**, 948–955 (1999)

Belin, T.: Missing data: what a little can do and what researchers can do in response. Am. J. Opthalmology **148**(6), 820–822 (2009)

Bodner, T.E.: What improves with increased missing data imputations? Struct. Equ. Model. **15**(4), 651–675 (2008)

Cain, D., Pare, V., Kalichman, S.C., Harel, O., Mthembu, J., Carey, M.P., Carey, K.B., Mehlomakulu, V., Simbayi, L.C., Mwaba, K.: Hiv risks associated with patronizing alcohol serving establishments in south african townships, cape town. Prev. Sci. **13**(6), 627–634 (2012)

Chang, C.-C.H., Yang, H.-C. , Tang, G., Ganguli, M.: Minimizing attrition bias: a longitudinal study of depressive symptoms in an elderly cohort. Int. Psychogeriatr. **21**(05), 869–878 (2009)

Collins, L., Schafer, J., Kam, C.: A comparison of inclusive and restrictive strategies in modern missing data procedures. Psychol. Methods **6**, 330–351 (2001)

Dempster, A., Laird, A., Rubin, D.: Maximum likelihood from incomplete data via the em algorithm. J. R. Stat. Soc. Ser. B Methodol. **39**(1), 1–38 (1977)

Diggle, P., Kenward, M.G.: Informative drop-out in longitudinal data analysis. Appl. Stat., 49–93 (1994)

Fitzmaurice, G., Laird, N., Ware, J.: Applied Longitudinal Analysis. Wiley Series in Probability and Statistics. Wiley (2011)

Gelman, A., Carlin, J., Stern, H., Rubin, D.: Bayesian Data Analysis. Chapman and Hall/CRC, Boca Raton, FL (2003)

Graham, J.W., Hofer, S.M., MacKinnon, D.P.: Maximizing the usefulness of data obtained with planned missing value patterns: An application of maximum likelihood procedures. Multivar. Behav. Res. 31(2), 197–218 (1996)

Graham, J. W., Olchowski, A.E., Gilreath, T.D.: How many imputations are really needed? some practical clarifications of multiple imputation theory. Prev. Sci. 8(3), 206–213 (2007)

Harel, O.: Inferences on missing information under multiple imputation and two-stage multiple imputation. Stat. Methodol. 4, 75–89 (2007)

Harel, O., Pellowski, J., Kalichman, S.: Are we missing the importance of missing values in HIV prevention randomized clinical trials? Review and recommendations. AIDS Behav. 16, 1382–1393 (2012)

Jamshidian, M., Jalal, S.: Tests of homoscedasticity, normality, and missing completely at random for incomplete multivariate data. Psychometrika 75(4), 649–674 (2010)

Jamshidian, M., Jalal, S., Jansen, C.: MissMech: an R package for testing homoscedasticity, multivariate normality, and missing completely at random (mcar). J. Stat. Softw. 56(6), 1–31 (2014)

Little, R., Rubin, D.: Statistical Analysis with Missing Data, 2nd edn. Wiley, Hoboken, NJ (2002)

Little, R.J.: A test of missing completely at random for multivariate data with missing values. J. Am. Stat. Assoc. 83(404), 1198–1202 (1988)

Little, R.J., D'Agostino, R., Cohen, M.L., Dickersin, K., Emerson, S.S., Farrar, J.T., Frangakis, C., Hogan, J.W., Molenberghs, G., Murphy, S.A., et al.: The prevention and treatment of missing data in clinical trials. N. Engl. J. Med. 367(14), 1355–1360 (2012)

Marchenko, Y.V., Reiter, J.P.: Improved degrees of freedom for multivariate significance tests obtained from multiply imputed, small-sample data. Stata J. 9(3), 388–397 (2009)

Reiter, J.P.: Small-sample degrees of freedom for multi-component significance tests with multiple imputation for missing data. Biometrika 94, 502–508 (2007)

Rubin, D.: Inference and missing data. Biometrika 63(3), 581–592 (1976)

Rubin, D.: Multiple Imputation for Nonresponse in Surveys. Wiley, Hoboken, NJ (1987)

Schafer, J.: Analysis of Incomplete Multivariate Data. Chapman and Hall/CRC, Boca Raton, FL (1997)

Schafer, J., Graham, J.: Missing data: our view of the state of the art. Psychol. Methods 7, 147–177 (2002)

Schafer, J.L.: Norm: analysis of multivariate normal datasets with missing values. R package version 1.0-9.4 (2012)

Templ, M., Alfons, A., Kowarik, A., Prantner, B.: VIM: visualization and imputation of missing values. R package version 4.0.0. (2013)

van Buuren, S., Groothuis-Oudshoorn, K.: Mice: multivariate imputation by chained equations in r. J. Stat. Softw. 45(3), 1–67 (2011)

van Buuren, S., Oudshoorn, K.: Multivariate imputation by chained equations:mice v1.0 user's manual (2000)

Wagstaff, D.A., Harel, O.: A closer examination of three small-sample approximations to the multiple-imputation degrees of freedom. Stata J. 11(3), 403–419 (2011)

White, I., Carlin, J.: Bias and efficiency of multiple imputation compared with complete-case analysis for missing covariate values. Stat. Med. 28, 2920–2931 (2010)

White, I.R., Royston, P., Wood, A.M.: Multiple imputation using chained equations: Issues and guidance for practice. Stat. Med. 30(4), 377–399 (2011)

A Continuous Latent Factor Model
for Non-ignorable Missing Data

Jun Zhang and Mark Reiser

Abstract Many longitudinal studies, especially in clinical trials, suffer from missing data issues. Most estimation procedures assume that the missing values are ignorable. However, this assumption leads to unrealistic simplification and is implausible for many cases. When non-ignorable missingness is preferred, classical pattern-mixture models with the data stratified according to a variety of missing patterns and a model specified for each stratum are widely used for longitudinal data analysis. But this assumption usually results in under-identifiability because of the need to estimate many stratum-specific parameters. Further, pattern mixture models have the drawback that a large sample is usually required. In this paper, a continuous latent factor model is proposed and this novel approach overcomes limitations which exist in pattern mixture models by specifying a continuous latent factor. The advantages of this model, including small sample feasibility, are demonstrated by comparing with Roy's pattern mixture model using an application to a clinical study of AIDS patients with advanced immune suppression.

1 Introduction

Missing values in multivariate studies pose many challenges. The primary research of interest focuses on accurate and efficient estimation of means and covariance structure in the population. The assumption and estimation of the covariance structure provide the foundation of many statistical models, for instance, structural equation modeling, principle component analysis, and so on. Literature on multivariate missing data methods was reviewed by Little and Rubin (2002) and Schafer (1997). For some frequentist statistical procedures, we may generally ignore the distribution of missingness only when the missing data are missing completely at

J. Zhang
Bayer Healthcare Pharmaceuticals Inc., 100 Bayer Boulevard, Whippany, NJ 07981, USA
e-mail: jun.zhang4@bayer.com

M. Reiser (✉)
School of Mathematical and Statistical Sciences, Arizona State University,
Tempe, AZ 85260, USA
e-mail: mark.reiser@asu.edu

© Springer International Publishing Switzerland 2015
D.-G. Chen, J. Wilson (eds.), *Innovative Statistical Methods for Public Health Data*,
ICSA Book Series in Statistics, DOI 10.1007/978-3-319-18536-1_9

random (MCAR), such as in the generalized estimation equations (GEE) estimation procedure. For likelihood or Bayes procedures, however, we may ignore the missing values when the missing data are missing at random (MAR), as in for example, the estimation procedure for linear mixed models. However, if missing at random in the data is questioned, and one suspects that the missing mechanism is NMAR, i.e. missingness may depend on missing values, then the joint modeling of the complete data and the missing indicators is required. The reason to follow this modeling method is that the resulting estimates of population parameters may be biased (Pirie et al. 1988) unless these NMAR aspects of the data are taken into account in the analysis. Furthermore, the results of the study may not be feasible to generalize because the observed respondents may not represent the target population. From a practical aspect, investigators could not point out whether violations of the MAR assumption are severe enough to result in a conclusions that are not valid.

Models for NMAR data have been proposed for a few decades, including selection models (Diggle and Kenward 1994), pattern-mixture models (Little 1993), as well as shared-parameter models (Little 1993). The detailed review of these models will be given in Sect. 2. All of these forms lead to a rich class of models: latent class models are one of the prevalent members in longitudinal studies. However, the selection of number of latent classes, which is the key assumption for latent class modeling for missingness, is unstable due to many factors as shown by simulation studies (Zhang and Reiser 2012). This sensitivity hinders the direct application of the latent class modeling technique, and intensive simulation studies should be performed before applying it to application studies. The primary goal of this paper is to develop a general method for non-ignorable modeling of incomplete multivariate data based on the idea of a continuous latent variable (Lord 1952, 1953; Bock and Aitkin 1981). We will summarize the distribution of the missingness indicators through a continuous latent factor model, and then relate to the model of interests by including an association of latent traits with subject-specific parameters from the population. A specific description of this new model will be given below.

2 Models

In this section we review mixed models that incorporate unobserved responses and present a novel parametric approach to modeling longitudinal data when non-ignorable missing values are involved. Mixed effects modeling is one of the prevalent methods for the analysis of correlated data where correlation can arise from repeated measurements, longitudinal data or clustering. Since the foundation paper of Laird and Ware (1982), a vast amount of literature has developed that extends a range of model fitting techniques and applications (Diggle et al. 1994; McCulloch and Searle 2001; Fitzmaurice et al. 2004). These together provide a comprehensive description of methods for estimation and prediction of linear, generalized linear and nonlinear mixed-effects modeling.

Fig. 3 Nonlinear and
discrete paradigm

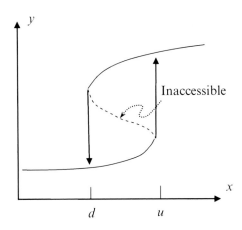

When the independent variable x declines from left to the right however, changes
in the dependent variabley y follow a different path. It declines gradually first also
following a nonlinear path; when x passes the threshold d (d for downward), y drops
suddenly with further declines in x resulting in not much change in y. We term this
as the *nonlinear discrete* (NLD) paradigm. If NLD data were analyzed using linear
regression method, the result would be "good", but the conclusion will be wrong.

Likewise, an NLD paradigm can be mathematically expressed as follows:

$$y = f_{nld}(x, u, d, c) \tag{3}$$

where x and y represent the independent and dependent variables, u and d are two
thresholds on x, c represents a set of covariates, and f_{nld} is a nonlinear and discrete
function characterize the relationship between x and y.

Up to date, no analytical method has been established in medical and health
research to simultaneously quantify a NLD relationship. Adaptation of the *bifurcation analysis* (Chitnis et al. 2006) to establish new statistical methods may represent
a promising approach to advance medical and health research. Bifurcation analysis
has been widely used in physics and engineering and has not been used in medical
and health research.

4 Quantum Paradigm and Cusp Modeling

Similar to the dual-characteristics of wave and particle of light ray, the dynamics of
many medical and health phenomenon may also contain a continuous component
and a discontinuous or quantum component. For example, the occurrence of a
disease (e.g., heart disease) contains (1) a continuous and accumulative exposure
to the disease-causing risk factors (e.g., fat and salt intake and lack of exercise)
and (2) a sudden process (e.g., a trigger, such as stress). Another example is the

process by which a smoker determines to quit smoking. He or she may make the decision based on (1) a careful assessment of the pros and cons of continuous smoking and quit and conclude that the pros are much greater than the cons if quit, or (2) simply quit "cold turkey" without effortful assessment, or simply decided after watching a movie on smoking and cancer, or mimic a role model who quit smoking. A conceptual framework that is capable of guiding new methodologies to characterize this type of change can be termed as *quantum* (Q) *paradigm*. Certainly a Q paradigm will be more close to the truth than any of the LC, NLC, and NLD paradigms introduced above to reflect the reality of a medical or health issues. More research effort is needed to develop this paradigm, including the establishment of analytical methodologies for use in medical and health research. Both authors of this chapter have collaborated since 2010 to work on this line of methodological research. Recently, they received 5 years of funding through a research grant (Awards #: R01HD075635, period: 2013–2018) from the National Institute of Health to establish a set of Quantum paradigm-based methodologies for health behavior research.

Along with the development of social and behavioral research, catastrophe modeling approach emerges. Catastrophe theory was established by Thom (1973, 1975) and Gilmore (1993) to describe complex phenomenon in science. According to Thom, many seemingly very complex systems in the universe, such as severe weather, earthquake, and social turmoil, is, in fact determined by a small number of factors. He termed these factors as control variables. According to the number of control variables and the complex of the relationship, seven elementary catastrophe models are developed, these models from simple to complex are (1) Fold (one control variable), (2) Cusp (two control variables), (3) Swallowtail (three control variables), (4) Butterfly (four control variables), (5) Hyperbolic Umbilic (three control variables), (6) Elliptic Umbilic (three control variables), and (7) Parabolic Umbilic (four control variables). The application of the catastrophe modeling methods in the physical science is well accepted, this method has not been widely used in medical health research. Readers who are interested in the catastrophe models can consult the related books.

Among the seven elementary catastrophe models described above, the cusp is more widely used in research probably due to the effort of a number of researchers, particularly Zeeman (Zeeman 1973, 1974, 1976), Guastello (Guastello 1982, 1989; Guastello et al. 2008, 2012), and others (Stewart and Peregoy 1983; Poston and Stewart 1996). Inspired and encouraged by the reported researches, the two authors of this chapter started to use the cusp modeling method in health and behavior research since 2009. In addition to application of the methods, the two authors also developed methods to determine sample size and statistical power for cusp catastrophe modeling (Chen et al. 2014a).

In the cusp catastrophe model, the dynamics of a disease or a health behavior z is presented as a function of two control factors (i.e., independent or predictor variables in statistical terminology) x and y as follows:

$$V(z, x, y) = \frac{1}{4}z^4 + \frac{1}{2}z^2 y + zx \qquad (4)$$

In the model, the variable x is termed as *asymmetry* and the variable y as *bifurcation*.

Figure 4 depicts the first derivative of the cusp model (Eq. 4). It is a curved equilibrium plane that determines the dynamic change in z along with change in x and y. The two control variables x and y form a control plane (see Fig. 5), governing the dynamics of the dependent variable z.

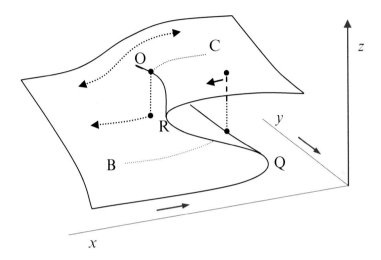

Fig. 4 An illustration of the cusp catastrophe model

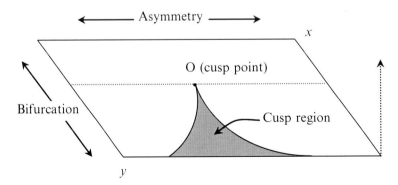

Fig. 5 Illustration of the control plane of cusp catastrophe (with reference to Fig. 4)

From Figs. 4 and 5, it can be seen that the cusp model contains two threshold lines O-Q (ascending) and O-R (descending), one continuous changing region (behind point O), two stable regions (bottom front and upper front) and one unstable region between O-Q and O-R. When a behavior z moves within the two stable regions, changes in either x and y results in little change in z; however, when z moves into the unstable region between O-Q and O-R, small changes in either x and/or y will result in phase change in z.

The three paths in Fig. 4 further illustrate how the cusp catastrophe model works. When the bifurcation variable $y < O$, Path A represents the linear and continuous relationship between x and z. This relationship is familiar with most researchers and can be adequately quantified with many conventional methods, including linear and nonlinear regression analyses. When $y > O$, the relationship between x and z can take two very different paths. Path B represents the process of sudden occurrence of a behavior. As x increases, z will experience little change; however, just as x passes O-Q, z will experience a sudden increase.

Likewise, Path C represents a relapse/recovery of a behavior with sudden change occurring along with the descending threshold O-R. In addition, in the unstable region, z can take two different values with opposite status at the same value of x and y. This phenomenon cannot be directly captured by the traditional continuous statistical approaches based on LC and NLC paradigms as shown in Figs. 1 and 2; however, it does reflect the NLD paradigm as shown in Fig. 3.

5   Do Current Research Need More Complex Analytical Paradigm?

Despite the widely acceptance of the LC and NLC paradigms, the large number of analytical and statistical methods guided by these two analytical paradigms, and great success of these methodologies in medical and health research, a further investigation of the research findings using these methodologies reveals obvious limitations. In most if not all reported etiological research, analytical models based linear and continuous (i.e., linear regression models) or nonlinear and continuous (i.e., logistic regression models) hypotheses can only explain a small proportion of the variance. This issue is much more significant in studies with focus on health related attitudes and behaviors. In such studies, a theory-guided linear model can only explain 15–25 % of the variance of a variable of interest in etiological research and a small to moderate effect in intervention trials (Godin and Kok 1996; Armitage and Conner 2001; Wu et al. 2005). The solid theoretical basis of these research studies and the high quality of data strongly suggest the limitations of the analytical paradigm.

Theoretically, from Figs. 1, 2, and 3 it can be seen what happens when a linear or a curve linear continuous method is used to analyze a phenomena that are nonlinear and discrete. Although these models may fit the data well if judged by the criteria for significant test established for the method, including the significance tests for the model parameters and R^2 for data-model fit. However, such models can hardly explain a large amount of variance because these linear and nonlinear continuous models only pick up a part of the underlying relationship between the predictor variables and the outcome variables, based on incorrect assumptions of linear/curve linear and continuous relationship. Therefore, findings from such analyses may also be misleading by presenting nonlinear and discrete relationships as linear/curve linear and continuous. Analytical methodology must consider these limitations and provide better analytical tools to the research community to advance medical and health research.

In addition to the theoretical analysis and empirical evidence regarding the limitations of the LC paradigm and NLC paradigm, reported studies reflecting the Quantum paradigm, particularly results from cusp catastrophic modeling analyses, provide additional data supporting the need for new and more complex analytical paradigm. A number of studies have used Q-paradigm based cusp modeling methods in medical and public health research to investigate fatigue (Guastello et al. 2012; Chen et al. 2014b), accident process (Guastello 1989), attitude change (Flay 1978; van der Maas et al. 2003), alcohol consumption and abuse (Clair 2004; Guastello et al. 2008; Smerz and Guastello 2008), substance use (Mazanov and Byrne 2006), tobacco use (Byrne 2001; Mazanov and Byrne 2006; Chen et al. 2012), smoking cessation (Mazanov and Byrne 2006; West and Sohal 2006), sexual risk behaviors (Chen et al. 2010a, 2013), and randomized controlled behavioral intervention trials (Chen et al. 2013). One characteristic common to these studies is that with exactly the same predictor variables, the data-model fit as measured by the amount of variance explained or R^2 varied from 0.4 to 0.9 for the Q-paradigm based models while the R^2 varied from <0.1 to 0.15 for linear models and from 0.15 to 2.2 for logistic regression models.

6 Polynomial Regression Approach

6.1 Introduction to the Polynomial Cusp Catastrophe Modeling

The lack of tools to solve the cusp model has prevented the application of the method in medical and health behavior research (Chen 1989). Solving the cusp model statistically as described by Eq. (4) is a challenge (Cobb and Ragade 1978; Guastello 1982). Through the effort of a group of scientist, a polynomial regression approach was established (Guastello 1982). This approach is to take the first derivative of Eq. (4) with regard to z:

$$\partial V / \partial z = z^3 + zy + x \tag{5}$$

Let x_1, y_1 and z_1 be the variables observed at time 1, and use the difference Δz of the observed values of the dependent variable z at two consecutive times as a numerical proxy of the derivative, and insert regression β coefficients to the related variables, re-arrange the term to obtain the following:

$$\Delta z = \beta_0 + \beta_1 z_1^3 + \beta_2 z_1^2 + \beta_3 y_1 z_1 + \beta_4 x_1 + \beta_5 y_1 \tag{6}$$

where $\Delta z = z_2 - z_1$, the differences in the outcome variable z measured at two consecutive time points. Additional terms (e.g., $\beta_2 z_1^2$, $\beta_4 x_1$ and $\beta_5 y_1$) are added to capture variations that may not be fully represented by the cusp model. With this specification, many statistical software packages with multiple regression can be used to evaluate this polynomial statistical cusp catastrophe model.

6.2 Assessment of the Polynomial Cusp Catastrophe Modeling Method

Two methods have been established to assess if the study variable follows a cusp catastrophe. Each method provides unique evidence.

6.2.1 Method 1: Significance of the Key Model Coefficients

According to the characteristics of cusp catastrophe (Cobb and Ragade 1978; Gilmore 1993), some statistical criteria have been established to assess if z is a cusp process (Guastello 1982). According to Guastello, if z follows cusp model, the following two conditions must be satisfied: (1) the coefficients β_1 must be statistically significant, and (2) either β_3 or β_4 must be statistically significant at $p < 0.05$ level.

6.2.2 Method 2: Assessment of Alternative Models

In this method, a number of models similar to the polynomial cusp model not containing the higher-orders of the outcome variable z are used to assess if the cusp model is superior to these alternative models (Guastello 1982; Chen et al. 2010a). Four alternative regression models are often used to model the same data. These four alternative models often take the following forms:

$$\Delta z = \beta_0 + \beta_1 z_1 + \beta_4 x_1 + \beta_5 y_1 \tag{7}$$

$$\Delta z = \beta_0 + \beta_1 z_1 + \beta_3 y_1 z_1 + \beta_4 x_1 + \beta_5 y_1 \tag{8}$$

$$z_2 = \beta_0 + \beta_1 z_1 + \beta_4 x_1 + \beta_5 y_1 \tag{9}$$

$$z_2 = \beta_0 + \beta_1 z_1 + \beta_3 y_1 z_1 + \beta_4 x_1 + \beta_5 y_1 \tag{10}$$

Among these four models, the first two are deferential linear regression models and the second two are pre-post linear regression models. The second and the fourth models contain an interaction term between y_1 and z_1, more close to the polynomial cusp model.

In modeling analysis, the R^2 of these alternative models and a cusp model are obtained and compared. If R^2 for the cusp model is greater than for the four alternative models, it will provide data supporting the superiority of the cusp model over the alternative models.

6.3   Procedure of Modeling Analysis

The following five steps are to be followed for polynomial cusp modeling analysis.

Step 1   Tabulation of the dependent variable to see if it shows a bimodal with two peaks. If not, cusp catastrophe model may not be relevant.

Step 2   Standardize all variables, including x, y, and x to create a new dataset. Making the standardization by subtracting the mean and then dividing by the standard deviation to create a set of new standardized x, y and z .

Step 3   Create new variables $z_1{}^3$, $z_1{}^2$, and yz_1 through simple arithmetic computing and add them into the dataset.

Step 4   Conduct regression analysis using the standardized and the newly created variables and the five linear equations from (6) to (10). In the modeling analysis, ask the program to output R^2 for all five models. These R^2 will be used later for comparison purposes to determine which model is superior than others in reporting results.

Step 5   Reporting

6.4   An Empirical Example

Data used in this example were derived from a randomized controlled trial conducted in the Bahamas to test a program in encourage HIV protective behaviors (e.g., use condom) and discourage HIV risk behaviors (e.g., engage in risky sex). A total of 1,360 middle school students from 15 government-run schools were randomized into three groups: the first group (n = 427) with only students receiving intervention, the second group (n = 436) with both students and their parents receiving intervention, and the third group (n = 497) receiving environmental conservation intervention as the intentional control. Among the total, 366 (85.7 %) participants in group one, 389 (89.2 %) in group two, and 417 (83.9) in group three participated in follow-up assessment 24 months post-intervention. The program showed significant effect at multiple follow-up assessments (Chen et al. 2009, 2010b; Gong et al. 2009). To assess factors associated with sexual initiation, we included only students who reported never engaged in sexual intercourse in a lifetime. To illustrate the polynomial cusp catastrophe approach, we used the following three key variables.

The dependent variable z *Sexual progression index* (SPI): This variable was assessed based on self-reported data. SPI was set to "1" for participants who reported never having had sexual intercourse and also claimed that they not likely to have sex in the next 6 months (e.g., responded "very unlikely" to the question "how likely is it you will have sex in the next 6 months"); SPI was set to "2" for participants who reported never having had sex but unsure if they were going to have sex in the next 6 months (e.g., responded "likely," "neutral," and "unlikely"); SPI was set to "3" for participants who never had sex and claimed that they were going to have sex in the next 6 months (e.g., responded "very likely"); and lastly SPI was set to "4" for participants who initiated sexual intercourse regardless of their planning to have sex in the future. We then $z_1 =$ SPI assessed at the baseline and $z_2 =$ SPI assessed at the 24-month post-intervention.

The asymmetry variable x_1: *Chronological age* (in years) at the baseline was used as the asymmetry variable. It is a common knowledge that as age increases, the likelihood to have sex increases.

The bifurcation variable y_1, the *perceived rewards from sex* (scores) at the baseline: This variable was used as the bifurcation variable. This variable was assessed using the question, "How would you feel if you were to have sex in the next six months?" Answer options to this question were "Very bad" (scored 1), "Somewhat bad" (scored 2), "Neither good nor bad" (scored 3), "Good" (scored 4), and "Very good" (scored 5).

After standardization of the four variables z_1, z_2, x_1, and y_1, four new variables were generated as delta $z = z_2 - z_1$; the squared term: $z_1^2 = z_1 \times z_1$; the cubic term $z_1^3 = z_1^2 \times z_1$; and the cross term $y_1 z_1 = y_1 \times z_1$. These four newly generated variables were used in analysis using Eqs. (6)–(10). Among the 1,360 subjects at baseline, data for 1,241 students were included; others 119 who reported ever had sexual intercourse at the baseline were excluded. The average age of the sample was 10.05 (SD = 0.7) with an age range of 9–12, and 47.0 % were boys.

Table 1 presents the results from the polynomial cusp catastrophe modeling (Eq. 6). The beta coefficients for the cubic term ($\beta = 0.1116$, $p = 0.000$) and the

Table 1 Results from polynomial cusp modeling of sexual initiation among Bahamian students, N = 1,240

Variables/terms	Beta coefficients	t-Value	p-Value
z_1^3: Cubic of SPI assessed at baseline	0.1116	6.00	0.000
z_1^2: Square of SPI assessed at baseline	−0.7319	12.10	0.000
$y z_1$: Cross-term	0.0824	1.80	0.073
y_1: Chronic age (years)	0.0613	1.20	0.231
x_1: Perceived rewards from having sex	0.2767	3.94	0.000
R^2: Proportions of variance explained	0.51	–	–

bifurcation term ($\beta = 0.2767$, $p = 0.000$) were both statistically highly significant, indicating that the sexual progression from no intention to have sex to actual sexual initiation follows the cusp model (with reference to Fig. 4). As age increases, the likelihood to initiate sex increases. The perceived reward from having sex serves as an influential factor to bifurcate the impact of age. When the level of perceived reward is low, the likelihood to initiate sex will be governed mainly by age. However, at the same age, if a student perceives the reward from having sex, he or she may start to engage in sex; if a student does not come to assess rewards from sex or perceived no rewards from having sex, this student may not initiate sex even though he or she may be at the age to initiate sex. At the bottom of the table, it can be seen that the R^2 of this model was 0.51, indicating that this simple two-predictor variable model can explain more than 50 % of the variance in sexual initiation.

Table 2 Comparison of the R^2 of the four alternative models with the cusp model

Model name	Expression	R^2
Polynomial cusp	$\Delta z = \beta_0 + \beta_1 z_1^3 + \beta_2 z_1^2 + \beta_3 y_1 z_1 + \beta_4 x_1 + \beta_5 y_1$	0.51
Differential linear model	$\Delta z = \beta_0 + \beta_1 z_1 + \beta_4 x_1 + \beta_5 y_1$	0.20
Differential linear model with interaction term	$\Delta z = \beta_0 + \beta_1 z_1 + \beta_3 y_1 z_1 + \beta_4 x_1 + \beta_5 y_1$	0.21
Pre-post model	$z_2 = \beta_0 + \beta_1 z_1 + \beta_4 x_1 + \beta_5 y_1$	0.14
Pre-post model with interaction	$z_2 = \beta_0 + \beta_1 z_1 + \beta_3 y_1 z_1 + \beta_4 x_1 + \beta_5 y_1$	0.14

Results in Table 2 indicate that with exact the same variables, the polynomial cusp model performed significantly better than the other four alternative models with regard to the amount of variances explained by a model.

6.5 Allocation of Contrail Variables as Asymmetry and Bifurcation

One unanswered question in cusp modeling analysis for medical and health behavior study among the potential control variables is: which should be tested as asymmetry and which as bifurcation? More research is needed to develop guidelines and standard regarding the variable selection (Guastello 1982; Stewart and Peregoy 1983; Chen et al. 2010a, 2013). The following are a couple of experience-based and commonly accepted rules.

Variables more likely to be modeled as asymmetry are those that are relatively stable and their development is gradual, their dynamic changes overtime are smooth, and they reflect primarily intra-personal characteristics. Typical examples include chronological age, knowledge, skills, hormone levels, cognitive function. Often the relationship between the asymmetry variable and the outcome variable is stable and robust without the impact of the bifurcation variable.

Bifurcation variables on the other hand, are rather volatile; they reflect either contextual factors or a perception of situational conditions, or emotion-related factors. One characteristic common to these variables is that they change more rapidly than the asymmetry variables. Typical examples include stress, peer pressure, self-efficacy, beliefs, and attitudes.

It is worth noting that the whether a variable is asymmetry or bifurcation is also relative. For example, in a study to investigate the role of inflammation and cognitive functioning on fatigue, a model with inflammation as asymmetry and the cognitive functioning as bifurcation fit the data well (Chen et al. 2014b). Here the cognitive function is also an intrapersonal factor that is relatively stable. However, it was used as a bifurcation. The reason for this selection is that relative to the process of inflammation, cognitive function is more volatile and less stable. Executive function is situational and can be affected also by emotions, while neuromuscular inflammation follows specific pathological processes.

7 Likelihood Approach with Stochastic Cusp Catastrophe Model

7.1 Introduction to the Likelihood Stochastic Approach

Although the polynomial approach introduced in the previous section is straight-forward and can be executed with many software packages that can be used for regression analysis, it needs longitudinal data. This has limited researchers to use the cusp catastrophic modeling method in research. In addition, the polynomial method allows the use of only one single variable to assess either the asymmetry or the bifurcation control variables, preventing researchers from exploring more complex research questions. To overcome these limitations, another approach, the stochastic likelihood estimation to test cusp catastrophe models has been established.

This approach was first explored since 1978 by a number of researchers, including Cobb et al. (Cobb and Ragade 1978; Cobb and Watson 1980; Cobb and Zacks 1985), Oliva et al. (1987) and Lange et al. (2000). This approach has been established taking the advantage of likelihood estimate in statistics. It has been achieved by taking the first derivative of Eq. (4) described in Sect. 4, and then adding a random Weiner process $W(t)$ with variance σ^2:

$$dz = \frac{\partial V(z, x, y)}{\partial z} dt + dW(t) \tag{11}$$

With this stochastic cusp model, the probability distribution of the dependent variable (z) under the equilibrium can be expressed as:

$$f(z) = \frac{\psi}{\sigma^2} exp\left[\frac{\alpha(z - \lambda) + \frac{1}{2}\beta(z - \lambda)^2 - \frac{1}{4}(z - \lambda)^4}{\sigma^2}\right] \tag{12}$$

where ψ is a normalizing constant and λ is to determine the origin of z.

Figure 6 illustrates the density distribution of the cusp model (Eq. 12). It is worth noting that at different regions of the x-y control plane, the density function of Eq. (12) takes different forms. (1) When the bifurcation variables y is above zero, the density distribution is bimodal with two peaks when x and y vary within the cusp region (the gray area); (2) in the rest of the control plane, the density function is unimodal with only one peak; and (3) the density distribution tends to be symmetrical toward the center where $x = 0$, skewed to the right when $x < 0$ and skewed to the left when $x > 0$.

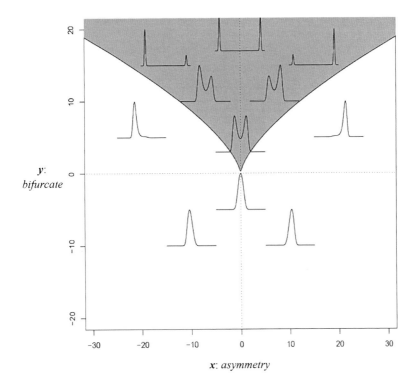

Fig. 6 Density distribution of a cusp catastrophe model at different regions of the x-y control plane

With density function of Eq. (12) of the stochastic cusp model, the theory of maximum likelihood can be employed for estimating parameters and statistical inference. For a study with n subjects, the following likelihood function can be established:

$$l\left(z, \alpha, \beta \middle| Z, X, Y\right) = \sum_{i=1}^{n} \log \psi_i - \sum_{i=1}^{n} \left(\alpha_i z_i + \frac{1}{2}\beta_i z_i^2 - \frac{1}{4}z_i^4\right) \quad (13)$$

With the likelihood function of Eq. (13), the model parameters can be estimated by applying the powerful likelihood theory when data are available from a randomly selected sample.

7.2 Advantages of the Likelihood Stochastic Cusp Modeling Approach

7.2.1 Modeling Cross-Sectional Data

The likelihood function of Eq. (13) in Sect. 7.1 above indicates that the likelihood stochastic cusp approach does not require longitudinal data. Instead of modeling changes as in the polynomial regression approach, the likelihood function only requires the measurement of the observed variables at a time point for all subjects in a study. This greatly increases the opportunity to apply the cusp catastrophe modeling method in medical and health research. Collecting cross-sectional data is much more cost-effective. In addition, a lot of existing data that are available for modeling analysis are cross-sectional in nature, including both medical (e.g., many datasets from clinical records) and health behavior research data (such as the National Health and Nutrition Examination Survey, the National Survey on Drug Use and Health, the National Health Interview Survey).

In addition to cross-sectional data, longitudinal models can also be tested by selecting the control variables x and y assessed at an earlier period to predict the outcome variable z at the subsequent times. This approach has also been used in reported studies to assess HIV risk behaviors and tobacco use among adolescents (Chen et al. 2010a, 2012, 2013).

7.2.2 Modeling More Than One Observed Variable

One limitation for the polynomial regression it described in Sect. 6 is that it only allows for one observed variable for each of the three model variables x, y, and z. With the specification of the stochastic model by Eq. (12), it removes this limitation of the polynomial regression approach. For example, in a study with n participants, researchers often measure more than one variable for each underlying (latent) constructs, such as cognitive functioning, self-efficacy, health literature, etc. Assume p's dependent variables Z_p, q's asymmetry variables X_q, and r's bifurcation variables Y_r are observed. Assuming a linear relationship between a group of observed variables and the corresponding latent construct, the following linear combinations for each of the three subconstructs can be used for stochastic cusp modeling:

$$z = w_0 + w_1 Z_1 + w_2 Z_2 + \cdots + w_p Z_p \qquad (14)$$

$$x = \alpha_0 + \alpha_1 X_1 + \alpha_2 X_2 + \cdots + \alpha_p X_q \qquad (15)$$

$$y = \beta_0 + \beta_1 Y_1 + \beta_2 Y_2 + \cdots + \alpha_r Y_r \qquad (16)$$

where X, Y, and Z are observed variables and w, α, β are model parameters to be estimated.

It is worth noting here that since x and y are specified independently, this will make it possible for researchers to test the same variable as both asymmetry and bifurcation variables simultaneously, which no previous methods are possible, including the methods by Cobb (Cobb and Watson 1980; Cobb and Zacks 1985) and Lange and Olivia (Lange et al. 2000).

7.3 The R-Based Cusp Package for Modeling Analysis

With the multivariate specification of a cusp model, the statistical solution becomes much more complex, as compared with the polynomial regression method as previously described in Sect. 6. Several researchers, including Oliva (Oliva et al. 1987), Lange and Oliva (Lange et al. 2000), and Cobb (Cobb and Ragade 1978; Cobb 1981; Cobb and Zacks 1985) have proposed and tested various statistical methods based on the likelihood theory with cross-sectional data and multivariate predictor variables. Assuming that only the two control variables are multivariates, Cobb has established a set of computing methods for parameter estimation (Cobb and Ragade 1978; Cobb 1981; Cobb and Zacks 1985). But no computing software was developed. Following Cobb's approach, Lange and Oliva (Lange et al. 2000) developed the software GEMCAT II and used in research (Lange et al. 2000, 2004). However, this method only allows for the two control variables to be multivariate.

Based on previous work (Flay 1978; Cobb and Watson 1980; Cobb 1981; Cobb et al. 1983; Cobb and Zacks 1985), Oliva (Oliva et al. 1987), and van der Mass et al. (2003), the R Package "Cusp" was developed and reported by Grassmen and colleagues (2009). In developing the software, the Broyden–Fletcher–Goldfarb–Shanno algorithm with bounds (Zhu et al. 1997) was used to minimize the likelihood function for optimal solution of the cusp model. The package is very efficient for modeling analysis. In addition to fitting the cusp catastrophe with data, this R-based cusp package contains a number of functions for modeling analysis, including utility functions to generate observations from the estimated cusp density, to evaluate the density and cumulative distribution function, to evaluate data-model fit, and to display the modeling results, including plots. Different from the polynomial regression method, there is no need for researchers to convert the data, the cusp package has the function to normalize the data using a QR decomposition approach before modeling analysis.

7.4 Assessment of Data-Model Fit

The data-model fit can be assessed in the following four aspects.

First, to draw conclusion that the dependent variable z is cusp, the estimated parameters for the α's and β's must be statistically significant at a pre-determined level of type I error.

Second, the negative log-likelihood value and chi-square test. The R-based cusp package produces outputs of the negative likelihood value and the associated likelihood-ratio Chi-square test. Statistically, models with smaller the negative log-likelihood values are better than those with larger values. The associated likelihood-ratio Chi-square test is defined as twice the difference of the negative log-likelihood values between the cusp and the comparison models (e.g., linear and nonlinear logistic regression models). Chi-square test with p-value <0.05 indicates that the cusp model is a better fit than a comparison model. Otherwise, it cannot be determined if the cusp model is a better fit than the comparison model.

Third, the alternative models and pseudo-R^2. To assess if cusp model is superior to other models, the R-based cusp package includes (1) linear multiple regression model and (2) nonlinear logistic regression models as alternatives. Given the multivariate nature of both the predictor and the outcome variables, the following logistic model is proposed for comparison purpose (Hartelman et al. 1998; van der Maas et al. 2003):

$$z_i = \left(1 + e^{\frac{-x_i}{y_i^2}}\right)^{-1} + e_i \tag{17}$$

Pseudo-R^2 is thus computed for the alternative models.
R^2 is conceptually defined as:

$$R^2 = 1 - \frac{Var(error)}{Var(z)} \tag{18}$$

However since the relationship between the predictors and the outcome variables is implicitly expressed in a cusp model, we cannot use the method as in linear regression models where the relationship between the predictor and the outcome variables is explicitly specified. Therefore the methods used to compute the variance of error for linear regression method cannot be used to determine the variance of error for cusp models. To estimate R^2 conceptually similar, the cusp package adapted two different methods to evaluate the variances: the *delay convention (with mode of the density closest to the cusp state plane as the expected value)* and the *Maxwell convention (with the mode at which the density is the highest as expected value)*. To distinguish the R^2 computed in linear regression, the R^2 in this cusp package is termed as pseudo-R^2. As usual, a larger R^2 indicates a better data-model fit.

Fourth, the Akaike Information Criterion *(AIC) (Akaike, 1974)* and Bayesian Information Criterion *(BIC) (Gelfand and Dey, 1994)* are computed for cusp models as well as the corresponding linear and logistic regression models. Statistically, a model with a small AIC or BIC indicates a better data-model fit.

7.5   Steps to Use R-Based Cusp Package

The R-based Cusp package is relatively easy to use, following the steps we described below.

Step 1: Prepare data and save it in .csv format for R modeling
You can prepare your data using any software, including excel sheet, SAS, SPSS, and name the variables as usual. After quality check, save the data into ".csv" format (also known as comma-separated values). CSV is one of the most commonly used data formats for R to read for analysis.

Step 2: Install R and the Cusp Package
R is a free software environment for statistical computing and graphics created through the Comprehensive R Achieve Network (CRAN) (http://www.r-project.org/). You can install the software on your computer by:

(1) Searching the web using the key phrase "download r," find the link, download and install R on your computer; or
(2) Go to the official website for R is: http://cran.r-project.org/.

   After the R is installed/or if your computer has R ready installed, then you can install the "Cusp Package" to your computer.

(1) Run R on your computer
(2) Click the tap "Package" on top of the screen "R Console," then click "install package," a list of countries/regions appear. Select one location near to your physical location by clicking on it. You will then see a long list of numerous statistical packages. Scroll down the list to locate the word "cusp," which is the name for the cusp analysis package.
(3) Click on "cusp." In a little while, this package will be automatically installed on your computer.

Step 3: Develop your R Codes for Analysis
The R codes include the following key components: (a) read in data; (b) specify the model, (c) instruct for modeling fitting, (d) output modeling results, (e) output for graphic results.

7.6   An Empirical Example

In the following example, we demonstrate how to conduct cusp catastrophe modeling with the likelihood estimation approach and cross-sectional data with a clinical example. Data for this example were obtained from the second wave of data on Survey of Midlife Development in the United States (MIDUS II), an on-going nationally representative longitudinal survey dataset. MIDUS II is the 10-year follow-up study of MIDUS I (a longitudinal study of physical and psychological health of adults in the United States). Among the 4,963 participants in MIDUS I, 75 % were retained at MIDUS II. Additional studies were included in MIDUS II, including the daily dairies to track stressors, the assessment of cognitive functioning, the collection of biomarkers and physical assessments, and the brain functioning assessments. A total of 935 subjects who participated in the cross-sectional assessment for cognition and biomarker study were included. Data used in this example have already been published (Chen et al. 2014b). The original data can be obtained free of charge from the Inter-University Consortium for Political and Social Research (ICPSR).

As an illustration, the grip strength was used as the outcome variable Z, the biomarker pro-inflammatory cytokine II-6 was used as the asymmetry variable X, and the executive functioning was used as the bifurcation variables Y. Inflammation is known to have degrading effects on bone and muscle mass. Such effects are thought to contribute to muscle weakness by accelerated protein loss and contractile dysfunction (Beyer et al. 2011). Since muscle strength often relies on brain control, especially the cognitive operation on executive function, it may interact with levels of inflammation as indicated by IL-6, to explain individuals' differences in grip strength (MacDonald et al. 2011).

Variable X: IL-6 was measured using Quantikine® high-sensitivity enzyme linked immunosorbent assay kits (R&D Systems, Minneapolis, MN). The laboratory intra-assay coefficient of variance was 13 % for IL-6. Grip strength was assessed using a handheld dynamometer. The average of three trials in the dominant hand was used for modeling analysis.

Variable Y: The executive functioning was measured using five tests: working memory span (Digits Backward); verbal fluency (Category Fluency); inductive reasoning (Number Series); processing speed (Backward Counting) from the Brief Test of Adult Cognition by Telephone (BTACT); attention switching and inhibitory control from the Stop and Go Switch Task (SGST). An average of z-scores for all tests was used as a composite score (Lachman et al. 2011) and used in modeling analysis.

Variable Z: Grip strength was measured with a handheld dynamometer. The average of three trials in the dominant hand was used for analysis

Step 1: Data preparation

In this section, all the texts with font Arial are R codes that can be directly used for analysis. The text with "#" indicates descriptive text and the rest are executable R codes.

For simplicity, we assume that the obtained data are manually entered into computer, and then save as: "data4cusp.csv" on drive C with the path "C:\cusp\data\". Three variables in the data4cusp.csv are: gripstrength (scores ranging from 1 to 10), cytokine (a proxy of inflammation), and cognition (scale scores assessing executive functioning)

Step 2: Read data into R and obtain basic statistics of the data

```
## read in saved data set into R dataset,
#   rename it as "datcusp"
# header = "T" indicating the first raw of the data
#   contains variable names
# na.strangs = "." indicating the blank space is
# used  for missing data
datcusp = read.csv("C:\cusp\data\data4cusp.csv",
   header="T", na.strings = ".")
## check data
# list variables in the dataset datcusp
names (datcusp)
#compute basic statistics of all variables in the
data summary (datcusp)
```

Step 3: Prepare a dataset "datcusp" for modeling

In actual data analysis, researchers may have a larger number of variables included in the csv dataset. After reading in data in step 2 above, these variables will all be available in the computer for analysis. R package has a data function for researchers to select specific variables from the long list of variables for modeling with the following data.frame statement:

```
datmodel = data.frame (z = datcusp$fatigue,
   y= datcusp$cognition, x= datcusp$cytokine)
```

Step 4: Modeling analysis

The following R statement will conduct cusp modeling analysis using the dataset "datmodel" created in the previous step. y z is equivalent to Eq. (14): $z = w_0 + w_1$ *gripstrength*; likewise, x is equivalent to Eq. (15) and beta y is equivalent to Eq. (16).

```
# fit cusp model
fit < - cusp (y ~ z, alpha ~ x, beta ~y,
   data = datmodel)
```

Step 5: Modeling results

Result from the cusp catastrophe modeling can be obtained by calling the following summary statements from the cusp package. The first one gives the general results, and the second one produces results of alternative models for comparison, including results from logistic regression models.

```
# cusp modeling results that can be formatted
for better presentation
summary (fit)
```

Table 3 Comparison of the cusp catastrophe modeling with multiple linear regression modeling and nonlinear logistic regression modeling

Model	Model coefficients		Data-model fit			
	Cytokine	Cognition	−log likelihood	R^2	AIC	BIC
Cusp	−0.1349 (<0.001)	−0.1599 (0.013)	1,145.84	0.7918	2,303	2,332
Linear	1.0481 (0.020)	2.3129 (<0.001)	3,408.94	0.0543	6,825	6,845
Logistic	−0.0573 (<0.001)	−0.1153 (0.003)	3,408.11	0.0559	6,826	2,332

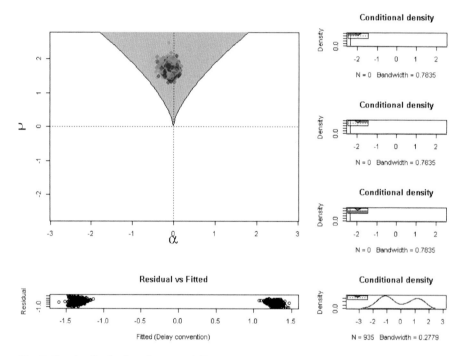

Fig. 7 Density distribution of cusp modeling

Table 3 summarizes the results from the cusp modeling analysis. First of all, the model coefficients for cusp were all statistically significant. Second, among the three models, the −log likelihood and the AIC were the smallest and the R^2 was the largest for the cusp model. Evidence from these results suggests that the grip strength follows a cusp process. However, since the BIC was the same for both cusp and logistic regression model and the model coefficients are also pointed to the same direction; this evidence suggests that if we do not consider variances explained by a model, logistic regression may also provide an approach to assess factors related to grip strengths.

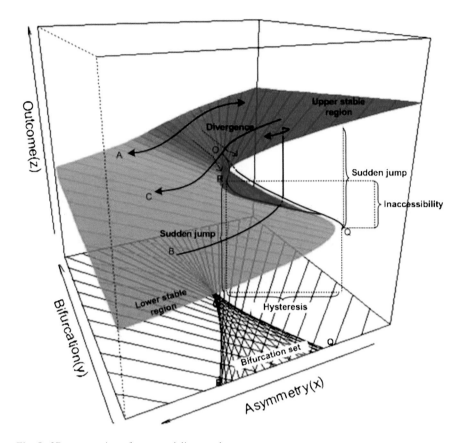

Fig. 8 3D presentation of cusp modeling result

Step 6. Graphic presentation.

Graphic presentation can be obtained using the following statements, including 2-D description of the density function (Fig. 7) and 3-D presentation (Fig. 8) of the cusp equilibrium plane.

```
# general 2-D graphic presentation
Plot (fit)
# advanced 3-D graphic presentation
Cusp3d(fit)
```

7.7   Additional Notes

7.7.1   Modeling Analysis

In the previous section, we demonstrated step by step the procedure to conduct cusp modeling using the R package. For those who are not familiar with R, as an exercise, you can type in these codes one at a time to learn how to conduct the modeling analysis. For experienced researchers, you can compile your R codes and save them as script file, and execute them. This script file also serves as a records of your modeling analysis.

7.7.2   Results Interpretation

Since cusp modeling analysis is still in its early stage, it is likely that you may find strange results. For example, you may find a very good data-model fit, but the results may not be consistent with the graphic presentation. We are investigating these inconsistencies in the funded project.

References

Armitage, C.J., Conner, M.: Efficacy of the theory of planned behaviour: a meta-analytic review. Br. J. Soc. Psychol. **40**(Pt 4), 471–499 (2001)

Barnes, R.D., Blomquist, K.K., et al.: Exploring pretreatment weight trajectories in obese patients with binge eating disorder. Compr. Psychiatry **52**(3), 312–318 (2011)

Beyer, I., Bautmans, I., et al.: Effects on muscle performance of NSAID treatment with piroxicam versus placebo in geriatric patients with acute infection-induced inflammation. A double blind randomized controlled trial. BMC Musculoskelet. Disord. **12**, 292 (2011)

Byrne, D.G.: A cusp catastrophe analysis of changes to adolescent smoking behaviour in response to smoking prevention programs. Nonlinear Dynamics Psychol. Life Sci. **5**, 115–137 (2001)

Chen, X., Brogan, K.: Developmental trajectories of overweight and obesity of US youth through the life course of adolescence to young adulthood. Adolesc. Health Med. Ther. **3**, 33–42 (2012)

Chen, X., Jacques-Tiura, A.J.: Smoking initiation associated with specific periods in the life course from birth to young adulthood: data from the National Longitudinal Survey of Youth 1997. Am. J. Public Health **104**(2), e119–e126 (2014)

Chen, X.: [Xin Wei Yi Xue] Behavioral Medicine. Shanghai Scientific Publication House, Shanghai (1989)

Chen, X., Lunn, S., et al.: A cluster randomized controlled trial of an adolescent HIV prevention program among Bahamian youth: effect at 12 months post-intervention. AIDS Behav. **13**(3), 499–508 (2009)

Chen, X., Lunn, S., et al.: Modeling early sexual initiation among young adolescents using quantum and continuous behavior change methods: implications for HIV prevention. Nonlinear Dynamics Psychol. Life Sci. **14**(4), 491–509 (2010a)

Chen, X., Stanton, B., et al.: Effects on condom use of an HIV prevention programme 36 months postintervention: a cluster randomized controlled trial among Bahamian youth. Int. J. STD AIDS **21**(9), 622–630 (2010b)

Chen, X., Gong, J., et al.: Cusp catastrophe modeling of cigarette smoking among vocational high school students. Conference Paper on the 140th American Public Health Association Meeting (2012)

Chen, X., Stanton, B., et al.: Intention to use condom, cusp modeling, and evaluation of an HIV prevention intervention trial. Nonlinear Dynamics Psychol. Life Sci. **17**(3), 385–403 (2013)

Chen, D., Chen, X., et al.: Cusp catastrophe polynomial model: power and sample size. Open J. Stat. **4**(4), 803–813 (2014a)

Chen, D.G., Lin, F., et al.: Cusp catastrophe model: a nonlinear model for health outcomes in nursing research. Nurs. Res. **63**(3), 211–220 (2014b)

Chitnis, M., Cushing, J.M., et al.: Bifurcation analysis of a mathematical model for malaria transmission. J. SIAM Appl. Math. **67**(1), 24–45 (2006)

Clair, S.: A cusp catastrophe model for adolescent alcohol use: an empirical test. Nonlinear Dynamics Psychol. Life Sci. **2**(3), 217–241 (2004)

Cobb, L.: Stochastic differential equations for social sciences. In: Cobb, L., Thrall, R.M. (eds.) Mathematical Frontiers of the Social and Policy Sciences. Westview Press, Boulder (1981)

Cobb, L., Ragade, R.K.: Applications of catastrophe theory in the behavioral and life sciences. Behav. Sci. **23**, 291–419 (1978)

Cobb, L., Watson, B.: Statistical catastrophe theory: an overview. Math. Model. **1**(4), 311–317 (1980)

Cobb, L., Zacks, S.: Applications of catastrophe theory for statistical modeling in the biosciences. J. Am. Stat. Assoc. **80**(392), 793–802 (1985)

Cobb, L., Koppstein, P., et al.: Estimation and moment recursion relations for multimodal distributions of the exponential family. J. Am. Stat. Assoc. **78**(381), 124–130 (1983)

Flay, B.R.: Catastrophe theory in social psychology: some applications to attitudes and social behavior. Behav. Sci. **23**(5), 335–350 (1978)

Gilmore, R.: Catastrophe Theory for Scientists and Engineers. Dover Publications, New York (1993)

Godin, G., Kok, G.: The theory of planned behavior: a review of its applications to health-related behaviors. Am. J. Health Promot. **11**(2), 87–98 (1996)

Gong, J., Stanton, B., et al.: Effects through 24 months of an HIV/AIDS prevention intervention program based on protection motivation theory among preadolescents in the Bahamas. Pediatrics **123**(5), e917–e928 (2009)

Grasman, R.P., Mass, H.J., et al.: Fitting the cusp catastrophe in R: a cusp package primer. J. Stat. Softw. **32**(8), 1–27 (2009)

Guastello, S.J.: Moderator regression and the cusp catastrophe: an application of two-stage personal selection, training, therapy and policy evaluation. Behav. Sci. **27**, 259–272 (1982)

Guastello, S.J.: Catastrophe modeling of the accident processes: evaluation of an accident reduction program using the occupational hazards survey. Accid. Anal. **21**, 17–28 (1989)

Guastello, S.J., Aruka, Y., et al.: Cross-cultural generalizability of a cusp catastrophe model for binge drinking among college students. Nonlinear Dynamics Psychol. Life Sci. **12**(4), 397–407 (2008)

Guastello, S.J., Boeh, H., et al.: Cusp catastrophe models for cognitive workload and fatigue in a verbally cued pictorial memory task. Hum. Factors **54**(5), 811–825 (2012)

Hartelman, P.A., et al.: Detecting and modelling developmental transitions. Br. J. Dev. Psychol. **16**, 97–122 (1998)

Jones, B.L., Nagin, D.S.: Advances in group-based trajectory modeling and an SAS procedure for estimating them. Sociol. Methods Res. **35**(4), 542–571 (2007)

Lachman, M.E., Agrigoroaei, S., et al.: Frequent cognitive activity compensates for education differences in episodic memory. Am. J. Geriatr. Psychiatry **18**(1), 4–10 (2011)

Lange, R., Oliva, T.A., et al.: An algorithm for estimating multivariate catastrophe models: GEMCAT II. Stud. Nonlinear Dyn. Econ. **4**(3), 137–168 (2000)

Lange, R., McDade, S.R., et al.: The estimation of a cusp model to describe the adoption of word for windows. J. Prod. Innov. Manag. **21**(1), 15–32 (2004)

MacDonald, S.W., DeCarlo, C.A., et al.: Linking biological and cognitive aging: toward improving characterizations of developmental time. J. Gerontol. B Psychol. Sci. Soc. Sci. **66**(Suppl. 1), i59–i70 (2011)

Mazanov, J., Byrne, D.G.: A cusp catastrophe model analysis of changes in adolescent substance use: assessment of behavioural intention as a bifurcation variable. Nonlinear Dynamics Psychol. Life Sci. **10**(4), 445–470 (2006)

Muthen, B., Muthen, L.K.: Integrating person-centered and variable-centered analyses: growth mixture modeling with latent trajectory classes. Alcohol. Clin. Exp. Res. **24**(6), 882–891 (2000)

Nagin, D.S.: Group-Based Modeling of Development. Harvard University Press, Cambridge (2005)

Oliva, T.A., Desarbo, W.S., et al.: GEMCAT – a general multivariate methodology for estimating catastrophe models. Behav. Sci. **32**(2), 121–137 (1987)

Poston, T., Stewart, I.N.: Catastrophe Theory and Its Applications. Dover, New York (1996)

Smerz, K.E., Guastello, S.J.: Cusp catastrophe model for binge drinking in a college population. Nonlinear Dynamics Psychol. Life Sci. **12**(2), 205–224 (2008)

Stewart, I.N., Peregoy, P.L.: Catastrophe theory modeling in psychology. Psychol. Bull. **94**(2), 336–362 (1983)

Thom, R.: Structural Stability and Morphogenesis: Essai D'une Theorie Generale Des Modeles. W. A. Benjamin, California (1973)

Thom, R.: Structural Stability and Morphogenesis. Benjamin-Addison-Wesley, New York (1975)

van der Maas, H.L., Kolstein, R., et al.: Sudden transitions in attitudes. Sociol. Methods Res. **23**(2), 125–152 (2003)

West, R., Sohal, T.: "Catastrophic" pathways to smoking cessation: findings from national survey. BMJ **332**(7539), 458–460 (2006)

Wong, E.S., Wang, B.C., et al.: BMI trajectories among the severely obese: results from an electronic medical record population. Obesity (Silver Spring) **20**(10), 2107–2112 (2012)

Wu, Y., Stanton, B.F., et al.: Protection motivation theory and adolescent drug trafficking: relationship between health motivation and longitudinal risk involvement. J. Pediatr. Psychol. **30**(2), 127–137 (2005)

Zeeman, E.: Catastrophe theory in brain modelling. Int. J. Neurosci. **6**, 39–41 (1973)

Zeeman, E.: On the unstable behavior of the stock exchanges. J. Math. Econ. **1**, 39–44 (1974)

Zeeman, E.C.: Catastrophe theory. Scientific American. **234**(4), 65–83 (1976).

Zhu, C., Byrd, R., et al.: L-BFGS-B: Fortran subroutines for large-scale bound constrained optimization. ACM Trans. Math. Softw. **23**(4), 550–560 (1997)

On Ranked Set Sampling Variation and Its Applications to Public Health Research

Hani Samawi and Robert Vogel

Abstract The foundation of any statistical inference depends on the collection of required data through some formal mechanism that should be able to capture the distinct characteristics of the population. One of the most common mechanisms to obtain such data is the simple random sample (SRS). In practice, a more structured sampling mechanism, such as stratified sampling, cluster sampling or systematic sampling, may be obtained to achieve a representative sample of the population of interest. A cost effective alternative approach to the aforementioned sampling techniques is the ranked set sampling (RSS). This approach to data collection was first proposed by McIntyre (Aust. J. Agr. Res. 3:385–390, 1952) as a method to improve the precision of estimated pasture yield. In RSS the desired information is obtained from a small fraction of the available units.

Keywords Ranked set sample (RSS) • Extreme ranked set sample (ERSS) • Median ranked set sample (MRSS) • Simple random sample (SRS) • Simulation • Naive estimator • Regression estimator • Ratio estimator • Normal data • Concomitant variable • Varied set size ranked set sampling (VSRSS) • Bilirubin • Quantiles • Bivariate ranked set sampling (BVRSS) • Clinical trials

1 Introduction

In many agricultural and environmental studies and recently in human populations, quantification of a sampling unit can be more costly than the physical acquisition of the unit. For example, the level of bilirubin in the blood of infants can be ranked

H. Samawi (✉)
Department of Biostatistics, Jiann-Ping Hsu College of Public Health, Georgia Southern University, Hendricks Hall, Room 1006, Statesboro, GA 30460, USA
e-mail: hsamawi@georgiasouthern.edu

R. Vogel (✉)
Department of Biostatistics, Jiann-Ping Hsu College of Public Health, Georgia Southern University, Hendricks Hall, Room 1013, Statesboro, GA 30460, USA
e-mail: rvogel@georgiasouthern.edu

© Springer International Publishing Switzerland 2015
D.-G. Chen, J. Wilson (eds.), *Innovative Statistical Methods for Public Health Data*,
ICSA Book Series in Statistics, DOI 10.1007/978-3-319-18536-1_13

visually by observing Color of the face, Color of the chest, Color of lower part of the body, and Color of terminal parts of the whole body. Then, as the yellowing goes from face to terminal parts, the level of bilirubin in the blood increases (Nelson et al. 1992; Samawi and Al-Sageer 2001).

In some circumstances, considerable cost savings can be achieved if the number of measured sampling units is only small fraction of the number of available units but all units contribute to the information content of the measured units. Ranked set sampling (RSS) is a method of sampling that can achieve this goal. RSS was first introduced by McIntyre (1952). The use of RSS is highly powerful and superior to the standard simple random sampling (SRS) for estimating some of the population parameters. The RSS procedure can be obtained by selecting r random sets each of size r from the target population. In most practical situations, the size r will be 2, 3, or 4. Rank each set by a suitable method of ranking, such as prior information or visual inspection. In sampling notation, let X_{ij} denote the jth observation in the ith set and $X_{i(j)}$ is the jth ordered statistic in the ith set. $X_{1(1)}, X_{2(2)}, \ldots, X_{r(r)}$ are quantified by obtaining the element with the smallest rank from the first set, the second smallest from the second set, and so on until the largest unit from the rth set is measured, then this represents one cycle of RSS. We can repeat the whole procedure m times to get an RSS of size $n = mr$.

A variety of extreme ranked set sample (ERSS) procedures have been introduced and investigated by Samawi et al. (1996) to estimate the population mean. Similar to RSS, in ERSS, we only quantify the minimum and the maximum ranked observation. In the case of symmetric populations, Samawi et al. (1996) showed that the ERSS procedure gives an unbiased estimate of the population mean and it is more efficient than the SRS mean, using the same number of quantified units. Recently, ERSS applied to genetics for quantitative trait loci (QTL) mapping (see Chen 2007). He indicated that since the frequency of the Q allele, in the general population, is small therefore, instead of drawing a simple random sample (SRS) from the population, one of the approaches adopted for detecting QTL using population data is to truncate the population at a certain quantile of the distribution of Y and take a random sample from the truncated portion and a random sample from the whole population. The two samples drawn are genotyped and compared on the number of Q-alleles. Then if a significant difference exists, the candidate QTL is claimed as a true QTL (see Slatkin 1999; Xu et al. 1999; Chen 2007). However, this approach needs a large number of individuals have to be screened before a sample can be taken from the truncated portion and hence it is not practical. Alternatively, the ERSS can be used as follows: Individuals are taken in sets and the individuals within each set are ranked according to their trait values. The one with the largest trait value is put into an upper sample and the one with the smallest trait value is put into a lower sample. Then the two samples obtained this way are then genotyped and compared. Also, ERSS approach has been applied for linkage disequilibrium mapping of QTL recently by Chen et al. (2005).

The ERSS has been applied to a sib-pair regression model where extremely concordant and/or discordant sib-pairs are selected by the ERSS (see Zheng et al. 2006). As indicated by Chen (2007), the ERSS approach can be applied also to many other genetic problems such as the transmission disequilibrium test (TDT) (Spielman et al. 1993) and the gamete competition model (Sinsheimer et al. 2000).

Another variation of RSS is the median ranked set sampling (MRSS) investigated by Muttlak (1997). The ratio estimator using RSS is investigated by Samawi and Muttlak (1996). The ratio estimator is used to obtain increased precision for estimating the population mean or total by taking the advantage of the correlation between an auxiliary variable X and the variable of interest Y. Samawi and Muttlak (2001) used MRSS in ratio estimation. They showed that MRSS gives approximately an unbiased estimate of a population ratio in case of symmetric populations and it is more efficient than SRS, using the same number of quantified units. Moreover, Al-Saleh and AL-Kadiri (2000) showed that the efficiency in estimating the populations mean can be improved even more by using a double ranked set sampling technique (DRSS). Samawi (2002) suggested a double extreme ranked set sampling (DERSS) for the mean and ratio estimators. Additional information about RSS and its application can be found in Kaur et al. (1995) and Patil et al. (1999).

Stratified RSS was introduced by Samawi (1996) and used to improve ratio estimation by Samawi and Siam (2003). A varied set size RSS (VSRSS) has been introduced and investigated by Samawi (2011) for estimating a population means and ratios. This approach can be useful in queuing and epidemiology studies where cases come in different size batches.

Research in multiple characteristics estimation has been performed by Patil et al. (1993, 1994) and Norris et al. (1995). They used a bivariate ranked set sampling (BVRSS) procedure ranking on only one of the characteristics (X or Y). However, BVRSS, ranking on both characteristics (X or Y), was introduced by Al-Saleh and Zheng (2002). They indicated that BVRSS procedure could easily be extended to a multivariate one. The performance of BVRSS in comparison with RSS and SRS for estimating the population means, using ratio and regression estimators, is considered by Samawi and Al-Saleh (2007).

Another attempted application of RSS is in treatment comparison experiments including some clinical trials. In RSS, many more sampling units are sampled and discarded than those eventually fully measured. This might not be desirable in the situation where sampling units are not easy to obtain, which is especially the case in clinical trials. Ozturk and MacEachern (2004) and Zheng et al. (2006) separately considered an RSS approach which generates RSSs for each treatment but without discarding any sampling units (see Chen 2007). The approach as described by Zheng et al. (2006) is as follows: Assume that the response variable (Y) is correlated with a common concomitant variable (X). Let the set size k in RSS be even. The RSS is carried out two sets at a time. That is, each time two random sets of experimental units are taken and ranked separately according to the values of X. For the first ranked set, units with odd ranks are assigned to treatment 1 and units with even ranks are assigned to treatment 2. For the second ranked set, units with odd ranks are assigned to treatment 2 and units with even ranks are assigned to treatment 1. This process produces two correlated general RSS samples, each for each treatment. It does not discard any experimental units. It is shown in Zheng et al. (2006) that this method of treatment assignment is much more efficient than a simple random assignment. They have applied the above method retrospectively to a well-known randomized double-blind multi-center clinical trial called ACTG 320 to compare the effects of the three-drug combination of IDV+ZDV+3TC and the two-drug combination of ZDV+3TC on an AIDS-defining event. They use the RSS protocol with r = 4 is applied (see Chen 2007).

2 RSS for a Univariate Population

The RSS procedure can be obtained by selecting r random sets each of size r from the target population. In most practical situations, the size r will be 2, 3, or 4. Rank each set by a suitable method of ranking, such as prior information, visual inspection or by an experimenter himself. In sampling notation, let X_{ij} denote the jth observation in the ith set and $X_{i(j)}$ is the jth ordered statistic in the ith set. If only $X_{1(1)}, X_{2(2)}, \ldots, X_{r(r)}$ quantified by obtaining the element with the smallest rank from the first set, the second smallest from the second set, and so on until the largest unit from the rth set is measured, then this represents one cycle of RSS. We can repeat the whole procedure m times to get an RSS of size $n = mr$.

2.1 Naive Estimation for the Population Mean

Let X_{ij} denote the jth observation in the ith set and $X_{i(j)}$ is the jth ordered statistic in the ith Let $\{X_{1(1)k}, X_{2(2)k}, \ldots, X_{r(r)k}; k = 1, 2, \ldots, m\}$ be the quantified RSS of size $n = mr$. Under RSS scheme, the sample mean $\overline{X}_{RSS} = \frac{1}{rm} \sum_{i=1}^{r} \sum_{k=1}^{m} X_{(i)k}$ is an unbiased estimator of the population mean (μ) and

$$Var\left(\overline{X}_{RSS}\right) = \frac{\sigma^2}{n} - \frac{1}{mr^2} \sum_{i=1}^{r} \left(\mu_{(i)} - \mu\right)^2, \tag{1}$$

where $\mu_{(i)} = E\left(X_{(i)}\right)$, and σ^2 is the population variance of X. See Takahasi and Wakimoto (1968).

2.2 Quantiles and Distribution Function Estimation

For $0 < p < 1$, the population pth quantile is defined as $\xi_p = \inf\{x : F(x) \geq p\}$ and is denoted by $F^{-1}(p)$. Suppose $X_1, X_2, \ldots, X_n$ is an SRS of size n from a population. Then for a given t, $F(t)$ can be estimated by

$$\hat{F}(t) = \frac{1}{n} \sum_{i=1}^{n} I\,(X_i \le t),\tag{2}$$

where $I(.)$ is an indicator function. Clearly, $E\left(\hat{F}(t)\right) = F(x)$ and var $\left(\hat{F}(t)\right) = \frac{1}{n}F(t)\,(1 - F(t))$.

Let $X_{(1)}, X_{(2)}, \ldots, X_{(n)}$ be the order statistics of an SRS of size n. Then ξ_p can be estimated by the sample pth quantile which is defined as follows:

$$\hat{\xi}_p = \begin{cases} X_{(np)}, & \text{if } np \text{ is an integer} \\ X_{([np]+1)}, & \text{if } np \text{ is not an integer} \end{cases}\tag{3}$$

see Serfling (1980). Under some mild conditions about $F(t)$, Bahadur (1966) showed that $\sqrt{n}\left(\hat{\xi}_p - \xi_p\right)$ converges in distribution to $N\left(0, \frac{p(1-p)}{f^2(\xi_p)}\right)$.

Now, let $X_{(1)k}, X_{(2)k}, \ldots, X_{(r)k}$, $k = 1, 2, \ldots, m$ be an RSS of size $n = ms$ from $F(x)$. Then for fixed t, Stokes and Sager (1988) defined the empirical cdf of the RSS by

$$F*(t) = \frac{1}{n} \sum_{i=1}^{r} \sum_{k=1}^{m} I\left(X_{(i)k} \le t\right)\tag{4}$$

with variance

$$\text{var}\,(F*(t)) = \frac{1}{n}\left\{F(t) - \sum_{i=1}^{r}[I_{F(t)}\,(i, r - i + 1)]^2/r\right\},\tag{5}$$

where $I_{F(t)}\,(i, r - i + 1)$ is the incomplete Beta function. Also, if $f_{(i)}(x)$, $i = 1, 2, \ldots, r$, is positive in a neighborhood of ξ_p and is continuous at ξ_p, Samawi (2001) and Chen (2000) showed that $\sqrt{n}\left(\tilde{\xi}_p - \xi_p\right)$ converge in distribution to

$$N\left(0, \frac{p - \sum_{i=1}^{r}[I_{p(i,r-i+1)}]^2/r}{f^2(\xi_p)}\right), \text{ where } \tilde{\xi}_p \text{ is the sample quantile based on the RSS.}$$

Samawi (2001) showed that the relative efficiency of using RSS relative to SRS, by estimation of the quantiles for different values of p, ranging from 1.05 to 1.77 for $r = 3$ and the efficiency increases asset size r increases. As an application to quantiles estimation using RSS Samawi (2001) illustrated the method by using the data from Iowa 65+ Rural Health Study. He found the normal ranges ($p = 0.05$ and $p = 0.95$) of hemoglobin level in the blood of the women aged 70+ were disease free.

2.3   Ratio Estimation

The ratio estimator is used to improve precision of estimating the population mean of a variable of interest (Y) using some concomitant variable (X). Let (X,Y) have the c.d.f. F(x, y) with mean μ_x and μ_y, variances σ_x^2 and σ_y^2 correlation coefficient ρ, then $R = \frac{\mu_y}{\mu_x}$ denotes the ratio of means. Using a simple bivariate random sample from F(x, y), the estimator of R is given by:

$\hat{R}_{SRS} = \frac{\overline{Y}}{\overline{X}}$, where $\overline{X}$ and $\overline{Y}$ are the sample means of X and Y, respectively.

Hansen et al. (1953) showed that the variance of $\hat{R}_{SRS}$ can be approximated by:

$$\text{Var}\left(\hat{R}_{SRS}\right) \cong \frac{R^2}{n}\left(V_x^2 + V_y^2 - 2\rho V_x V_y\right),\tag{6}$$

where $V_x = \frac{\sigma_x}{\mu_x}$, $V_y = \frac{\sigma_y}{\mu_y}$, and $\rho = \frac{E\left[(X-\mu_x)(Y-\mu_y)\right]}{\sigma_x \sigma_y}$.

The ratio estimator using RSS data, if ranking is on the variable X, with errors in ranking for the variable Y is given by Samawi and Muttlak (1996) as $\hat{R}_{RSS} = \frac{\overline{Y}_{[r]}}{\overline{X}_{(r)}}$,

where $\overline{Y}_{[r]} = \frac{1}{n}\sum_{k=1}^{m}\sum_{i=1}^{r} Y_{i[i]k}$ and $\overline{X}_{(r)} = \frac{1}{n}\sum_{k=1}^{m}\sum_{i=1}^{r} X_{i(i)k}$ are the sample means using RSS and n = mr. Note that, () denotes perfect ranking while [] denotes ranking with error. Also, they showed that the approximate variance of $\hat{R}_{RSS}$ is given by:

$$\text{Var}\left(\hat{R}_{RSS1}\right) \cong \frac{R^2}{n}\left\{\left(V_x^2 + V_y^2 - 2\rho V_x V_y\right) - \frac{1}{r}\left[\sum_{i=1}^{r}\left(M_{x(i)} - M_{y[i]}\right)^2\right]\right\},\tag{7}$$

where $M_{x(i)} = \frac{\mu_{x(i)}-\mu_x}{\mu_x}$ and $M_{y[i]} = \frac{\mu_{y[i]}-\mu_y}{\mu_y}$.

Moreover, Samawi and Muttlak (1996) show that if ranking on X is perfect and ranking on Y is with error in the ranking, then this ratio estimator is more efficient than when ranking on Y is perfect and ranking on X is with error in the ranking. They showed that the relative efficiency of using RSS relative to SRS for estimating the ratio (population mean using the ratio estimate), when ranking on X, ranges from 1.62 to 1.88 for r = 3 and the efficiency increases as r increases.

2.4   Regression Estimation for the Population Mean

As in ratio estimation, the linear regression estimator is used to increase the precision of estimating the population mean by using extra information in an auxiliary variable X that is correlated with Y. When the relation is approximately linear, and the line does not go through the origin, an estimate of the population mean based on the linear regression of Y on X is suggested rather than using the ratio of the two variables. Regression estimators using SRS and RSS are investigated by Sukhatme and Sukhatme (1970) and Yu and Lam (1997), respectively.

Let (X_i, Y_i), $i = 1,2,\ldots,n$, be a bivariate sample from $F(x, y)$, and

$$Y_i = \mu_y + \beta (X_i - \mu_x) + \varepsilon_i \tag{8}$$

where μ_x and μ_y are the means of X and Y, respectively, and for fixed X_i, ε_i, $i = 1,2,\ldots,n$ are i.i.d. with mean zero and variance σ_ε^2.

When μ_x is unknown, the method of double sampling can be used to obtain an estimate of μ_x. This involves drawing of a large random sample of size n', which is used to estimate μ_x. Then a sub-sample of size n is selected from the original selected units to study the primary characteristic of Y. Set $n' = r^3m$ and $n = r$ $(rm) = r^2m$, when the first and the second-phase samples are both conducted by SRS scheme. Then the double-sampling regression estimator $\overline{Y}_{ds}$ is given by

$$\overline{Y}_{ds} = \overline{Y}_{SRS} + \widehat{\beta} \left(\overline{X}' - \overline{X}_{SRS} \right), \tag{9}$$

where $\overline{X}_{SRS} = \frac{1}{n}\sum X_i$, $\overline{Y}_{SRS} = \frac{1}{n}\sum Y_i$, $\overline{X}'$ is the sample mean of X based on r^3m observations from the first phase and

$$\widehat{\beta} = \frac{\sum (X_i - \overline{X}_{SRS}) (Y_i - \overline{Y}_{SRS})}{\sum (X_i - \overline{X}_{SRS})^2}.$$

When the underlying distribution of (X, Y) is assumed to be bivariate normal, then the regression estimator (Sukhatme and Sukhatme 1970) $\overline{Y}_{ds}$ is an unbiased estimator for μ_y and its variance is given by

$$Var \left(\overline{Y}_{ds} \right) = \frac{\sigma_\varepsilon^2}{n} \left(1 + \frac{r-1}{r(n-3)} \right) + \frac{1}{rm} \rho^2 \sigma_y^2. \tag{10}$$

If the assumption of the linear relationship in (8) is invalid, then the SRS regression estimator in (9) is in general a biased estimator for μ_y.

Using the bivariate RSS, ranking only on X, assume that the relationship between $Y_{[i]k}$ and $X_{(i)k}$ is

$$Y_{[i]k} = \mu_y + \beta \left(X_{(i)k} - \mu_x \right) + \varepsilon_{[i]k}, \tag{11}$$

$i = 1,2,\ldots,r$ and $k = 1,2,\ldots,rm$. Again, when μ_x is unknown the method of double sampling (two-phase sampling) can be used to obtain an estimate of μ_x. Set $n' = r^3m$ and $n = r$ $(rm) = r^2m$, and when the first-phase sampling is an SRS and the second-phase sampling is an RSS. Then the double-sampling regression estimator $\overline{Y}_{Rds}$ based on RSS is given by Yu and Lam (1997) as:

$$\overline{Y}_{Rds} = \overline{Y}_{RSS} + \widehat{\beta}_{RSS}\left(\overline{X}' - \overline{X}_{RSS}\right), \tag{12}$$

where $\overline{X}' = \frac{1}{n'}\sum_{i=1}^{n'} X_i$ is the sample mean of X based on the r^3m observations

of the first phase, $\overline{X}_{RSS} = \frac{1}{n}\sum_{k=1}^{rm}\sum_{i=1}^{r} X_{(i)k}$, $\overline{Y}_{RSS} = \frac{1}{n}\sum_{k=1}^{rm}\sum_{i=1}^{r} Y_{[i]k}$ and $\widehat{\beta}_{RSS} =$

$$\frac{\sum_{k=1}^{rm}\sum_{i=1}^{r}\left(X_{(i)k} - \overline{X}_{RSS}\right)\left(Y_{[i]k} - \overline{Y}_{RSS}\right)}{\sum_{k=1}^{rm}\sum_{i=1}^{r}\left(X_{(i)k} - \overline{X}_{RSS}\right)^2}.$$

By using the basic properties of conditional moments, Yu and Lam (1997) showed that, under (12), $\overline{Y}_{Rds}$ is an unbiased estimator of μ_y and the variance is given by:

$$Var\left(\overline{Y}_{Rds}\right) = \frac{\sigma_\varepsilon^2}{n}\left(1 + E\left[\frac{\left(\overline{Z}_{RSS} - \overline{Z}\right)^2}{S_{zR}^2}\right]\right) + \frac{1}{rn}\rho^2\sigma_y^2, \tag{13}$$

where $\overline{Z} = \frac{\overline{X}' - \mu_x}{\sigma_x}$, $Z_{(i)k} = \frac{X_{(i)k} - \mu_x}{\sigma_x}$, $\overline{Z}_{RSS} = \frac{1}{n}\sum_{k=1}^{rm}\sum_{i=1}^{r} Z_{(i)k}$, $S_{zR}^2 = \frac{1}{n}\sum_{k}\sum_{i}\left(Z_{(i)k} - \overline{Z}_{RSS}\right)^2$ and $n = r^2m$.

Moreover, if the assumption of linear relationship is invalid, the RSS regression estimator in (12) is in general a biased estimator for μ_y.

3 Varied Set Size RSS

The varied set size ranked set sample (VSRSS) is investigated by Samawi (2011). The VSRSS is obtained by randomly selecting c sets of different sizes, respectively, say, $\{k_1^2, k_2^2, \ldots, k_c^2\}$. Apply the scheme of RSS on each set separately to obtain c RSSs of sizes $\{k_1, k_2, \ldots, k_c\}$ respectively. This will produce a VSRSS of size $n = \sum_{l=1}^{c} k_l$. Then $\{X_{1(1):k_1}, \ldots, X_{k_1(k_1):k_1}; X_{1(1):k_2}, \ldots, X_{k_2(k_2):k_2}; \ldots; X_{1(1):k_c}, \ldots, X_{k_c(k_c):k_c}\}$ denotes by VSRSS. Note that $X_{j(j)k_l}$ is the jth order statistics of the jth sample of the lth set, $l = 1, 2, \ldots, c$. Let X have a probability density function (p.d.f.), $f(x)$, and a cumulative distribution function (c.d.f.), $F(x)$, with mean μ and variance σ^2. Let $X_{(j):s}$ denotes the jth order statistic from a sample of size s. Furthermore, let $\mu_{(j):s} = E\left(X_{(j):s}\right)$, $\sigma_{(j):s}^2 = Var\left(X_{(j):s}\right)$ and $f_{(j):s}(x)$ and $F_{(j):s}(x)$ are the p.d.f. and c.d.f. of $X_{(j):s}$, respectively.

Theorem 1 (Samawi 2011) Let X have a probability density function (p.d.f.), $f(x)$, and a cumulative distribution function (c.d.f.), $F(x)$, with mean μ and variance σ^2, then:

(1)

$$\sum_{i=1}^{c}\sum_{j=1}^{k_i} f_{(j):k_i}(x) = f(x)\sum_{i=1}^{c} k_i, \tag{14}$$

where $f_{(j):k_i}(x) = \frac{k_i!}{(j-1)!(k_i-j)!}[F(x)]^{j-1}[1-F(x)]^{k_i-j}f(x)$.

(2)

$$\sum_{i=1}^{c}\sum_{j=1}^{k_i} F_{(j):k_i}(x) = F(x)\sum_{i=1}^{c} k_i. \tag{15}$$

(3)

$$\sum_{i=1}^{c}\sum_{j=1}^{k_i} \mu_{(j):k_i} = \mu\sum_{i=1}^{c} k_i. \tag{16}$$

(4)

$$\sum_{i=1}^{c}\sum_{j=1}^{k_i} \sigma^2_{(j):k_i} = \sigma^2\sum_{i=1}^{c} k_i - \sum_{i=1}^{c}\sum_{j=1}^{k_i} \left(\mu_{(j):k_i} - \mu\right)^2 \tag{17}$$

3.1 Naive Estimator of Population Means Using VSRSS

Using VSRSS scheme, a population mean μ can be estimated by: $\overline{X}_{VSRSS} = \frac{1}{n}\sum_{i=1}^{c}\sum_{j=1}^{k_i} X_{j(j):k_i}$, where $n = \sum_{i=1}^{c} k_i$. Also, using the SRS, $X_1, X_2, \ldots, X_n$, the sample mean denoted by: $\overline{X}_{SRS} = \frac{1}{n}\sum_{i=1}^{n} X_i$. Note that $E\left(\overline{X}_{SRS}\right) = \mu$ and $Var\left(\overline{X}_{SRS}\right) = \frac{\sigma^2}{n}$.

Theorem 2 (Samawi 2011). Under VSRSS scheme

1. $\overline{X}_{VSRSS}$ is an unbiased estimator of μ.
2.

$$Var\left(\overline{X}_{VSRSS}\right) = \frac{\sigma^2}{n} - \frac{1}{n^2}\sum_{i=1}^{c}\sum_{j=1}^{k_i} \left(\mu_{(j):k_i} - \mu\right)^2; \ n = \sum_{i=1}^{c} k_i. \tag{18}$$

Theorem 3 Samawi (2011)

$$Var\left(\overline{X}_{VSRSS}\right) \leq Var\left(\overline{X}_{SRS}\right)$$

Special case when $c = r$ and $k_i = i$, $i = 1, 2, \ldots, r$. Then $n = \frac{r(r+1)}{2}$.

The performance of the estimators is investigated for different set sizes and $c = 3$, and 4.

Samawi (2011) showed that VSRSS is more efficient than SRS for estimating the population mean, for all of the proposed cases and distributions. Also, in some cases VSRSS is more efficient than the RSS. However, VSRSS is more practical than RSS in some situations when equal set size of RSS cannot be obtained.

3.2 Ratio Estimation

Let the ranking be performed on the variable X. Let () denote perfect ranking while [] denote ranking with error. We assume ranking on X is perfect while ranking on Y is with error. Let

$$\left\{ \left(X_{1(1):k_1}, Y_{1[1]k_1}\right), \ldots, \left(X_{k_1(k_1):k_1}, Y_{k_1[k_1]:k_1}\right) ; \left(X_{1(1):k_2}, Y_{1[1]k_2}\right), \ldots, \left(X_{k_2(k_2):k_2}, \right.\right.$$
$$\left.\left. Y_{k_2[k_2]:k_2}\right) ; \ldots ; \left(X_{1(1):k_c}, Y_{1[1]k_c}\right), \ldots, \left(X_{k_c(k_c):k_c}, Y_{k_c[k_c]:k_c}\right) \right\}$$

be the VSRSS, where $X_{j(j)k_i}$ is the jth smallest X unit in the jth bivariate RSS of set size k_i and $Y_{j[j]k_i}$ is the jth corresponding Y observation, $i = 1, 2, \ldots, c$.

Let $\hat{\mu}_x = \overline{X}_{(VSRSS)}$ and $\hat{\mu}_y = \overline{Y}_{[VSRSS]}$, where $\overline{X}_{(VSRSS)} = \frac{1}{n}\sum_{i=1}^{c}\sum_{j=1}^{k_i} X_{j(j)k_i}$,

$\overline{Y}_{[VSRSS]} = \frac{1}{n}\sum_{i=1}^{c}\sum_{j=1}^{k_i} Y_{j[j]k_i}$ and $n = \sum_{i=1}^{c} k_i$. Also, let $\sigma_x^2 = Var(X)$, $\sigma_y^2 = Var(Y)$,

$\sigma_{x(j):k_i}^2 = Var\left(X_{j(j)k_i}\right)$, $\sigma_{y[j]:k_i}^2 = Var\left(Y_{j[j]k_i}\right)$ and $\sigma_{x(j)y[j]:k_i} = Cov\left(X_{j(j):k_i}, Y_{j[j]:k_i}\right)$.

The estimator of the population ratio R using VSRSS is given by

$$\hat{R}_{VSRSS} = \frac{\overline{Y}_{[VSRSS]}}{\overline{X}_{(VSRSS)}}. \tag{19}$$

Assume that the population is large enough so that the sample fraction $\frac{n}{N}$ is negligible. Then by using a Taylor series expansion, $\hat{R}_{VSRSS}$ the variance of $\hat{R}_{VSRSS}$ can be approximated by:For large population size

$$Var\left(\hat{R}_{VSRSS}\right) \cong \frac{R^2}{n}\left[V_x^2 + V_y^2 - 2\rho\,V_x V_y - \frac{1}{n}\left[\sum_{i=1}^{c}\sum_{j=1}^{k_i}\left(M_{x(j):k_i} - M_{y[j]:k_i}\right)^2\right]\right],$$

(20)

where $M_{x(j):k_i} = \frac{(\mu_{x(j):k_i} - \mu_x)}{\mu_x}$, $M_{y[j]:k_i} = \frac{(\mu_{y[j]:k_i} - \mu_y)}{\mu_y}$, $M_{x(j):k_i}M_{y[j]:k_i} = \frac{(\mu_{x(j):k_i} - \mu_x)(\mu_{y[j]:k_i} - \mu_{[y]})}{\mu_x\mu_y}$, $V_x = \frac{\sigma_x}{\mu_x}$, $V_y = \frac{\sigma_y}{\mu_y}$ and ρ is the correlation coefficient between X and Y.

Samawi (2011) showed that using VSRSS for estimating the ratio is more efficient than using SRS for the same size. This will result in large savings in sample size and hence in time and money. Furthermore, he showed by simulation that negative values of ρ give higher efficiencies than the positive values of ρ in most of the cases.

Samawi (2011) illustrated the use of VSRSS on date palm tree in Oman. In the illustration he indicated that date palm is considered the most important fruit crop in the Sultanate of Oman and occupying nearly 50 % of the cultivated land in Oman. It is estimated that 35,000 ha of land are planted with date palms and 28,000 ha with other crops, including 11,000 ha planted with rotation crops. These statistics reflect the importance of date palm tree to the Omani people who have lived with this tree for centuries. The date palm has retained its value for the dwellers of the desert because of its adaptive characteristics to the environment and the wide range of its benefits. It provides the family with many of life's necessities.

Different literature at different times has cited variable estimation of the number of palm trees and yield quantity. The total number of date palm trees currently is estimated to be around seven million with a wide range of varieties. FAO (1982) report indicated that the estimated annual production of Omani dates was 50,000 tons and the number of date palm trees was 1 million for the period 1961–1978. Currently the numbers of date palm trees are estimated to be higher than before due to the introduction of new and easier production practices along with a new cultivar, which has increased the large scale farming of date palms. The number has now risen to seven million trees. Due to the variety of different types of palm trees in each farm, we use VSRSS in one of the farms in Muscat (capital of Oman) area to produce an efficient sample to estimate the total amount of date that farms could produce in 2003. The total number of farms in Oman is about 9,476 in 2003. We used the naive estimator of mean and the ratio estimation procedure using VSRSS. The ranking was performed on the height of those palm trees. The data set consists of (Y) the amount of date, in kilograms, the palm tree produces and the height (X), in meters, of the tree. Table 1 consists of the selected samples. Table 2 contains all the proposed estimators. The total number of tree in that farm is 250 and the total height of all the trees is 800 m.

The total production of dates, per farm, using naive SRS estimator is 22,650 kg and using VSRSS naive estimator is 25,250 kg. However, using SRS ratio estimate of the total is 22,416 kg, while using VSRSS ratio estimator is 25,968 kg. The total production of dates in Oman can be estimated by using VSRS as 239,269 tons and

Table 1 Oman palm trees data (2003)

Type of the tree	VSRSS sample (2,3,2,2,1,2,1,2), n = 15		SRS sample, n = 15	
	Height (X m)	Amount of date (Y kg)	Height (X m)	Amount of date (Y kg)
Khalas	0.50	30.00	2.00	65.00
Khalas	6.00	204.00	3.64	99.00
Khosab	1.20	72.00	1.200	40.00
Khosab	5.00	132.00	5.60	150.00
Khosab	6.00	195.00	5.30	130.00
Hilali	5.50	200.00	0.40	65.00
Hilali	1.85	4.50	1.85	4.50
Khunaizi	1.00	52.00	1.75	85.00
Khunaizi	3.00	60.00	4.00	52.00
Jibreen	3.33	120.00	8.00	240
Fardh	0.50	42.00	1.15	14.00
Fardh	1.50	36.00	1.50	36.00
Kharmah	5.00	156.00	5.30	187.00
Tabaq	0.50	72.00	1.00	52.50
Tabaq	5.80	140.00	5.80	140.00

Table 2 Results of estimating μ_x, μ_y and R using SRS and VSRSS (standard deviations)

Sample	Estimator		
	Naive mean of X	Naive mean of $Y(\overline{Y})$	Ratio estimator $\hat{R}$
SRS	3.23 (2.31)	90.70(66.70)	28.08
VSRSS	3.11 (2.23)	101.00(67.00)	32.48

by using SRS as 214631.4 tons. However, as in William et al. (2004) was 238,600. This indicates that using VSRSS is more accurate than using SRS in this case.

4 Stratified Ranked Set Sample

Stratified simple random sampling (SSRS) is used in certain types of surveys because it combines the conceptual simplicity of SRS with potentially significant gains in efficiency. It is a convenient technique to use whenever we wish to ensure that our sample is representative of the population and also to obtain separate estimates for parameters of each strata of the population. In this section we introduce the concept of stratified ranked set sample (SRSS) for estimating the population mean. SRSS combines the advantages of stratification and RSS to obtain an unbiased estimator for the population mean, with potentially significant gains in efficiency.

An SSRS (for example, see Hansen et al. 1953) is a sampling plan in which a population is divided into L mutually exclusive and exhaustive strata, and an SRS of n_h elements is taken and quantified within each stratum h. The sampling is performed independently across the strata. In essence, we can think of an SSRS scheme as one consisting of L separate simple random samples.

An SRSS is a sampling plan in which a population is divided into L mutually exclusive and exhaustive strata, and an RSS of n_h elements is quantified within each stratum, $h = 1, 2, \ldots, L$. The sampling is performed independently across the strata. Therefore, we can think of an SRSS scheme as a collection of L separate ranked set samples.

Suppose that the population is divided into L mutually exclusive and exhaustive strata. Let $X_{h11}^*, X_{h12}^*, \ldots, X_{h1n_h}^*; X_{h21}^*, X_{h22}^*, \ldots, X_{h2n_h}^*; \ldots; X_{hn_h1}^*, X_{hn_h2}^*, \ldots, X_{hn_hn_h}^*$ be n_h independent random samples of size n_h each one is taken from each stratum $(h = 1, 2, \ldots, L)$. Assume that each element X_{hij}^* in the sample has the same distribution function $F_h(x)$ and density function $f_h(x)$ with mean μ_h and variance σ_h^2. For simplicity of notation, we will assume that X_{hij} denotes the quantitative measure of the unit X_{hij}^*. Then, according to our description $X_{h11}, X_{h21}, \ldots, X_{hn_h1}$ could be considered as the SRS from the h-th stratum. Let $X_{hi(1)}^*, X_{hi(2)}^*, \ldots, X_{hi(n_h)}^*$ be the ordered statistics of the i-th sample $X_{hi1}^*, X_{hi2}^*, \ldots, X_{hin_k}^*$ $(i = 1, 2, \ldots. n_k)$ taken from the h-th stratum. Then, $X_{h1(1)}, X_{h1(2)}, \ldots, X_{hn_h(n_h)}$ denotes the RSS for the h-th stratum. If $N_1, N_2, \ldots, N_L$ represent the number of sampling units within respective strata, and $n_1, n_2, \ldots, n_L$ represent the number of sampling units measured within each stratum, then $N = \sum_{h=1}^{L} N_h$ will be the total population size, and $n = \sum_{h=1}^{L} n_h$ will be the total sample size.

The following notations and results will be used throughout this section. For all $i, i = 1, 2, \ldots, n_h$ and $h = 1, 2, \ldots, L$, let $\mu_h = E\left(X_{hij}\right), \sigma_h^2 = Var\left(X_{hij}\right), \mu_{h(i)} = E\left(X_{hi(i)}\right), \sigma_{h(i)}^2 = Var\left(X_{hi(i)}\right)$, for all $j = 1, 2, \ldots, n_h$ and let $T_{h(i)} = \mu_{h(i)} - \mu_h$.

As in Dell and Clutter (1972), one can show easily that for a particular stratum $h, (1 = 1, 2, \ldots, L), f_h(x) = \frac{1}{n_h} \sum_{i=1}^{n_h} f_{h(i)}(x)$, and hence $\sum_{i=1}^{n_h} \mu_{h(i)} = n_h \mu_h, \sum_{i=1}^{n_h} T_{h(i)} = 0$ and $\sum_{i=1}^{n_h} \sigma_{h(i)}^2 = n_h \sigma_h^2 - \sum_{i=1}^{n_h} T_{h(i)}^2$.

The mean μ of the variable X for the entire population is given by

$$\mu = \frac{1}{N} \sum_{h=1}^{L} N_h \mu_h = \sum_{h=1}^{L} W_h \mu_h \qquad (21)$$

where $W_h = \frac{N_h}{N}$.

If within a particular stratum, h, we supposed to have selected SRS of n_h elements from N_h elements in the stratum and each sample element is measured with respect to some variable X, then the estimate of the mean μ_h using SRS of size n_h is given by

$$\overline{X}_h = \frac{1}{n_h} \sum_{i=1}^{n_h} X_{hi1}. \tag{22}$$

The mean and variance of $\overline{X}_h$ are known to be $E\left(\overline{X}_h\right) = \mu_h$ and $Var\left(\overline{X}_h\right) = \frac{\sigma_h^2}{n_h}$, respectively, assuming N_h's are large enough. The estimate of the population mean μ using SSRS of size n is defined by

$$\overline{X}_{SSRS} = \frac{1}{N} \sum_{h=1}^{L} N_h \overline{X}_h = \sum_{h=1}^{L} W_h \overline{X}_h \tag{23}$$

The mean and the variance of $\overline{X}_{SSRS}$ are known to be $E\left(\overline{X}_{SSRS}\right) = \mu$ and

$$Var\left(\overline{X}_{SSRS}\right) = \sum_{h=1}^{L} W_h^2 \left(\frac{\sigma_h^2}{n_h}\right) \tag{24}$$

respectively, assuming N_h's are large enough.

If within a particular stratum h, we supposed to have selected RSS of n_h elements from N_h elements in the stratum and each sample element is measured with respect to some variable X, then the estimate of the mean μ_h using RSS of size μ_h is given by

$$\overline{X}_h = \frac{1}{n_h} \sum_{i=1}^{n_h} X_{hi(i)} \tag{25}$$

It can be shown that the mean and variance of $\overline{X}_{h(n_h)}$ are $E\left(\overline{X}_{h(n_h)}\right) = \mu_h$ and

$$Var\left(\overline{X}_{h(n_h)}\right) = \frac{\sigma_h^2}{n_h} - \frac{1}{n_h^2} \sum_{i=1}^{n_h} T_{h(i)}^2, \tag{26}$$

respectively, assuming N_h's are large enough. Therefore, the estimate of the population mean μ using SRSS of size n is defined by

$$\overline{X}_{SRSS} = \frac{1}{N} \sum_{h=1}^{L} N_h \overline{X}_{h(n_h)} = \sum_{h=1}^{L} W_h \overline{X}_{h(n_h)}. \tag{27}$$

Algebraically, it can be shown that the mean and the variance of $\overline{X}_{SRSS}$ are $E\left(\overline{X}_{SRSS}\right) = \mu$ (i.e., and unbiased estimator) and

$$Var\left(\overline{X}_{SRSS}\right) = \sum_{h=1}^{L} W_h^2 \left(\frac{\sigma_h^2}{n_h} - \frac{1}{n_h^2} \sum_{i=1}^{n_h} T_{h(i)}^2\right), \tag{28}$$

	SRS	RSS		SSRS	SRSS
Table 3 Body mass index samples of diabetic women aged 80–85 years with and without urinary incontinence	18.88	18.88	Stratum 1	23.45	23.45
	19.76	22.88	28.95	23.46	
	20.57	23.45	30.17	30.10	
	25.66	24.38	Stratum 2	19.61	19.61
	26.01	26.30	24.07	24.38	
	28.95	27.31	27.49	31.31	
	33.52	36.65		33.52	31.95
Estimated mean	24.77	25.69		26.95	26.15
Standard error	2.03	2.06		1.72	1.67

respectively, assuming N_h's are large enough. Samawi (1996) showed that using SRSS for estimating the population mean is more efficient than using SSRS. As an illustration to this method Samawi (1996) used Iowa 65+ Rural Health Study. In Table 3 he presented three samples of size 7 each, from baseline interview data for the (RHS), which is a longitudinal cohort study of 3,673 individuals (1,420 men arid 2,253 women) ages 65 or older living in Washington and Iowa countries of the State of Iowa in 1982. In the Iowa 65+ RHS there were 33 diabetic women aged 80–85, of whom 14 reported urinary incontinence. The question of interest is to estimate the mean body mass index (BMI) of diabetic women. BMI may be different for diabetic women with or without urinary incontinence. Thus, here is a situation where stratification might work well. The 33 women were divided into two strata, the first consists of those women without urinary incontinence and the second consists of those 14 women with urinary incontinence. Four samples of size ($n = 7$) each were drawn from those women using SSRS, SRSS, RSS, and SRS. Note that in case of SRSS and RSS the selecting samples are drawn with replacement. The calculated values of BMI are given in Table 2. These calculations indicate the same pattern of conclusions that were obtained earlier, and illustrate the method described in Sect. 2.

The BMI data are a good example where we need stratification to find an unbiased estimator for the population mean of those diabetic women aged 80–85 years. Since the 33 women were divided into two strata, the first consists of those women without urinary incontinence and the second consists of those women with urinary incontinence. It is clear that the mean of the BMI in each stratum will be different. Also, there is potential that women can be ranked visually according to their BMI. In this situation using SRSS to estimate the mean BMI is recommended of those women. SRSS will give an unbiased and more efficient estimate of the BMI mean. Moreover, SRSS can provide an unbiased and more efficient estimate for the mean of each stratum.

5   Bivariate Population

Samawi and Muttlak (1996) used a modification of the RSS procedure in case of
bivariate distributions to estimate a population ratio. The procedure is described as
follows:

First choose r^2 independent bivariate elements from a population that has a
bivariate distribution function F(x, y) with parameters μ_x, μ_y, σ_x^2, σ_y^2 and correlation
coefficient ρ. Rank each set with respect to one of the variables Y or X. Suppose
ranking is on variable X. Then divide the elements into r sets. From the first set
obtain the element with the smallest rank of X, together with the associated value
of the variable Y. From the second set obtain the second smallest element of X,
together with the associated value of the variable Y. The procedure is continued
until the element with the largest ranking observation of X is measured from the rth
set. The whole procedure can be repeated m times to get a bivariate RSS sample of
size n = mr ranking only on one variable. In Sampling notation $\{(X_{i(i)k}, Y_{i[i]k}), i = 1,$
2, ..., r; k = 1,2, ...,m} will denote the bivariate RSS. However, ranking on both
variables X and Y is introduced by Al-Saleh and Zheng (2002). Based on Al-Saleh
and Zheng (2002) description, a BVRSS can be obtained as follows: Suppose *(X, Y)*
is a bivariate random vector with the joint probability density function (p.d.f.) *f(x, y)*.

Step 1. A random sample of size r^4 is identified from the population and randomly
allocated into r^2 pools of size r^2 each so that each pool is a square matrix with r
rows and r columns.

Step 2. In the first pool, rank each set (row) by a suitable method of ranking with
respect to (w.r.t.) the first characteristics (X). Then from each row identify the
unit with the smallest rank w.r.t. X.

Step 3. Rank the r minima obtained in Step 2, in a similar manner but w.r.t. the
second characteristic (Y). Then identify and measure the unit with the smallest
rank w.r.t. Y. This pair of measurements (x, y), which is resembled by the label
(1, 1), is the first element of the BVRSS sample.

Step 4. Repeat Steps 2 and 3 for the second pool, but in Step 3, the pair that
corresponds to the second smallest rank w.r.t. the second characteristic (Y) is
chosen for actual measurement (quantification). This pair resembled by the label
(1, 2).

Step 5. The process continues until the label (r, r) is resembled from the r^2th (last)
pool.

The above procedure produces a BVRSS of size r^2. The procedure can be
repeated *m* times to obtain a sample of size $n = mr^2$. In sampling notation,
assume that a random sample of size mr^4 is identified (no measurements
were taken) from a bivariate probability density function, say *f(x, y); (x, y)*
$\in$ R^2, with means μ_x and μ_y, variances σ_x^2 and σ_y^2 and correlation coefficient
ρ. Following the Al-Saleh and Zheng (2002) definition of BVRSS, then
$$\left[\left(X_{[i](j)k}, Y_{(i)[j]k}\right), i = 1, 2, \ldots, r; \ j = 1, 2, \ldots, r; \ and \ k = 1, 2, \ldots, m\right]$$

denotes the BVRSS. Now, let $f_{X_{[i](j)}, Y_{(i)[j]}}(x, y)$ be the joint p.d.f. of $\left(X_{[i](j)\,k}, Y_{(i)[j]k} \right)$, $k = 1, 2, \ldots, m$. Al-Saleh and Zheng (2002), with $m = 1$, showed that

(1) $\frac{1}{r^2} \sum\limits_{j=1}^{r} \sum\limits_{i=1}^{r} f_{[i](j),\, (i)[j]}(x, y) = f(x, y)$,

(2) $\frac{1}{r^2} \sum\limits_{j=1}^{r} \sum\limits_{i=1}^{r} f_{X_{[i](j)}}(x) = f_X(x)$, and

(3) $\frac{1}{r^2} \sum\limits_{j=1}^{r} \sum\limits_{i=1}^{r} f_{Y_{(i)[j]}}(y) = f_Y(y)$.

5.1   Ratio Estimators

It is common in practice to estimate the ratio of two means of two correlated variables, says X and Y, where both X and Y vary from one unit to another. For example, in a household survey, the average expenditure on cosmetics per an adult female could be estimated. Example of this kind occurs frequently when the sampling unit (the household) comprises a group or a cluster of elements and the interest is in the population mean per element. Moreover, a ratio estimator is used to obtain increased precision of estimating the population mean or total by taking advantage of the correlation between an auxiliary variable X and the variable of interest Y.

Now let the bivariate random variable (X, Y) has c.d.f. $F(x, y)$ with means μ_x and μ_y, variances σ_x^2 and σ_y^2, and correlation coefficient ρ, then $R = \frac{\mu_y}{\mu_x}$ will denote the population ratio. Using the notations of Sect. 2, assume that the BVRSS $[(X_{[i](j)k}, Y_{(i)[j]k}), k = 1, 2, \ldots, m; i, j = 1, 2, \ldots, r]$ is measured. Let $\overline{X}_{BVRSS} = \frac{1}{r^2 m} \sum\limits_{i=1}^{r} \sum\limits_{j=1}^{r} \sum\limits_{k=1}^{m} X_{[i](j)k}$, and $\overline{Y}_{BVRSS} = \frac{1}{r^2 m} \sum\limits_{i=1}^{r} \sum\limits_{j=1}^{r} \sum\limits_{k=1}^{m} Y_{(i)[j]k}$, then the population ratio R can be estimated, using BVRSS, by

$$\widehat{R}_{BVRSS} = \frac{\overline{Y}_{BVRSS}}{\overline{X}_{BVRSS}}. \tag{29}$$

By using Taylor expansion (see, for example, Bickel and Doksum 1977) and assuming large population size, it is easy to show that $E\left(\widehat{R}_{BVRSS} \right) = \frac{\mu_y}{\mu_x} + O\left(\frac{1}{n} \right)$, and the variance of R_{BVRSS} is approximated by

$$Var\left(\widehat{R}_{BVRSS} \right) \cong \frac{R^2}{n}$$

$$\left(V_x^2 + V_y^2 - 2\rho V_x V_y - m \left(\frac{\sum_{i=1}^{r}\sum_{j=1}^{r} T_{x[i](j)}^{**2}}{n\mu_x^2} + \frac{\sum_{i=1}^{r}\sum_{j=1}^{r} T_{y(i)[j]}^{**2}}{n\mu_y^2} - 2\frac{\sum_{i=1}^{r}\sum_{j=1}^{r} T_{x[i](j)y(i)[j]}^{**}}{n\mu_x\mu_y} \right) \right)$$

(30)

where V_x^2 and V_y^2 are as in Eq. (20), $T_{x[i](j)}^{**} = \mu_{x[i](j)} - \mu_x$, $T_{y(i)[j]}^{**} = \mu_{y(i)[j]} - \mu_y$ and
$T_{x[i](j)y(i)[j]}^{**} = \left(\mu_{x[i](j)} - \mu_x\right)\left(\mu_{y(i)[j]} - \mu_y\right)$. However, in case of SRS

$$Var\left(\widehat{R}_{BVSRS}\right) \cong \frac{R^2}{n}\left(V_x^2 + V_y^2 - 2\rho V_x V_y\right).$$

Hence,

$$Var\left(\hat{R}_{BVSRS}\right) - Var\left(\widehat{R}_{BVRSS}\right)$$

$$= m\left(\frac{\sum_{i=1}^{r}\sum_{j=1}^{r} T_{x[i](j)}^{**2}}{n\mu_x^2} + \frac{\sum_{i=1}^{r}\sum_{j=1}^{r} T_{y(i)[j]}^{**2}}{n\mu_y^2} - 2\frac{\sum_{i=1}^{r}\sum_{j=1}^{r} T_{x[i](j)y(i)[j]}^{**}}{n\mu_x\mu_y} \right)$$

(31)

$$= \frac{m}{n}\sum_{i=1}^{r}\sum_{j=1}^{r}\left(\frac{T_{x[i](j)}^{**}}{\mu_x} - \frac{T_{y(i)[j]}^{**}}{\mu_x} \right)^2 \geq 0.$$

Now when $\rho > 0$, $\sum_{i=1}^{r} T_{x[i](j)y(i)[j]}^{**}$ tends to be positive because X tends to increase

as Y increases and since $\frac{1}{r}\sum_{i=1}^{r}\mu_{x[i](j)} = \mu_x$ and $\frac{1}{r}\sum_{i=1}^{r}\mu_{y(i)[j]} = \mu_y$. Also, $\rho < 0$,

$\sum_{i=1}^{r} T_{x[i](j)y(i)[j]}^{**}$ tends to be negative because X tends to decrease as Y increases.

Therefore, from (31) $Var\left(\hat{R}_{BVSRS}\right) - Var\left(\widehat{R}_{BVRSS}\right)$ when $\rho < 0$ is much larger
than when $\rho > 0$. Hence, the relative efficiency of R_{BVRSS} relative to $\hat{R}_{BVSRS}$ is much
higher when $\rho < 0$ than when $\rho > 0$.

Thee simulation from the bivariate normal and Plackett's distributions, respectively, showed that in all cases estimating the population ratio using BVRSS is more efficient than using BVSRS and RSS. Also, the asymptotic relative efficiency increases as the set size r increases for any given positive or negative value of ρ. The performance of the ratio estimator using BVRSS is improved over SRS when the absolute value of ρ increases.

5.2 *Regression Estimator Using BVRSS*

In the two-phase regression estimator using BVRSS, for the kth cycle, $k = 1, 2, \ldots,$ m, in the first stage, suppose that (X, Y) is a bivariate random vector with the joint p.d.f.

$f(x, y)$. A random sample of size r^4 is identified from the population and randomly allocated into r^2 pools of size r^2 each, where each pool is a square matrix with r rows and r columns then proceed as follows:

Step (a): From the first r pools, rank each set (row) in each pool by a suitable method of ranking like prior information, visual inspection or by the experimenter himself, ... etc. w.r.t. the first characteristics (X), and then from each row identify and get the actual measurement of the units with the smallest rank w.r.t. X.

From each row in each of the second r pools, identify and get the actual measurement (in the same way as in Step 1) of the second minimum w.r.t. the first characteristic (X), and so on until you identify and get the actual measurements of the rth smallest unit (maximum), from each row of each of the last r pools.

Note that there will be r pools of quantified samples (w.r.t the variable X) each of size r^2. Repeat this m times. Used the quantified sample of size n = r3 m to estimate μ_x. Then proceed as follows:

Step (b): For a fixed k

From any given produced pool (produced in Step (a)), identify the ith minimum value by judgment w.r.t. the second characteristic (Y), from the ith row, of that pool, and quantify the second characteristic only as the first characteristic is already quantified in Step (a).

Steps (a) and (b) describe a procedure to produce a BVRSS of size n $= r^2$m, for regression estimators.

Using the BVRSS sample, $\left[\left(X_{[i](j)\,k}, Y_{(i)[j]k} \right), i = 1, 2, \ldots, r; \; j = 1, 2, \ldots, \right.$ $r; \; and \; k = 1, 2, \ldots, m]$ and assume that

$$Y_{(i)[j]k} = \mu_y + \beta \left(X_{[i](j)k} - \mu_x \right) + \varepsilon_{ijk}, \quad i, j = 1, 2, \ldots, r, \; k = 1, 2, \ldots, m, \quad (32)$$

where β is the model slope, and ε_{ijk} are the random errors with $E\left(\varepsilon_{ijk}\right) = 0$, var $\left(\varepsilon_{ijk}\right) = \sigma_e^2$, $Cov\left(\varepsilon_{ijk}, \varepsilon_{lst}\right) = 0$, $i \neq l$, $j \neq s$ and/ or $k \neq t$. Also, assume that $X_{[i](j)k}$ and ε_{ijk} are independent. From the first stage, let $\bar{X}_{RSS}$ be the sample mean based on RSS samples of size r^3m, i.e., $\bar{X}_{RSS} = \frac{1}{r^3m} \sum_{k=1}^{m} \sum_{z=1}^{r} \sum_{j=1}^{r} \sum_{i=1}^{r} X_{i(j)k}$. Note that,

by Al-Saleh and Zheng (2002)

$$E\left(\bar{X}_{RSS}\right) = \mu_x \qquad (33)$$

$$Var\left(\overline{X}_{RSS}\right) = \frac{\sigma^2}{r^3 m} - \frac{1}{r^4 m}\sum \left(\mu_{x(j)} - \mu_x\right)^2 \qquad (34)$$

Using BVRSS sample, the regression estimator of the population mean μ_y can be defined as

$$\overline{Y}_{RegBVRSS} = \overline{Y}_{BVRSS} + \hat{\beta}_{BVRSS}\left(\overline{X}_{RSS} - \overline{X}_{BVRSS}\right), \qquad (35)$$

where
$$\hat{\beta}_{BVRSS} = \frac{\sum\limits_{k=1}^{m}\sum\limits_{i=1}^{r}\sum\limits_{j=1}^{r}\left(X_{[i](j)k} - \overline{X}_{BVRSS}\right)Y_{(i)[j]k}}{\sum\limits_{k=1}^{m}\sum\limits_{i=1}^{r}\sum\limits_{j=1}^{r}\left(X_{[i](j)k} - \overline{X}_{BVRSS}\right)^2}, \quad \overline{X}_{BVRSS} = \frac{1}{r^2 m}\sum\limits_{k=1}^{m}\sum\limits_{i=1}^{r}\sum\limits_{j=1}^{r}X_{[i](j)k},$$

and $\overline{Y}_{BVRSS} = \frac{1}{r^2 m}\sum\limits_{k=1}^{m}\sum\limits_{i=1}^{r}\sum\limits_{j=1}^{r}Y_{(i)[j]k}$.

Using the basic properties of conditional moments the following results can easily be proven.

Proposition 1 (Samawi and Al-Saleh 2007) Under the assumptions of (32), $E\left(\hat{\beta}_{BVRSS}\right) = \beta.$

Proposition 2 (Samawi and Al-Saleh 2007) $Var\left(\hat{\beta}_{BVRSS}\Big| X\right) =$

$$\frac{\sigma_e^2}{\sum\limits_{k=1}^{m}\sum\limits_{i=1}^{r}\sum\limits_{j=1}^{r}\left(X_{[i](j)k} - \overline{X}_{BVRSS}\right)^2}.$$

Theorem 4 (Samawi and Al-Saleh 2007) Under the assumptions of (32):

$$E\left(\overline{Y}_{RegBVRSS}\right) = \mu_y.$$

$$Var\left(\overline{Y}_{RegBVRSS}\right) = \left(1 - \rho^2\right)\frac{\sigma_y^2}{n}\left[1 + E\left(\frac{\left(\overline{Z}^*_{RSS} - \overline{Z}_{BVRSS}\right)^2}{S_{BVRSS}^2}\right)\right] + \frac{\beta^2}{r^2 n}\sum\limits_{i=1}^{r}\sigma_{x(j)}^2,$$

where $n = r2\,m$,

$$Z_{[i](j)k} = \frac{X_{[i](j)k} - \mu_x}{\sigma_x}, \quad S_B^2 = \frac{1}{n}\sum\limits_{k=1}^{m}\sum\limits_{j}^{r}\sum\limits_{i=1}^{r}\left(Z_{[i](j)k} - \overline{Z}_{BVRSS}\right)^2,$$

$$\overline{Z}_{BVRSS} = \frac{\overline{X}_{BVRSS} - \mu_x}{\sigma_x} \quad \text{and} \quad \overline{Z}^*_{RSS} = \frac{\overline{X}_{RSS} - \mu_x}{\sigma_x}.$$

Simulation studies conducted by Samawi and Al-Saleh (2007) show that the regression estimator based on BVRSS, from bivariate normal distribution, is more efficient than the naive estimator using BVRSS only whenever $|\rho| > 0.90$ and the set size is small. This is always the case when using RSS technique for regression estimator (Yu and Lam 1997.) Clearly, the relative efficiency is affected only slightly by the number of cycles m. However, regression estimator using BVRSS, from bivariate normal distribution is more efficient than naïve estimators based on SRS and RSS whenever $|\rho| > 0.4$.

In addition they showed that the regression estimator using BVRSS is always superior to double sampling regression estimators using SRS and RSS. Although, the efficiency is affected by the value of ρ and the sample size, $\overline{Y}_{RegBVRSS}$ is still more efficient than using other sampling methods. Even with departures from the normality assumption, they showed that $\overline{Y}_{RegBVRSS}$ is still more efficient than other regression estimators based on SRS and RSS.

In order to investigate the performance of the methods introduced in this section to a real data set we compare the BVRSS regression estimation to BVSRS regression to data collected from trauma victims in a hospital setting. Each observation consists of the patients' age, bd score, and gender. The bd score is a measure indicating the level of blunt force trauma as reported by the administering doctor. The data contains $N = 1{,}480$ female. For the analysis we treat the data as the population and resample it 5,000 times under the various sampling mechanisms (i.e., BVRSS and BVSRS) to estimate the mean bd (Y) score using the covariate age (X). The following are the exact population values of the data:

For Females it was found that the mean age $(\mu_x) = 35.44$, Variance $(\sigma_x^2) = 412.58$ the mean bd score $(\mu_y) = -2.25$, Variance $(\sigma_y^2) = 12.19$, $\rho = 0.21$. Using BVSRS, estimator has mean -2.41 with variance 0.21. Using BVRSS, estimator has a mean -2.48, with variance 0.20. From the results above we conclude that both sampling techniques exhibit similar performance in terms of bias with BVRSS performing better in terms of variance.

Finally, whenever BVRSS is possible to be conducted and the relationship between X and Y is approximately linear, ratio and regression estimators, using BVRSS, are recommended.

References

Al-Saleh, M.F., Al-Kadiri, M.A.: Double ranked set sampling. Stat. Probab. Lett. **48**(2), 205–212 (2000)

Al-Saleh, M.F., Zheng, G.: Estimation of bivariate characteristics using ranked set sampling. Aust. N. Z. J. Stat. **44**, 221–232 (2002)

Bahadur, R.R.: A note on quantiles in large samples. Ann. Math. Stat. **37**, 577–590 (1966)

Bickel, P.J., Doksum, K.A.: Mathematical Statistics. Holden-Day, Inc., Oakland (1977)

Chen, Z.: On ranked-set sample quantiles and their application. J. Stat. Plan. Inference **83**, 125–135 (2000)

Chen, Z., Zheng, G., Ghosh, K., Li, Z.: Linkage disequilibrium mapping of quantitative trait loci by selective genotyping. Am. J. Hum. Genet. **77**, 661–669 (2005)

Chen, Z.: Ranked set sampling: Its essence and new applications. Environ. Ecol. Stat. **14**, 355–363 (2007)

Dell, T.R., Clutter, J.L.: Ranked set sampling theory with order statistics background. Biometrics **28**, 545–555 (1972)

Food and Agriculture Organization (FAO): Date Production and Protection. FAO Plant Production and Protection Paper 35. FAO (1982)

Hansen, M.H., Hurwitz, W.N., Madow, W.G.: Sampling Survey Methods and Theory, vol. 2. Wiley, New York (1953)

Kaur, A., Patil, G.P., Sinha, A.K., Tailie, C.: Ranked set sampling: an annotated bibliography. Environ. Ecol. Stat. **2**, 25–54 (1995)

McIntyre, G.A.: A method for unbiased selective sampling using ranked set. Aust. J. Agr. Res. **3**, 385–390 (1952)

Muttlak, H.A.: Median ranked set sampling. J. Appl. Stat. Sci. **6**(4), 245–255 (1997)

Nelson, W.E., Behrman, R.E., Kliegman, R.M., Vaughan, V.C.: Textbook of Pediatrics, 4th edn. W. B. Saunders Company Harcourt Barace Jovanovich, Inc, Philadelphia (1992)

Norris, R.C., Patil, G.P., Sinha, A.K.: Estimation of multiple characteristics by ranked set sampling methods. COENOSES **10**(2&3), 95–111 (1995)

Ozturk, O., MacEachern, S.N.: Order restricted randomized designs for control versus treatment comparison. Ann. Inst. Stat. Math. **56**, 701–720 (2004)

Patil, G.P., Sinha, A.K., Taillie, C.: Relative efficiency of ranked set sampling: comparison with regression estimator. Environmetrics **4**, 399–412 (1993)

Patil, G.P., Sinha, A.K., Taillie, C.: Ranked set sampling for multiple characteristics. Int. J. Ecol. Environ. Sci. **20**, 94–109 (1994)

Patil, G.P., Sinha, A.K., Taillie, C.: Ranked set sampling: a bibliography. Environ. Ecol. Stat. **6**, 91–98 (1999)

Samawi, H.M.: Stratified ranked set sample. Pak. J. Stat. **12**(1), 9–16 (1996)

Samawi, H.M.: On quantiles estimation using ranked samples with some applications. JKSS **30**(4), 667–678 (2001)

Samawi, H.M.: Varied set size ranked set sampling with application to mean and ratio estimation. Int. J. Model. Simul. **32**(1), 6–13 (2011)

Samawi, H.M., Al-Sageer, O.A.: On the estimation of the distribution function using extreme and median ranked set sampling. Biom. J. **43**(3), 357–373 (2001)

Samawi, H.M., Al-Saleh, M.F.: On bivariate ranked set sampling for ratio and regression estimators. Int. J. Model. Simul. **27**(4), 1–7 (2007)

Samawi, H.M.: On double extreme ranked set sample with application to regression estimator. Metron **LX**(1–2), 53–66 (2002)

Samawi, H.M., Muttlak, H.A.: Estimation of ratio using ranked set sampling. Biom. J. **38**(6), 753–764 (1996)

Samawi, H.M., Muttlak, H.A.: On ratio estimation using median ranked set sampling. J. Appl. Stat. Sci. **10**(2), 89–98 (2001)

Samawi, H.M., Siam, M.I.: Ratio estimation using stratified ranked set sample. Metron **LXI**(1), 75–90 (2003)

Samawi, H.M., Ahmed, M.S., Abu Dayyeh, W.: Estimating the population mean using extreme ranked set sampling. Biom. J. **38**(5), 577–586 (1996)

Serfling, R.J.: Approximation Theorems of Mathematical Statistics. Wiley, New York (1980)

Sinsheimer, J.S., Blangero, J., Lange, K.: Gamete competition models. Am. J. Hum. Genet. **66**, 1168–1172 (2000)

Slatkin, M.: Disequilibrium mapping of a quantitative-trait locus in an expanding population. Am. J. Hum. Genet. **64**, 1765–1773 (1999)

Spielman, R.S., McGinnis, R.E., Ewens, W.J.: Transmission test for linkage disequilibrium: the insulin gene region and insulin-dependent diabetes mellitus (IDDM). Am. J. Hum. Genet. **52**, 506–516 (1993)

Stokes, S.L., Sager, T.W.: Characterization of a ranked set sample with application to estimating distribution functions. J. Am. Stat. Assoc. **83**, 374–381 (1988)

Sukhatme, P.V., Sukhatme, B.V.: Sampling Theory of Surveys with Applications. Iowa State University Press, Ames (1970)

Takahasi, K., Wakimoto, K.: On unbiased estimates of the population mean based on the stratified sampling by means of ordering. Ann. Inst. Stat. Math. **20**, 1–31 (1968)

William, E., Ahmed, M., Ahmed, O., Zaki, L., Arash, N., Tamer, B., Subhy, R.: Date Palm in the GCC countries of the Arabian Peninsula. http://www.icarda.org/aprp/datepalm/introduction/intro-body.htm (2004)

Xu, X.P., Rogus, J.J., Terwedom, H.A., et al.: An extreme-sib-pair genome scan for genes regulating blood pressure. Am. J. Hum. Genet. **64**, 1694–1701 (1999)

Yu, L.H., Lam, K.: Regression estimator in ranked set sampling. Biometrics **53**, 1070–1080 (1997)

Zheng, G., Ghosh, K., Chen, Z., Li, Z.: Extreme rank selections for linkage analysis of quantitative trait loci using selected sibpairs. Ann. Hum. Genet. **70**, 857–866 (2006)

Weighted Multiple Testing Correction for Correlated Endpoints in Survival Data

Changchun Xie, Enas Ghulam, Aimin Chen, Kesheng Wang, Susan M. Pinney, and Christopher Lindsell

Abstract Multiple correlated time-to-event endpoints often occur in clinical trials and some time-to-event endpoints are more important than others. Most weighted multiple testing adjustment methods have been proposed to control family-wise type I error rates either only consider the correlation among continuous or binary endpoints or totally disregard the correlation among the endpoints. For continuous or binary endpoints, the correlation matrix can be directly estimated from the corresponding correlated endpoints. However, it is challenging to directly estimate the correlation matrix from the multiple endpoints in survival data since censoring is involved. In this chapter, we propose a weighted multiple testing correction method for correlated time-to-event endpoints in survival data, based on the correlation matrix estimated from the WLW method proposed by Wei, Lin, and Weissfeld. Simulations are conducted to study the family-wise type I error rate of the proposed method and to compare the power performance of the proposed method to the nonparametric multiple testing methods such as the alpha-exhaustive fallback (AEF), fixed-sequence (FS), and the weighted Holm-Bonferroni method when used for the correlated time-to-event endpoints. The proposed method and others are illustrated using a real dataset from Fernald Community Cohort (formerly known as the Fernald Medical Monitoring Program).

C. Xie (✉) • E. Ghulam • A. Chen • S.M. Pinney
Division of Epidemiology and Biostatistics, Department of Environmental Health, University of Cincinnati, Cincinnati, OH, USA
e-mail: xiecn@ucmail.uc.edu; ghulamem@mail.uc.edu; chenai@ucmail.uc.edu; pinneysm@ucmail.uc.edu

K. Wang
Department of Biostatistics and Epidemiology, East Tennessee State University, Johnson City, TN, USA
e-mail: wangk@mail.etsu.edu

C. Lindsell
Department of Emergency Medicine, University of Cincinnati, Cincinnati, OH, USA
e-mail: lindsecj@ucmail.uc.edu

© Springer International Publishing Switzerland 2015
D.-G. Chen, J. Wilson (eds.), *Innovative Statistical Methods for Public Health Data*, ICSA Book Series in Statistics, DOI 10.1007/978-3-319-18536-1_14

1 Introduction

Multiple correlated time-to-event endpoints are often collected to test the treatment effect in clinical trials. For example, the Outcome Reduction with an Initial Glargine Intervention (ORIGIN) trial (The ORIGIN Trial Investigators 2008) has two co-primary endpoints: the first is a composite of cardiovascular death, non-fatal myocardial infarction (MI), or non-fatal stroke; the second is a composite of these three events plus revascularization or hospitalization for heart failure. These two endpoints are correlated. Also, the first endpoint is considered more important than the second endpoint. The issue of multiplicity occurs when multiple hypotheses are tested in this way. Ignoring multiplicity can cause false positive results. Many statistical methods have been proposed to control family-wise error rate (FWER), which is the probability of rejecting at least one true null hypothesis. When some hypotheses are more important than others, weighted multiple testing correction methods may be useful. Commonly used weighted multiple testing correction methods to control FWER include the weighted Bonferroni correction, the Bonferroni fixed sequence (BFS), the alpha-exhaustive fallback (AEF), and the weighted Holm procedure. The weighted Bonferroni correction computes the adjusted P-value for p_i as $p_{adji} = min(1, p_i/w_i)$, where $w_i > 0, i = 1, \ldots, m$ are the weights with $\sum_{i=1}^{m} w_i = 1$ (m is the total number of tests performed) and rejects the null hypothesis, H_i if the adjusted p-value $p_{adji} \leq \alpha$ (or $p_i \leq w_i\alpha$). Combining a Bonferroni adjustment and the fixed sequence (FS) testing procedure, Wiens (2003) proposed a Bonferroni fixed sequence (BFS) procedure, where each of the null hypotheses is given a certain significance level and a pre-specified testing sequence that allows the significance level to accumulate for later testing when the null hypotheses are rejected. Wiens and Dmitrienko (2005, 2010) developed this method further to use more available alpha to provide an alpha-exhaustive fallback (AEF) procedure with more power than the original BFS. Holm (Holm 1979; Westfall et al. 2004) presented a weighted Holm method as follows. Let $q_i = p_i/w_i, i = 1, \ldots, m$. Without loss of generality, suppose $q_1 \leq q_2 \leq \cdots \leq q_m$. Then the adjusted p-value for the first hypothesis is $p_{adj_1} = min(1, q_1)$. Inductively, the adjusted p-value for the jth hypothesis is $p_{adj_j} = min(1, max(p_{adj(j-1)}, (w_j + \ldots + w_m)q_i)), j = 2, \ldots, m$. The method rejects a hypothesis if the adjusted p-value is less than the FWER, α.

It is notable that all these weighted multiple testing methods disregard the correlation among the endpoints and they are therefore appropriately called weighted nonparametric multiple testing methods. They are conservative if test statistics are correlated leading to false negative results. In other words, ignoring the correlation when correcting for multiple testing can lower the power of a study. Recently, weighted parametric multiple testing methods have been proposed to take into account correlations among the test statistics. These methods require the correlation matrix for the correlated tests related to the corresponding correlated endpoints. For continuous data or binary data, the correlation matrix can be directly estimated from the corresponding correlated endpoints (Conneely et al. 2007; Xie 2012; Xie et al. 2013; Xie 2014). However, it is challenging to directly estimate the correlation matrix from the multiple time-to-event endpoints in survival data since censoring is involved. Pocock et al. (1987) discussed the analysis of multiple endpoints in survival data using log-rank tests and gave the normal approximation to the log-rank test. However, the correlation matrix was not given despite being specified for other situations such as binary data. Alosh and Huque (2009) considered the correlation of a survival endpoint between the overall population and a subgroup. Their method was based on the proportion of subjects in the subgroup, which is not suitable for the estimation of the correlations between different survival endpoints measured in the same population. Wei et al. (1989) proposed a method called the WLW method to analyze multiple endpoints in survival data using the marginal Cox models. Instead of estimating the correlation matrix from the multiple time-to-event endpoints directly, they proposed a robust sandwich covariance matrix estimate for the maximum partial likelihood estimates for the event-specific regression coefficients. Neither Pocock's method nor the WLW method considered giving different weights to different endpoints. In this chapter, we will use the WLW method to estimate the correlations among the test statistics. With the estimated correlation matrix, we propose a weighted multiple testing correction for correlated endpoints, WTMCc, which can be used to apply different weights to hypotheses when conducting multiple testing for correlated time-to-event endpoints. Simulations are conducted to study the family-wise type I error rate of the proposed method and compare the power performance of the proposed method to the power performance of the alpha-exhaustive fallback (AEF), the fixed-sequence (FS), and the weighted Holm-Bonferroni method when used for the correlated time-to-event endpoints. One might consider other parametric methods such as Huque and Alosh (2008) flexible fixed-sequence (FFS) testing method and Li and Mehrotra's adaptive α allocation approach (4A), using the estimated correlation matrix from the WLW method. However, we previously compared the WMTCc method with both the FFS method and the 4A method and shown the WMTCc has its advantage (Xie 2014), and so we will not discuss the FFS method and the 4A method further in this chapter.

In the next section, the WMTCc method for correlated time-to-event endpoints is presented. In Sect. 3, simulations are conducted to evaluate the proposed method. A real example to illustrate use of the proposed method for correlated time-to-event endpoints is given in Sect. 4, followed by discussion and concluding remarks in Sect. 5.

2 Weighted Multiple Testing Correction for Correlated Time-to-Event Endpoints

Suppose there are n subjects and each subject can have up to K potential failure times (events). Let X_{ki} be the covariate process associated with the kth event for the ith subject. The marginal Cox models are given by

$$h_k(t) = h_{k0}(t)e^{\beta_k' X_{ki}(t)}, k = 1, \ldots, K \text{ and } i = 1, \ldots, n, \tag{1}$$

where $h_{k0}(t)$ is the event-specific baseline hazard function for the kth event and β_k is the (event-specific) column vector of regression coefficients for the kth event. The WLW estimates $\beta_1, \ldots, \beta_K$ by the maximum partial likelihood estimates $\hat{\beta}_1, \ldots, \hat{\beta}_K$, respectively, and uses a robust sandwich covariance matrix estimate, Σ for $(\hat{\beta}_1', \ldots, \hat{\beta}_K')'$ to account for the dependence of the multiple endpoints. This robust sandwich covariance matrix estimate can be obtained using the PHREG procedure in SAS. After we have the estimated robust sandwich covariance matrix, the WMTCc method is applied.

Assume that the test statistics follow a multivariate normal distribution with the estimated correlation matrix Σ, using the WLW method above. Let $p_1, \ldots, p_m$ be the observed p-values for null hypotheses $H_0^{(1)}, \ldots, H_0^{(m)}$, respectively, and $w_i > 0$, $i = 1, \ldots, m$ be the weight for null hypothesis $H_0^{(i)}$. Note that we do not require that $\sum_{i=1}^m w_i = 1$. It can be seen from Eqs. (3) or (4) below that the adjusted p-values depend only on the ratios of the weights. For each $i = 1, \ldots, m$, calculate $q_i = p_i/w_i$. Then the adjusted p-value for the null hypothesis $H_0^{(i)}$ is

$$p_{adj_i} = P(\min_j q_j \leq q_i)$$

$$= 1 - P(\text{all } q_j > q_i)$$

$$= 1 - P(\text{all} \quad p_j > p_i w_j/w_i) \tag{2}$$

$$= 1 - P\left(\bigcap_{j=1}^m a_j \leq X_j \leq b_j\right),$$

where $X_j, j = 1, \ldots, m$ are standardized multivariate normal with correlation matrix Σ and

$$a_j = \Phi^{-1}\left(\frac{p_i w_j}{2w_i}\right), \qquad b_j = \Phi^{-1}\left(1 - \frac{p_i w_j}{2w_i}\right) \tag{3}$$

for the two-sided case and

$$a_j = -\infty, \qquad b_j = \Phi^{-1}\left(1 - \frac{p_i w_j}{w_i}\right) \tag{4}$$

for the one-sided case.

Therefore the WMTCc method first adjusts the m observed p-values for multiple testing by computing m adjusted p-values in (2). If $p_{adj_i} \leq \alpha$, then reject the corresponding null hypothesis $H_0^{(i)}$. Suppose k_1 null hypotheses have been rejected, we then adjust the remaining $m - k_1$ observed p-values for multiple testing after removing the rejected k_1 null hypotheses, using the corresponding correlation matrix and weights. This procedure is continued until there is no null hypothesis left or there is no null hypothesis that can be rejected.

Computation of the adjusted p-values in (2) requires integration of the multivariate normal density function, which has no closed-form solution. However, Genz (1992, 1993) and Genz et al. (2014) have developed a computationally efficient method for numerical integration of the multivariate normal distribution and incorporated it into the package *mvtnorm* in the R software environment (R Development Core Team (2014). Based on the magnitude of the p-values and the nature of the analysis, one may choose the precision level to devote more computational resources to a high-precision analysis and improve computational efficiency.

3   Simulations

In this section, we present the results of simulations to estimate the family-wise type I error rate of the proposed method, and to compare the power performance of the proposed method with the alpha-exhaustive fallback (AEF), the fixed-sequence (FS), and the weighted Holm-Bonferroni method when used for the correlated time-to-event endpoints. The correlated time-to-event endpoints were generated using the following proportional hazards model

$$\lambda(t|X) = \lambda_0(t)exp(\beta'X), \tag{5}$$

where $\lambda_0(t)$ is the baseline hazard and X is a vector of covariates. This model is equivalent to the following transformed regression model (Fan et al. 1997):

$$\log(H_0(t)) = -\beta'X + \log(e), \tag{6}$$

where $e \sim exp(1)$ and $H_0(t)$ is the baseline cumulative hazard function. In order to obtain correlated survival data, we generated samples from a multi-exponential distribution with a given correlation matrix. This correlation matrix is the correlation of the different cumulative hazard functions, which is specifically designed for survival data to allow censoring. If the event times have an exponential distribution, this correlation matrix is the same as the correlation matrix of multivariate event times. This may not hold if the event times do not have exponential distribution.

We simulated a clinical trial with three correlated time-to-event endpoints and 240 individuals. Each individual had probability 0.5 to receive the active treatment and probability 0.5 to receive placebo. The baseline hazard $\lambda_0(t)$ was set to be $24t^2$. Equal correlation structure was used with ρ chosen as $0.0, 0.3, 0.5, 0.7$ and 0.9. The treatment effect size was assumed as $0.0, 0.05$, and 0.2. The survival times were censored by the uniform distribution $U(0, 3)$. The weights for the three endpoints were $(5, 4, 1)$, which corresponds to alpha allocations $(0.025, 0.02, 0.005)$.

The simulation results are summarized in Table 1. From these simulations, we can conclude the following:

1. The proposed method using estimated correlation matrices from the WLW method can control the family-wise type I error rate well (the first part of Table 1). Both the WMTCc and the FS can keep the family-wise type I error rate at 5 % level as the correlation, ρ, increases. However, the family-wise type I error rates for the AEF and the weighted Holm decreases as the correlation, ρ, increases, resulting in decreased power with increasing correlation.
2. The WMTCc method has higher power for testing the first hypothesis than the AEF and the weighted Holm methods (Table 1)
3. The WMTCc method has a power advantage over the weighted Holm method for each individual hypothesis, especially when the correlation, ρ, is high.
4. The WMTCc method has a higher chance of rejecting at least one hypothesis compared to the weighted Holm and the AEF methods, especially when the correlation, ρ, is high.
5. The FS method has the highest power for testing the first hypothesis. However, the WMTCc method can still have high power for testing other hypotheses when the power for testing the first hypothesis is very low, which is not true for the FS method.

4   Example: Modeling Correlated Time-to-Event Outcomes in the Fernald Community Cohort

To illustrate the proposed method, we analyze data from the Fernald Community Cohort (FCC). Community members of a small Ohio town, living near a uranium refinery, participated in a medical monitoring program from 1990 to 2008. The Fernald Medical Monitoring Program (FMMP) provided health screening and promotion services to 9,782 persons who resided within close proximity to the plant. For more details, see Wones et al. (2009) or the cohort website (Fernald Medical Monitoring Program website 2014). For illustration purposes, we considered four time-to-event outcomes among female participants: three types of incident cancers (colon cancer, lung cancer, and breast cancer) and their composite (any of the three cancers). We were interested in testing the association between smoking and the four outcomes after adjusting for age and uranium exposure. First, we tested one outcome at a time, the results are shown in Table 2. Although the two-tailed unadjusted p-values for colon cancer and breast cancer are large, the coefficients of smoking for all the four outcomes are positive, indicating their potential harmful associations of smoking. Since we have four tests, we need to consider adjusting for the multiple testing. To illustrate the weighted multiple testing methods, the weight $0.4, 0.2, 0.2, 0.2$ were given to the composite endpoint, lung cancer, colon cancer, and breast cancer separately. The corresponding α

Table 1 Three endpoints: simulated power (%) or significant level (%) based on 100,000 runs for selected treatment differences for the WMTCc method, AEF, FS and the weighted Holm-Bonferroni method (The first cell entry is for the first endpoint, the second entry is for the second endpoint, and the third entry is for the third endpoint. The probability (%) that at least one hypothesis is rejected is given in brackets)

α allocations or weight	Effect size	ρ	WMTCc	AEF	FS	Weighted Holm-Bonferroni
α allocations (0.025,0.02, 0.005) or weight (5,4,1)	0.0, 0.0, 0.0	0.0	2.6, 2.1, 0.5 (5.0)	2.5, 2.1, 0.6 (5.0)	5.0, 0.3, 0.01 (5.0)	2.5, 2.1, 0.05 (5.0)
		0.3	2.7, 2.2, 0.6 (5.0)	2.5, 2.1, 0.6 (4.8)	5.0, 0.5, 0.1 (5.0)	2.6, 2.1, 0.6 (4.8)
		0.5	3.0, 2.5, 0.8 (5.1)	2.6, 2.2, 0.8 (4.5)	5.1, 1.0, 0.3 (5.1)	2.7, 2.2, 0.8 (4.5)
		0.7	3.4, 2.9, 1.3 (5.0)	2.6, 2.4, 1.2 (4.1)	5.0, 1.7, 0.9 (5.0)	2.8, 2.4, 1.1 (4.1)
		0.9	4.2, 3.7, 2.4 (5.0)	2.7, 2.6, 1.9 (3.3)	5.0, 3.0, 2.3 (5.0)	2.8, 2.5, 1.9 (3.3)
	0.2, 0.05, 0.05	0.0	75.4, 8.6, 3.6 (76.9)	74.9, 9.2, 2.7 (76.7)	82.9, 9.3, 1.1 (82.9)	75.2, 8.6, 3.5 (76.7)
		0.3	75.7, 9.3, 4.6 (76.2)	74.8, 9.8, 3.6 (75.5)	83.0, 10.4, 2.5 (83.0)	75.0, 9.1, 4.5 (75.5)
		0.5	76.4, 9.8, 5.4 (76.6)	74.9, 10.0, 4.5 (75.1)	83.0, 10.8, 3.7 (83.0)	74.9, 9.3, 5.2 (75.1)
		0.7	77.7, 10.3, 6.4 (77.9)	74.9, 10.2, 5.6 (75.1)	83.1, 10.9, 5.3 (83.1)	74.9, 9.5, 6.0 (75.1)
		0.9	80.0, 11.0, 8.0 (80.3)	74.8, 10.2, 7.5 (74.9)	82.9, 10.9, 7.7 (82.9)	74.8, 9.5, 7.3 (74.9)
	0.05, 0.05, 0.2	0.0	7.3, 6.3, 55.4 (59.7)	7.2, 6.2, 55.3 (59.5)	11.3, 1.3, 1.1 (11.3)	7.2, 6.2, 55.2 (59.5)
		0.3	7.8, 6.8, 55.5 (57.7)	7.5, 5.5, 54.9 (56.9)	11.3, 2.6, 2.5 (11.3)	7.5, 6.6, 54.8 (56.9)
		0.5	8.2, 7.3, 56.0 (57.0)	7.7, 6.9, 54.4 (55.4)	11.2, 3.8, 3.7 (11.2)	7.7, 6.9, 54.4 (55.4)
		0.7	8.8, 8.0, 57.1 (57.6)	7.9, 7.3, 54.1 (54.5)	11.2, 5.3, 5.3 (11.2)	7.9, 7.3, 54.1 (54.5)
		0.9	9.9, 9.2, 59.7 (60.1)	8.0, 7.6, 54.0 (54.2)	11.3, 7.8, 7.6 (11.3)	8.0, 7.6, 54.0 (54.2)
	0.2, 0.2, 0.2	0.0	80.5, 79.9, 75.1 (96.9)	79.5, 80.1, 75.5 (96.8)	83.0, 68.9, 57.2 (83.0)	80.4, 79.8, 75.0 (96.8)
		0.3	80.1, 79.3, 74.0 (92.9)	78.8, 79.2, 74.2 (92.5)	82.9, 71.0, 62.2 (82.9)	79.7, 78.9, 73.6 (92.5)
		0.5	80.0, 79.3, 73.9 (90.0)	78.4, 78.7, 73.7 (89.1)	83.0, 73.0, 66.1 (83.0)	79.2, 78.4, 73.2 (89.1)
		0.7	80.3, 79.6, 74.5 (87.1)	77.8, 78.1, 73.5 (85.0)	83.0, 75.2, 70.3 (83.0)	78.5, 77.8, 73.0 (85.0)
		0.9	81.4, 80.6, 76.6 (84.2)	76.8, 77.0, 74.1 (79.5)	82.9, 78.5, 75.9 (82.9)	77.4, 76.6, 73.9 (79.5)

The total sample size is 240

Table 2 The results of analyzing each of the four endpoints: Cox model with smoking as covariate, adjusting for age and uranium exposure

Outcome	Coefficient of smoking	SE of coefficient	Hazard ratio	Unadjusted P-value
Composite of lung, colon and breast cancer	0.2947	0.1317	1.34	0.0252
Lung cancer	2.1997	0.4533	9.02	0.0000012
Colon cancer	0.1347	0.3771	1.14	0.72
Breast cancer	0.0288	0.1550	1.03	0.85

Table 3 The estimated correlation matrix of the test statistics for the four endpoints, using the WLW method

	The composite of lung, colon and breast cancer	Lung cancer	Colon cancer	Breast cancer
The composite of lung, colon, and breast cancer	1	0.290	0.342	0.838
Lung cancer	0.290	1	−0.004	0.040
Colon cancer	0.342	−0.004	1	−0.002
Breast cancer	0.838	0.040	−0.002	1

allocations are $0.02, 0.01, 0.01, 0.01$. The testing sequence for the AEF and the FS methods is the composite endpoint, lung cancer, colon cancer, breast cancer. In applying the WMTCc method, we estimated the correlation matrix of the test statistics for the four endpoints, using the WLW method. This estimated correlation matrix is given in Table 3. The adjusted p-values from the WMTCc method are $0.041, 0.000005, 0.92, 0.92$, respectively. The first and the second null hypothesis can be rejected, corresponding to the composite endpoint and lung cancer respectively. The weighted Holm-Bonferroni method gave the adjusted p-values as $0.051, 0.000005, 1.0, 1.0$ respectively. Only the second null hypothesis, corresponding to lung cancer, can be rejected. In this example, the AEF method has the same results as the weighted Holm-Bonferroni method. The FS method has the same results as the WMTCc method since we specified the right testing sequence. For illustration purposes, if we change the testing sequence to the composite endpoint, colon cancer, lung cancer, breast cancer, even the null hypothesis for lung cancer cannot be rejected. Although the AEF method depends on the testing sequence, it can still reject the null hypothesis, corresponding to lung cancer (since $0.0000012 < 0.01$), but not others. The WMTCc method and the weighted Holm-Bonferroni method do not depend on the testing sequence.

5 Discussions

In this chapter, we investigated the weighted multiple testing correction for correlated time-to-event endpoints. Extensive simulations were conducted to evaluate the WMTC method in comparison with three existing nonparametric methods. The simulations showed that the proposed method using estimated correlation matrices from the WLW method can control the family-wise type I error rate very well as summarized in the first part of Table 1. The proposed method has a power advantage over the weighted Holm method for each individual hypothesis, especially when the correlation ρ is high. It also has higher power for testing the first hypothesis (which is usually the most important hypothesis) than the AEF method. For the FS method, if we cannot reject the first hypothesis, the remaining hypotheses cannot be rejected even if their unadjusted p-values are very small. This is not true for the WMTCc method, which can still have high power for testing other hypotheses when the power for testing the first hypothesis is very low.

It should be noted that the WMTCc method assumes that test statistics are asymptotically distributed as multivariate normal with the estimated correlation matrix from the data, using the WLW method. The positive semi-definite assumption needs to be checked since the estimated correlation matrix from an inconsistent data set might not be positive semi-definite. If this is the case, the algorithm proposed by Higham (2002) can be used to compute the nearest correlation matrix.

In conclusion, the WMTCc method outperforms the existing nonparametric methods in multiple testing for correlated time-to-event multiple endpoints in clinical trials.

Acknowledgements This project was supported by the National Center for Research Resources and the National Center for Advancing Translational Sciences, National Institutes of Health, through Grant 8 UL1 TR000077-04 and National Institute for Environmental Health Sciences, Grant P30-ES006096 (UC Center for Environmental Genetics). The content is solely the responsibility of the authors and does not necessarily represent the official views of the NIH.

References

Alosh, M., Huque, M.F.: A flexible strategy for testing subgroups and overall population. Stat. Med. **28**, 3–23 (2009)

Conneely, K.N., Boehnke, M.: So many correlated tests, so little time! Rapid adjustment of p values for multiple correlated tests. Am. J. Hum. Genet. **81**, 1158–1168 (2007)

Fan, J., Gijbels, I., King, M.: Local likelihood and local partial likelihood in hazard regression. Ann. Stat. **25**(4), 1661–1690 (1997)

Fernald Medical Monitoring Program Website: https://urldefense.proofpoint.com/v2/url?u=http-3A__www.eh.uc.edu_fmmp&d=AAIGAQ&c=4sF48jRmVAe_CH-k9mXYXEGfSnM3bY53YSKuLUQRxhA&r=656gLa67DL3AtCWt3Jb0tIRzTwk1qCp1OB7YsvvcToI&m=6W9WCEZFMxFnHnV55uMK2eK2NDafDEWbmZP_2DcdldA&s=HjK4SFlUlSnSDz50bfhJBuDPUCEfjPDRzFZTbg0sAl0&e= (2014). Cited 15 Nov 2014

Genz, A.: Numerical computation of multivariate normal probabilities. J. Comput. Graph. Stat. **1**, 141–149 (1992)

Genz, A.: Comparison of methods for the computation of multivariate normal probabilities. Comput. Sci. Stat. **25**, 400–405 (1993)

Genz, A., Bretz, F., Hothorn, T.: mvtnorm: multivariate normal and t distribution. R package version 2.12.0. Available at https://urldefense.proofpoint.com/v2/url?u=http-3A__cran.r-2D project.org_web_packages_mvtnorm_&d=AAIGAQ&c=4sF48jRmVAe_CH-k9mXYXEGfSn M3bY53YSKuLUQRxhA&r=656gLa67DL3AtCWt3Jb0tIRzTwk1qCp1OB7YsvvcToI&m=6 W9WCEZFMxFnHnV55uMK2eK2NDafDEWbmZP_2DcdldA&s=4LjNlTNOcwwRiQYj7_ CHG0qMaZIphbnaImMOKgYfryk&e=\index.html (2014). Cited 15 Nov 2014

Higham, N.J.: Computing the nearest correlation matrix - A problem from finance. IMA J. Numer. Anal. **22**(3), 329–343 (2002)

Holm, S.: A simple sequentially rejective multiple test procedure. Scand. J. Stat. **6**, 65–70 (1979)

Huque, M.F., Alosh, M.: A flexible fixed-sequence testing method for hierarchically ordered correlated multiple endpoints in clinical trials. J. Stat. Plann. Inference **138**, 321–335 (2008)

Pocock, S.J., Geller, N.L., Tsiatis, A.A.: The analysis of multiple endpoints in clinical trials. Biometrics **43**, 487–498 (1987)

R Development Core Team: R: a language and environment for statistical computing. R Foundation for Statistical Computing. Aavailable at https://urldefense.proofpoint.com/v2/url?u=http-3A__ www.r-2Dproject.org_&d=AAIGAQ&c=4sF48jRmVAe_CH-k9mXYXEGfSnM3bY53YSKuL UQRxhA&r=656gLa67DL3AtCWt3Jb0tIRzTwk1qCp1OB7YsvvcToI&m=6W9WCEZFMxFn HnV55uMK2eK2NDafDEWbmZP_2DcdldA&s=k45dskHmTjrjhL-mG248jkpbB-Vc6UP2wX W0uveFHtw&e= (2014). Cited 15 Nov 2014

The ORIGIN Trial Investigators: Rationale, design and baseline characteristics for a large simple international trial of cardiovascular disease prevention in people with dysglycaemia: the ORIGIN trial. Am. Heart J. **155**, 26–32 (2008)

Wei, L.J., Lin, D.Y., Weissfeld, L.: Regression analysis of multivariate incomplete failure time data by modeling marginal distributions. J. Am. Stat. Assoc. **84**, 1065–1073 (1989)

Westfall, P.H., Kropf, S., Finos, L.: Weighted FWE-controlling methods in high-dimensional situations. In: Recent Developments in Multiple Comparison Procedures. IML Lecture Notes and Monograph Series, vol. 47, pp. 143–154. Institute of Mathematical Statistics, Beachwood (2004)

Wiens, B.L.: A fixed sequence Bonferroni procedure for testing multiple endpoints. Pharm. Stat. **2**, 211–215 (2003)

Wiens, B.L., Dmitrienko, A.: The fallback procedure for evaluating a single family of hypotheses. J. Biopharm. Stat. **15**, 929–942 (2005)

Wiens, B.L., Dmitrienko, A.: On selecting a multiple comparison procedure for analysis of a clinical trial: fallback, fixed sequence, and related procedures. Stat. Biopharm. Res. **2**, 22–32 (2010)

Wones, R., Pinney, S.M., Buckholz, J., Deck-Tebbe, C., Freyberg, R., Pesce, A.: Medical monitoring: a beneficial remedy for residents living near an environmental hazard site. J. Occup. Environ. Med. **51**(12), 1374–1383 (2009)

Xie, C.: Weighted multiple testing correction for correlated tests. Stat. Med. **31**, 341–352 (2012)

Xie, C., Lu, X., Pogue, J., Chen, D.: Weighted multiple testing corrections for correlated binary endpoints. Commun. Stat. Simul. Comput. **42**(8), 1693–1702 (2013)

Xie, C.: Relations among three parametric multiple testing methods for correlated tests. J. Stat. Comput. Simul. **84**(4), 812–818 (2014)

Meta-Analytic Methods for Public Health Research

Yan Ma, Wei Zhang, and Ding-Geng Chen

Abstract This chapter presents an overview on meta-analysis (MA) intended for public health researchers to understand and to apply the methods of MA. Emphasis is focused on classical statistical methods for estimation of the parameters of interest in MA as well as recent development in research in MA. Specifically, univariate and multivariate fixed- and random-effects MAs, as well as meta-regression are discussed. All methods are illustrated by examples of published MA in public health research. We demonstrate how these approaches can be implemented using software packages in R.

1 Introduction of Meta-Analysis for Evidence-Based Health Care

There has been an increasing interest in the adoption of evidence-based strategies to inform policy making for population health (Brownson et al. 2009; Fielding and Briss 2006; Glasziou and Longbottom 1999). Similar to evidence-based practice in other disciplines such as medicine, psychology, and education, evidence-based public health is an integration of (1) the best available research evidence, (2) practitioner's expertise, and (3) the expectations, preferences, and values of patients. Among these three components, the best available research evidence can be obtained through a systematic review (SR). An SR is a literature review focusing on a single question that tries to identify, appraise, select, and synthesize all high quality research evidence relevant to that question. Meta-analysis (MA) is the quantitative extension of SR and deals with statistical methods for examining the validity of the extracted summary statistics (effect size) from each component study, for quantifying the heterogeneity between the effect sizes, and at the end, for providing

Y. Ma (✉) • W. Zhang
Department of Epidemiology and Biostatistics, The George Washington University, Washington, DC, USA
e-mail: yanma@email.gwu.edu

D.-G. Chen
School of Social Work, University of North Carolina, Chapel Hill, NC 27599, USA
e-mail: dinchen@email.unc.edu

© Springer International Publishing Switzerland 2015
D.-G. Chen, J. Wilson (eds.), *Innovative Statistical Methods for Public Health Data*, ICSA Book Series in Statistics, DOI 10.1007/978-3-319-18536-1_15

an estimate of the overall pooled effect size with optimal precision. With rising cost of health research, many studies are carried out with small sample sizes resulting in low power for detecting useful effect size. This phenomenon has increased the chance of producing conflicting results from different studies. By pooling the estimated effect sizes from each of the component studies through meta-analytic methods, information from larger number of patients and increased power is expected (Peto 1987). More detailed discussions on meta-analysis for clinical trials can be found from Whitehead (2002) and the implementation of meta-analysis in *R* can be found in Chen and Peace (2013).

A typical MA deals with n independent studies in which a parameter of interest θ_i ($i = 1, 2, \ldots, n$) is estimated. It can be applied to a broad range of study designs such as single-arm or multiple-arm studies, randomized controlled studies, and observational studies. For illustrative purposes, we focus on MA of two-arm studies, where θ_i is some form of the effect size between the two groups. The most popular choice for θ_i is standardized mean difference for a continuous outcome, or odds ratio, risk ratio, and risk difference for dichotomous outcome. In most cases, an estimate $\hat{\theta}_i$ of the true θ_i and its associated standard error could be directly extracted from each study. The ultimate goal of meta-analysis is to produce an optimal estimate of the population effect size by pooling the estimates $\hat{\theta}_i$ ($i = 1, 2, \ldots, n$) from individual studies using appropriate statistical models.

This chapter presents an overview on MA intended for public health researchers to understand and to apply the methods of MA. Emphasis is focused on classical statistical methods for estimation of the parameters of interest in MA as well as recent development in research in MA. Specifically, univariate and multivariate fixed- and random-effects MAs, as well as meta-regression are discussed. All methods are illustrated by examples of published MAs in health research. We demonstrate how these approaches can be implemented in R.

2 Univariate Meta-Analysis

2.1 The Assumption of Homogeneity

In any MA the point estimates of the effect size $\hat{\theta}_i$ from different studies are inevitably different due to two sources of variation, within- and between-study variations. The within-study variation is caused by sampling error, which is random or non-systematic. In contrast, the between-study variation is resulted from the systematic differences among studies. If it is believed that between-study variation does not exist, the effect estimates $\hat{\theta}_i$ are considered homogeneous. Otherwise, they are heterogeneous. Underlying causes of heterogeneity may include differences across studies in patient characteristics, the specific interventions and design of the studies, or hidden factors. In MA, the assumption of homogeneity states that θ_i ($i = 1, 2, \ldots, n$) are the same in all studies, that is

$$\theta_1 = \theta_2 = \cdots = \theta_n = \theta. \tag{1}$$

Further, this assumption can be examined using a statistical test, known as Cochran's χ^2 test or the Q-test (Cochrane Injuries Group Albumin Reviewers 1998; Whitehead and Whitehead 1991). It indicates lack of homogeneity if the test is significant. However, it has been criticized for its low statistical power when the number of studies is small in an MA (Hardy and Thompson 1998). Higgins and Thompson (2002) developed a heterogeneity statistic I^2 to quantify heterogeneity in an MA. The I^2 $(0\% \le I^2 \le 100\%)$ has an interpretation as the proportion of total variation in the estimates of effect size that is due to heterogeneity between studies. For example, an I^2 of 0% (100%) implies that all variability in effect size estimates is due to sampling error (between-study heterogeneity).

2.2 Fixed Effects Univariate Meta-Analysis

Fixed effects univariate meta-analysis (F-UMA) assumes no heterogeneity, that is the underlying population effect sizes θ_i are constant across all studies as shown in Eq. (1). A typical fixed effects model is described as

$$Y_i = \theta + \epsilon_i; \ i = 1, 2, \ldots, n, \tag{2}$$

where for study i, Y_i represents the effect size, θ the population effect size, and ϵ_i the sampling error with mean 0 and variance σ_i^2. In general, the ϵ_i is assumed to follow a normal distribution $N(0, \sigma_i^2)$. A pooled estimate of θ is given by the weighted least square estimation

$$\hat{\theta} = \frac{\sum_{i=1}^{n} w_i Y_i}{\sum_{i=1}^{n} w_i},$$

and the variance of $\hat{\theta}$ can be expressed as

$$Var\left(\hat{\theta}\right) = 1 / \sum_{i=1}^{n} w_i$$

where a popular choice of weight is $w_i = 1/\sigma_i^2$ and variance σ_i^2 is estimated using sample variance $\hat{\sigma}_i^2$ of Y_i from study i. Hence, the 95 % confidence interval of θ is given by

$$\hat{\theta} - t_{0.025,(n-1)} \sqrt{Var\left(\hat{\theta}\right)} \le \theta \le \hat{\theta} + t_{0.025,(n-1)} \sqrt{Var\left(\hat{\theta}\right)},$$

where $t_{0.025,(n-1)}$ denotes the 0.025 percentile of a t–distribution with $(n-1)$ degrees of freedom.

2.3 Random Effects Meta-Analysis

The assumption of homogeneity is only an ideal situation since heterogeneity might still present even if the test of homogeneity is not significant. It is impossible for independent studies to be identical in every respect. Therefore heterogeneity should be very likely to exist in many MAs. The model that takes heterogeneity into account is the following random effects model:

$$Y_i = \theta + b_i + \epsilon_i, i = 1, 2, \ldots, n, \tag{3}$$

where for study i, Y_i represents the effect size, θ the population effect size, b_i the random effect with mean 0 and variance τ^2, and ϵ_i the sampling error with mean 0 and variance σ_i^2. It is assumed that b_i and ϵ_i are independent and follow normal distributions $N(0, \tau^2)$ and $N(0, \sigma_i^2)$, respectively. Let $\theta_i = \theta + b_i, i = 1, 2, \ldots, n$. Then the random effects model (3) can be simplified as

$$Y_i = \theta_i + \epsilon_i,$$

where θ_i represents the true effect size for study i. All θ_i ($i = 1, 2, \ldots, n$) are random samples from the same normal population

$$\theta_i \sim N(\theta, \tau^2)$$

rather than being a constant for F-UMA (1).Further, the marginal variance of Y_i is given by

$$Var(Y_i) = \tau^2 + \sigma_i^2,$$

which is composed of two sources of variation, the between-study variance τ^2 and within-study variance σ_i^2. If the between-study variance $\tau^2 = 0$, the random effects model (3) would reduce to the fixed effects model (2).

Similar to the fixed effects model, the within-study variance σ_i^2 can be estimated using the sample variance from study i ($i = 1, 2, \ldots, n$). However, information of between-study variance τ^2 is often not available and methods commonly used for assessing between-study heterogeneity include the DerSimonian and Laird's method of moments (MM) (DerSimonian and Laird 1986), the maximum likelihood estimation (MLE) method (Hardy and Thompson 1998), and the restricted maximum likelihood (REML) method (Raudenbush and Bryk 1985). MM is a distribution free and non-iterative approach whereas both MLE and REML are parametric methods and need iteration for estimating τ^2 and β. For MM, it utilizes the Q- statistic that is used for testing the assumption of homogeneity (Cochrane Injuries Group Albumin Reviewers 1998),

$$Q = \Sigma_{i=1}^n w_i \left(Y_i - \bar{Y} \right)^2$$

where $w_i = 1/\sigma_i^2$, $\overline{Y} = \Sigma_{i=1}^n w_i Y_i / \Sigma_{i=1}^n w_i$. Let $S_r = \Sigma_{i=1}^n w_i^r$, then the MM estimate of τ^2 is given by

$$\hat{\tau}^2 = \max\left(0, \frac{Q - (n-1)}{S_1 - \frac{S_2}{S_1}}\right) \qquad (4)$$

The truncation at zero in (4) is to ensure that the variance estimate is non-negative. Further, the estimate of the population effect size is given by

$$\hat{\theta} = \frac{\Sigma_{i=1}^n w_i^* Y_i}{\Sigma_{i=1}^n w_i^*} \qquad (5)$$

where $w_i^* = 1/\left(\sigma_i^2 + \hat{\tau}^2\right)$. The variance of $\hat{\theta}$ is simply

$$Var\left(\hat{\theta}\right) = 1/\Sigma_{i=1}^n w_i^*$$

and the 95 % confidence interval can be calculated by $\hat{\theta} - t_{0.025,(n-1)} \sqrt{Var\left(\hat{\theta}\right)} \leq \theta \leq \hat{\theta} + t_{0.025,(n-1)} \sqrt{Var\left(\hat{\theta}\right)}$.

The ML and REML estimates of τ^2 and θ do not have a closed form. In particular, the REML estimates are shown to be the iterative equivalent to the weighted estimators in (4) and (5) (Shadish and Haddock 2009).

2.4   Meta-Regression

Random effects univariate meta-analysis (R-UMA) takes into account between-study heterogeneity, but it is not a tool for exploring and explaining the reasons study results vary. Meta-regression, an approach for investigating the association between study or patient characteristics and outcome measure, can be used for this purpose. We introduce two types of meta-regressions, which are built on the fixed (2) and random (3) effects models, respectively.

Suppose that there are p predictors $X_1, X_2, \ldots, X_p$ and n independent studies. The fixed effects univariate meta-regression (F-UMR) model is given by

$$Y_i = \beta_0 + \beta_1 x_{i1} + \ldots + \beta_p x_{ip} + \epsilon_i \qquad (6)$$

where $x_{i1}, \ldots, x_{ip}$ $(i = 1, 2, \ldots, n)$ denote the observed values of the p predictor variables $X_1, X_2, \ldots, X_p$ for study i and $\beta_0, \beta_1, \ldots, \beta_p$ are regression coefficients. The effect size Y_i and sampling error ϵ_i have the same definitions as in F-UMA (2).

The model assumes that the variation in effect sizes can be completely explained by these predictors. In other words, the variation is predictable.

The random effects univariate meta-regression (R-UMR) model can be obtained by adding random effects b_i to the fixed model (6):

$$Y_i = \beta_0 + \beta_1 x_{i1} + \ldots + \beta_p x_{ip} + b_i + \epsilon_i, i = 1, 2, \ldots, n$$

where b_i is assumed independent with a mean 0 and variance τ^2. Unlike the F-UMR, where all variability in effect sizes can be explained by the predictors X_1, $X_2, \ldots, X_p$, the R-UMR assumes that the model can explain only part of the variation and random effects b_i account for the remainder.

It should be noted that the meta-regression technique is most appropriate when the number of studies in an MA is large. Furthermore, since the covariates and outcome in meta-regression are all study-level summary statistics (e.g., patient mean age, proportion of female patients), the relation between these covariates and outcome may not directly reflect the relation between subject scores and subjects' outcomes, causing aggregation bias. Therefore careful consideration and interpretation of the results are always recommended when performing meta-regression (Sutton et al. 2000).

3   Multivariate Meta-Analysis

3.1   Correlated Multiple Outcomes in Health Research

Medical research often compares multiple outcomes, frequently at multiple time points, between different intervention groups. The results of studies with multiple outcomes and/or endpoints are typically synthesized via conventional UMA on each outcome separately, ignoring the correlations between these outcomes measured on the same set of patients. For example, in the field of orthopedic surgery, when the effect of an antifibrinolytic agent on two outcomes of operative blood loss and blood transfusions is of interest, two univariate meta-analysis was utilized for pooling each effect size and for estimating their related precision. A joint synthesis of the amounts of blood loss and blood transfusions would, however, be more meaningful as the two outcomes are clearly correlated (higher amount of blood loss needing higher number of blood transfusions). The impact of ignoring the within-study correlation (WSC) has been explored extensively in the statistical literature, with issues including overestimated variance of the pooled effect size and biased estimates, which in turn may influence the statistical inferences (Riley 2009). Multivariate meta-analysis (MMA) was developed to synthesize multiple outcomes while taking into account their correlations, often resulting in superior parameter estimation. Although over the past two decades, MMA has become increasingly popular due to considerable advancements in statistical methodology and software, it is rarely considered in medical research. The goal of this section is therefore to increase awareness of the advantages of MMA and promote its use in health research.

3.2 Methods for Multivariate Meta-Analysis

Following the notations for UMA, the formulation for MMA, based on multivariate random-effects model, is written as

$$\mathbf{Y}_i = \boldsymbol{\beta} + \mathbf{b}_i + \boldsymbol{\varepsilon}_i; \ i = 1, 2, .., n,$$

$$\mathbf{Y}_i = (Y_{i1}, Y_{i2}, \ldots, Y_{iM})^\top ; \boldsymbol{\beta} = (\beta_1, \beta_2, \ldots, \beta_M)^\top ,$$

$$\mathbf{b}_i = (b_{i1}, b_{i2}, \ldots, b_{iM})^\top ; \boldsymbol{\varepsilon}_i = (\varepsilon_{i1}, \varepsilon_{i2}, \ldots, \varepsilon_{iM})^\top ,$$

where for the ith study, $\boldsymbol{\beta}$ describes the vector of population effect size of M outcomes, $\mathbf{b}_i$ the vector of between-study random effect, and $\boldsymbol{\varepsilon}_i$ the vector of within-study sampling error. It is often assumed that $\mathbf{b}_i$ and $\boldsymbol{\varepsilon}_i$ are independent, following multivariate normal distributions with zero means and $M \times M$ variance–covariance matrices $Var(\mathbf{b}_i) = \mathbf{D}$ and $Var(\boldsymbol{\varepsilon}_i) = \boldsymbol{\Omega}_i$, respectively.

For illustrative purposes, we focus on the simple case of meta-analysis with bivariate outcome variable $\mathbf{Y}_i = (Y_{i1}, Y_{i2})^\top ; i = 1, 2, \ldots, n$ as these methods can be easily extended to meta-analysis with $M > 2$ outcomes. With $M = 2$ in the random-effects model, the marginal variability in $\mathbf{Y}_i$ accounts for both between-study variation ($\mathbf{D}$) and within-study variation ($\boldsymbol{\Omega}_i$). In particular, the variance–covariance matrix for a bivariate meta-analysis (BMA) boils down to

$$Var(\mathbf{Y}_i) = \mathbf{D} + \boldsymbol{\Omega}_i,$$

$$\mathbf{D} = \begin{bmatrix} \tau_1^2 & \tau_{12} \\ \tau_{12} & \tau_2^2 \end{bmatrix}, \boldsymbol{\Omega}_i = \begin{bmatrix} \sigma_{i1}^2 & \sigma_{i12} \\ \sigma_{i12} & \sigma_{i2}^2 \end{bmatrix},$$

$$\tau_{12} = \tau_1 \tau_2 \rho_b, \sigma_{i12} = \sigma_{i1} \sigma_{i2} \rho_{iw},$$

where τ_1^2, τ_2^2 and ρ_b describe the between-study variation and correlation, whereas σ_{i1}^2, σ_{i2}^2, and ρ_{iw} capture the within-study variation and correlation. Similar to the UMA setting, the within-study variances σ_{i1}^2 and σ_{i2}^2 can be estimated using sample variances $\hat{\sigma}_{i1}^2$ and $\hat{\sigma}_{i2}^2$. Although the WSC ρ_{iw} is generally unknown, several approaches for addressing this issue have been discussed in Riley (2009). For simplicity, throughout this section, the within-study correlation is assumed equal across studies ($\rho_{iw} = \rho_w, i = 1, 2, \ldots, n$) and a sensitivity analysis for a wide range of ρ_w is conducted.

There are three major methods in the literature for MMA: Restricted maximum likelihood approach (Berkey et al. 1998) (REML), the multivariate extension of the

DerSimonian and Laird's method of moments (Jackson et al. 2010), and U-statistic based approach (Ma and Mazumdar 2011). Through extensive simulation studies, it is shown in Ma and Mazumdar (2011) that estimates from these three approaches are very similar. In addition, since REML was developed first, it has been the default approach for MMA. We introduce the statistical property and applications for REML next.

The REML approach has been widely used and is incorporated in most statistical software. By assuming the within-study variance matrix $\boldsymbol{\Omega}_i$ to be known, the remaining parameters of interest to be estimated include $\boldsymbol{\beta}$, τ_1^2, τ_2^2, and ρ_b. Under REML, $\mathbf{b}_i$ and $\boldsymbol{\varepsilon}_i$ are usually assumed to follow bivariate normal distributions, $\mathbf{b}_i \sim N(\mathbf{0}, \mathbf{D})$, $\boldsymbol{\varepsilon}_i \sim N(\mathbf{0}, \boldsymbol{\Omega}_i)$. The outcome variable $\mathbf{Y}_i$, as a result, follows a bivariate normal distribution with mean $\boldsymbol{\beta}$ and variance $\mathbf{D} + \boldsymbol{\Omega}_i$; $i = 1, 2, \ldots, n$.

Normal random effects and sampling errors are discussed as that is most commonly assumed. No closed form derivation for REML estimates exist and therefore iterative procedures (e.g. Newton-Raphson algorithm, E-M algorithm) have been developed for estimating $\boldsymbol{\beta}$ and variance $\mathbf{D}$. Briefly, the REML estimate of $\boldsymbol{\beta}$ can be derived as a function of $\hat{\mathbf{D}}$. This is equivalent to the Restricted Iterative Generalized Least Square (RIGLS) estimate

$$\hat{\boldsymbol{\beta}} = \left(\sum_{i=1}^{n} \left(\hat{\mathbf{D}} + \boldsymbol{\Omega}_i \right)^{-1} \right)^{-1} \left(\sum_{i=1}^{n} \left(\hat{\mathbf{D}} + \boldsymbol{\Omega}_i \right)^{-1} \mathbf{y}_i \right)$$

when outcomes are normally distributed (Riley et al. 2007). Asymptotically, the estimate $\hat{\boldsymbol{\beta}}$ above follows a normal distribution with mean $\boldsymbol{\beta}$ and variance

$$Var\left(\hat{\boldsymbol{\beta}} \right) = \left(\sum_{i=1}^{n} \left(\hat{\mathbf{D}} + \boldsymbol{\Omega}_i \right)^{-1} \right)^{-1} .$$

3.3 Multivariate Meta-Regression

When multiple outcomes is of interest, the univariate meta-regression (UMR) in Sect. 2.4 can be extended to a multivariate setting. It allows adjustment for study-level covariates, that may help explain between-study heterogeneity, when estimating effect sizes for multiple outcomes jointly. Similar to UMR, there are also fixed and random effects MMRs. For a bivariate outcome variable $\mathbf{Y}_i = (Y_{i1}, Y_{i2})^\top$; $i = 1, 2, \ldots, n$, a random effects multivariate meta-regression (R-MMR) model is given by

$$\mathbf{Y}_i = \mathbf{X}_i \boldsymbol{\beta} + \boldsymbol{b}_i + \boldsymbol{\epsilon}_i \tag{7}$$

where $\mathbf{Y}_i$ is a vector of 2 outcomes, $\mathbf{X}_i$ a matrix containing the study-level covariates for study i, $\boldsymbol{\beta}$ the regression coefficients associated with $\mathbf{X}_i$. The model (7) allows a separate intercept for each outcome and a separate slope measuring the association of each outcome and a specific covariate. The random effects $\mathbf{b}_i$ is also a vector, taking into account for each outcome the variation the cannot be explained by the model. The sampling error $\boldsymbol{\epsilon}_i$ and random effects $\mathbf{b}_i$ are assumed independent and follow multivariate normal distributions MVN$(0, \boldsymbol{\Omega}_i)$ and MVN$(0, D)$, respectively. Thus the marginal distribution of $\mathbf{Y}_i$ is MVN$(\mathbf{X}_i\boldsymbol{\beta}, \boldsymbol{\Omega}_i + D)$, where $\boldsymbol{\Omega}_i$ and D represent within- and between-study variance matrices, respectively. If $\mathbf{b}_i = 0$, then the R-MMR (7) reduces to fixed effects multivariate meta-regression (F-MMR). The commonly used estimation procedures for MMR include the generalized least squares, ML, and REML methods. Detailed information about these methods can be found in Berkey et al. (1998).

3.4   Univariate Versus Multivariate Meta-Analysis

There have been extensive debate regarding when, how, and why MMA can differ from two independent UMAs (Berkey et al. 1998; Riley et al. 2007; Sohn 2000). Since MMA is able to "borrow strength" across outcomes through the within-study correlations, this method is expected to produce increased precision of estimates compared to a UMA of each outcome separately. Riley et al. (2007) demonstrated that the completeness of data plays a role when assessing the benefits of using MMA. When all outcomes are available in each individual study (i.e., complete data), the advantages of MMA tend to be marginal. When at least one of the outcomes is unavailable for some studies (i.e., missing data), these advantages become more apparent. In particular, MMA can still incorporate those incomplete studies in analysis. However, studies with a missing outcome will be excluded in a UMA for the outcome. Therefore, Riley et al. (2007) recommended that MMA should be used if there are missing data and multiple separate UMAs are sufficient if there are complete data.

4   Applications

We apply the UMA and MMA to two published meta-analysis, one with complete data and the other one with missing data.

4.1   Example 1: A Meta-Analysis of Surgical Versus Non-surgical Procedure for Treating Periodontal Disease

A meta-analysis of five randomized controlled trials was conducted for comparing a surgical versus a non-surgical procedure for treating periodontal disease with two endpoints of probing depth (PD) and attachment level (AL) (Antczak-Bouckoms et al. 1993). The year of publication, sample size, summarized data in terms of mean differences of each endpoint between the two treatments (surgical minus non-surgical), and the within-study variances with known correlation are presented in Table 1.

We conducted fixed and random effects UMA and BMA using R package mvmeta (see the code in Appendix). The heterogeneity statistic I^2 is 69 % and 96 % for PD and AL, respectively, indicating that between-study variation accounts for the majority of the total variation in both PD and AL. Therefore random effects MA is more appropriate for this study than fixed effects MA.

The results from all methods indicate that the surgical procedure improved probing depth, whereas the non-surgical procedure improved attachment level and reveal a strong between-study correlation ($\hat{\rho}_b = 0.609$) across outcomes (Table 2). The most notable finding is that all the random effects standard errors (SEs) were considerably larger than the corresponding fixed effects SEs. For example, in the UMA setting, the random effects SE for PD is 0.0592, doubling that reported for the fixed effects SE (0.0289). This is not surprising since random effects MA accounts for between-study variation, which is ignored by fixed effects MA. In addition, the random effects point estimates of β_{PD} and β_{AL} were different from those produced by the fixed effects MAs. When comparing UMA with BMA, the BMA SEs were only slightly smaller than the corresponding UMA SEs for both fixed and random MAs, indicating little estimation precision was achieved by BMA. Hence, it confirmed that the advantage of BMA over UMA is not significant when the data are complete.

Table 1 Data of Example 1: surgical versus non-surgical procedure for treating periodontal disease

Study	Publication year	Number of patients	Outcome	Y_{ij}	s_{ij}^2	ρ_{wi}
1	1983	14	PD	0.47	0.0075	0.39
1	1983	14	AL	−0.32	0.0077	
2	1982	15	PD	0.20	0.0057	0.42
2	1982	15	AL	−0.60	0.0008	
3	1979	78	PD	0.40	0.0021	0.41
3	1979	78	AL	−0.12	0.0014	
4	1987	89	PD	0.26	0.0029	0.43
4	1987	89	AL	−0.31	0.0015	
5	1988	16	PD	0.56	0.0148	0.34
5	1988	16	AL	−0.39	0.0304	

Table 2 Bivariate and univariate meta-analysis results of Example 1: surgical versus non-surgical procedure for treating periodontal disease[a]

Method	$\hat{\beta}_{PD}$(s.e.)	95 % CI (PD)	$\hat{\tau}^2_{PD}$	$\hat{\beta}_{AL}$(s.e.)	95 % CI (AL)	$\hat{\tau}^2_{AL}$	$\hat{\rho}_b$
F-UMA	0.347(0.0289)	(0.267, 0.427)	–	−0.393(0.0189)	(−0.445, −0.340)	–	–
F-BMA	0.307(0.0286)	(0.228, 0.387)	–	−0.394(0.0186)	(−0.446, −0.343)	–	–
R-UMA	0.361(0.0592)	(0.196,0.525)	0.0119	−0.346(0.0885)	(−0.591,−0.100)	0.0331	–
R-BMA	0.353(0.0588)	(0.190,0.517)	0.0117	−0.339(0.0879)	(−0.583,−0.095)	0.0327	0.609

[a]*PD* probing depth, *AL* attachment level, *F-UMA* fixed effects univariate meta-analysis, *F-BMA* fixed effects bivariate meta-analysis, *R-UMA* random effects univariate meta-analysis, *R-BMA* random effects bivariate meta-analysis

In addition to MA, we also performed fixed and random UMR and BMR (Table 3). In these regression analyses, year of publication, a proxy for time of conducting of a study, was used as the predictor. Similar to the MAs in Table 2, we also found in MR analyses that all the random effects standard errors (SEs) were considerably larger than the corresponding fixed effects SEs. The year of publication was not a significant predictor in any of the analyses. The differences between UMR and BMR estimates (coefficients and SEs) were only marginal for both fixed and random effects MRs.

4.2   Example 2: A Meta-Analysis of Gamma Nail Versus Sliding Hip Screw for Extracapsular Hip Fractures in Adults

A systematic review was conducted for assessing comparative effect of cephalo-condylic intramedullary nails versus extramedullary fixation implants for treating extracapsular hip fractures in adults (Parker and Handoll 2008). Numerous endpoints included operative details, fractures fixation complications, and post-operative complications. Study results were integrated through multiple univariate meta-analysis. We performed a bivariate meta-analysis to compare Gamma nail (an intramedullary nail) and SHS (an extramedullary implant) with two outcome measures of length of surgery (in minutes) and amount of operative blood loss (in milliliters). Advantages of Gamma nail over SHS are hypothesized to be reduced blood loss and shorter operative time (Parker and Handoll 2008).

The data presented in Table 4 contains seven studies, among which four studies reported both outcomes, six reported length of surgery only, and five reported operative blood loss only. In this MA, the effect sizes of length of surgery (LOS) and operative blood loss (BL) were defined using Hedges' g (Hedges 1981). For illustrative purposes, data were analyzed under the following assumption: $\rho_w > 0$ in those four studies providing both outcomes as the amount of BL is likely to be positively associated with LOS. Three BMAs were performed with minor ($\rho_w = 0.2$), moderate ($\rho_w = 0.5$) and strong ($\rho_w = 0.8$) within-study correlations,

Table 3 Meta-regression analysis results of Example 1: surgical versus non-surgical procedure for treating periodontal disease[a]

	F-UMR (PD) $(Y_{PD} = b_1 + b_2 * year)$	F-UMR (AL) $(Y_{AL} = b_3 + b_4 * year)$	F-BMR	R-UMR (PD) $(Y_{PD} = b_1 + b_2 * year)$	R-UMR (AL) $(Y_{AL} = b_3 + b_4 * year)$	R-BMR
$\hat{b}_1 \left(\text{SE}\left(\hat{b}_1\right) \right)$	0.345(0.029)	–	0.305(0.029)	0.363(0.073)	–	0.359(0.073)
$\hat{b}_2 \left(\text{SE}\left(\hat{b}_2\right) \right)$	−0.008(0.008)	–	−0.005(0.008)	0.005(0.02)	–	0.005(0.022)
$\hat{\tau}_1^2$	–	–	–	0.019	–	0.02
$\hat{b}_3 \left(\text{SE}\left(\hat{b}_3\right) \right)$	–	−0.394(0.019)	−0.399(0.019)	–	−0.333(0.091)	−0.336(0.098)
$\hat{b}_4 \left(\text{SE}\left(\hat{b}_4\right) \right)$	–	−0.012(0.007)	−0.01(0.006)	–	−0.014(0.027)	−0.012(0.03)
$\hat{\tau}_2^2$	–	–	–	–	0.033	0.04
$\hat{\rho}_b$	–	–	–	–	–	0.561

[a]*PD* probing depth, *AL* attachment level, *F-UMR* fixed effects univariate meta-regression, *F-BMR* fixed effects bivariate meta-regression, *R-UMR* random effects univariate meta-regression, *R-BMA* random effects bivariate meta-regression

Table 4 Data of Example 2: Gamma nail versus sliding hip screw (SHS) for extracapsular hip fractures in adult[a]

	Sample size		Length of surgery (minutes)				Operative blood loss (ml)			
Study	G	S	Mean(G)	Std(G)	Mean(S)	Std(S)	Mean(G)	Std(G)	Mean(S)	Std(S)
1	203	197	55.4	20	61.3	22.2	244.4	384.9	260.4	325.5
2	60	60	47.1	20.8	53.4	8.3	152.3	130.7	160.3	110.8
3	73	73	65	29	51	22	240	190	280	280
4	53	49	59	23.9	47	13.3	258.7	145.4	259.2	137.5
5	104	106	46	11	44	15	NA	NA	NA	NA
6	31	36	56.7	17	54.3	16.4	NA	NA	NA	NA
7	93	93	NA	NA	NA	NA	814	548	1,043	508

[a] G=Gamma nail, S=SHS, NA=Not available

respectively. A UMA was also conducted for each outcome. Since nearly 85 % (I^2) of the total variation in LOS and 30 % in BL were from the between-study variation, we only conducted random effects MAs.

Shown in Table 5 are estimates of $(\beta_{LOS}, \beta_{BL}, \tau^2_{LOS}, \tau^2_{BL}, \rho_b)$ and the 95 % confidence interval of $\hat{\beta}$. Results of all four analyses imply Gamma nail was associated with longer LOS and less amount of BL, but these findings were not statistically significant. For all three BMAs, the effect size estimates (in absolute value) of LOS and BL were all greater than those of UMAs. Compared to UMA, in BMA, by modeling β_{LOS} and β_{BL} simultaneously, $\hat{\beta}_{LOS}$ $\left(\hat{\beta}_{BL}\right)$ "borrows strength" from the BL (LOS), despite the fact that the LOS (BL) is missing in few studies. This leads to more precise estimation with smaller standard errors and narrower confidence intervals under BMA. For example, when within-study correlation is moderate $(\rho_w = 0.5)$, the width of the 95 % CI in BMA was narrower by 2 % and 9 %, compared to that in UMA for LOS and BL, respectively.

Appendix

We performed all our analyses in R using the *mvmeta* package. In this appendix we provide the R code written for the meta-analysis and meta-regression in Example 1.
  ###R code for fixed effects UMA:

$$\text{mvmeta}(PD, S = \text{var.PD}, \text{data} = \text{ex.data}, \text{method} = \text{"fixed"})$$

where var.PD stands for the within-study variance of PD.
  ###R code for random effects UMA:

$$\text{mvmeta}(PD, S = \text{var.PD}, \text{data} = \text{ex.data}, \text{method} = \text{"REML"})$$

Table 5 Meta-analysis results of Example 2: Gamma nail versus sliding hip screw (SHS) for extracapsular hip fractures in adults[a]

Method	$\hat{\beta}_{LOS}$	$95\%CI_{LOS}$	Δ_{LOS}(CI)	$\hat{\tau}^2_{LOS}$	$\hat{\beta}_{BL}$	$95\%CI_{BL}$	Δ_{BL}(CI)	$\hat{\tau}^2_{BL}$	$\hat{\rho}_b$
UMA	0.117(0.1691)	(−0.318, 0.552)	−	0.141	−0.144(0.0811)	(−0.369, 0.082)	−	0.01	−
BMA(0.2)	0.160(0.1695)	(−0.275, 0.596)	0.11 %	0.147	−0.158(0.0737)	(−0.363, 0.047)	−6.65 %	0.007	−1
BMA(0.5)	0.148(0.1658)	(−0.278, 0.574)	−2.07 %	0.139	−0.160(0.0759)	(−0.371, 0.050)	−9.09 %	0.009	−1
BMA(0.8)	0.138(0.1640)	(−0.283, 0.560)	−3.10 %	0.136	−0.163(0.0779)	(−0.379, 0.054)	−3.99 %	0.01	−1

[a]LOS length of surgery, BL blood loss, UMA univariate meta-analysis, BMA bivariate meta-analysis, CI 95 % confidence interval, Δ(CI) the relative change in the width of CI, defined as (width of CI for the current BMA−width of CI for UMA)/(width of CI for UMA)∗100 %

###R code for fixed effects BMA:

```
mvmeta(cbind(PD, AL), S = cbind(var.PD, cov.PD.AL, var.AL), data = ex.data, method = "fixed")
```

where cov.PD.AL stands for the within-study covariance of PD and AL.
###R code for random effects BMA:

```
mvmeta(cbind(PD, AL), S = cbind(var.PD, cov.PD.AL, var.AL), data = ex.data, method = "REML")
```

###R code for fixed effects univariate MR:

```
mvmeta(PD~year, S = var.PD, data = ex.data, method = "fixed")
```

###R code for random effects univariate MR:

```
mvmeta(PD~year, S = var.PD, data = ex.data, method = "REML")
```

###R code for fixed effects bivariate MR:

```
mvmeta(cbind(PD, AL)~year, S = cbind(var.PD, cov.PD.AL, var.AL), data = ex.data, method = "fixed")
```

###R code for random effects bivariate MR:

```
mvmeta(cbind(PD, AL)~year, S = cbind(var.PD, cov.PD.AL, var.AL), data = ex.data, method = "REML")
```

References

Antczak-Bouckoms, A., Joshipura, K., Burdick, E., Tulloch, J.F.C.: Meta-analysis of surgical versus non-surgical method of treatment for periodontal disease. J. Clin. Periodontol. **20**, 259–68 (1993)

Berkey, C.S., Hoaglin, D.C., Antczak-Bouckoms, A., Mosteller, F., Colditz, G.A.: Meta-analysis of multiple outcomes by regression with random effects. Stat. Med. **17**, 2537–2550 (1998)

Brownson, R.C., Fielding, J.E., Maylahn, C.M., Evidence-based public health: a fundamental concept for public health practice. Annu. Rev. Public Health. **30**, 175–201 (2009)

Chen, D.G., Peace, K.E.: Applied Meta-Analysis with R. Chapman and Hall/CRC Biostatistics Series. Chapman and Hall/CRC, Boca Raton (2013)

Cochrane Injuries Group Albumin Reviewers: Human albumin administration in critically ill patients: systematic review of randomised controlled trials. Br. Med. J. **317**, 235–240 (1998)

DerSimonian, R., Laird, N.: Meta-analysis in clinical trials. Control. Clin. Trials **7**, 177–188 (1986)

Fielding, J.E., Briss, P.A.: Promoting evidence-based public health policy: Can we have better evidence and more action? Health Aff. Millwood **25**, 969–78 (2006)

Glasziou, P, Longbottom, H.: Evidence-based public health practice. Aust. N. Z. J. Public Health **23**, 436–40 (1999)

Hardy, R.J., Thompson, S.G.: Detecting and describing heterogeneity in meta-analysis. Stat. Med. **17**, 841–856 (1998)

Hedges, L.V.: Distribution theory for glass's estimator of effect size and related estimators. J. Educ. Stat. **6**, 107–28 (1981)

Higgins, J.P.T., Thompson, S.G.: Quantifying heterogeneity in a meta-analysis. Stat. Med. **21**, 1539–1558 (2002)

Jackson, D., White, I.R., Thompson, S.G.: Extending DerSimonian and Laird's methodology to perform multivariate random effects meta-analysis. Stat. Med. **29**, 1282–1297 (2010)

Ma, Y., Mazumdar, M.: Multivariate meta-analysis: a robust approach based on the theory of U-statistic. Stat. Med. **30**, 2911–2929 (2011)

Parker, M.J., Handoll, H.H.G.: Gamma and other cephalocondylic intramedullary nails versus extramedullary implants for extracapsular hip fractures in adults. Cochrane Database Syst. Rev. **16**(3), CD000093 (2008)

Peto, R.: Why do we need systematic overviews of randomized trials? Stat. Med. **6**, 233–240 (1987)

Raudenbush, S.W., Bryk, A.S.: Empirical Bayes meta-analysis. J. Educ. Stat. **10**(2), 75–98 (1985)

Riley RD, Abrams, K.R., Lambert, P.C., Sutton, A.J., Thompson, J.R.: An evaluation of bivariate random-effects meta-analysis for the joint synthesis of two correlated outcomes. Stat. Med. **26**, 78–97 (2007)

Riley, R.D.: Multivariate meta-analysis: the effect of ignoring within-study correlation. J. R. Stat Soc. Ser. A. **172**(4), 789–811 (2009)

Shadish, W.R., Haddock, C.K.: Combining estimates of effect size. In: Cooper, H., Hedges, L.V., (eds.) The Handbook of Research Synthesis, pp. 261–284. Russel Sage Foundation, New York (2009)

Sohn SY. Multivariate meta-analysis with potentially correlated marketing study results. Nav. Res. Logist. **47**, 500–510 (2000)

Sutton, A.J., Abrams, K.R., Jones, D.R., Sheldon, T.A., Song, F.: Methods for Meta-Analysis in Medical Research. Wiley, New York (2000)

Whitehead, A., Whitehead, J.: A general parametric approach to the meta-analysis of randomised clinical trials. Stat. Med. **10**, 1665–1677 (1991)

Whitehead, A.: Meta-Analysis of Controlled Clinical Trials. Wiley, Chichester (2002)

Index

© Springer International Publishing Switzerland 2015
D.-G. Chen, J. Wilson (eds.), *Innovative Statistical Methods for Public Health Data*,
ICSA Book Series in Statistics, DOI 10.1007/978-3-319-18536-1

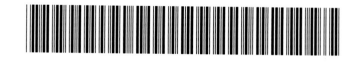